Current Topics in Pathology

Continuation of Ergebnisse der Pathologie

Edited by

E. Grundmann · W. H. Kirsten

Current Topics in Pathology
Volume 61

Glomerulonephritis

Contributors

J. Churg, H. Fischbach, E. Grishman, E. Heilmann,
U. Helmchen, U. Kneissler, Y. Kondo, H. Loew,
A. Okabayashi, A. Samizadeh, H. Shigematsu, G. H. Thoenes,
Ch. Witting

Editor

E. Grundmann

With 108 Figures and 9 Plates

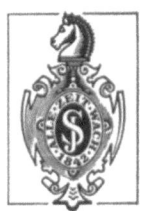

Springer-Verlag Berlin Heidelberg GmbH

E. Grundmann, Professor Dr.
Pathologisches Institut der Universität
Westring 17
D-4400 Münster/Westf., Germany

W. H. Kirsten, Professor Dr.
Department of Pathology
The University of Chicago
950 East 59th Street
Chicago, IL 60637, USA

ISBN 978-3-642-66223-2   ISBN 978-3-642-66221-8 (eBook)
DOI 10.1007/978-3-642-66221-8

Contents

OKABAYASHI, A., KONDO, Y., SHIGEMATSU, H.: Cellular and Histopathologic Consequences of Immunologically Induced Experimental Glomerulonephritis. With 14 Figures 1

WITTING, CH.: The Terminology of Glomerulonephritis—A Review. With 3 Figures 45

THOENES, G. H.: The Immunohistology of Glomerulonephritis—Distinctive Marks and Variability. With 10 Figures and 9 Plates 61

CHURG, J., GRISHMAN, E.: Electron Microscopy of Glomerulonephritis. With 24 Figures. 107

FISCHBACH, H.: The Morphologic Course of Different Glomerulonephritides (Examination of Repeat Biopsies in 264 Patients). With 25 Figures 155

HELMCHEN, U., KNEISSLER, U.: Role of the Renin-Angiotensin System in Renal Hypertension. An Experimental Approach. With 20 Figures . 203

LOEW, H., SAMIZADEH, A., HEILMANN, E.: New Clinical Syndromes under Regular Intermittent Hemodialysis. With 12 Figures. 239

Subject Index 277

List of Contributors

J. CHURG, Mount Sinai School of Medicine, Department of Pathology, Fifth Avenue and 100th Street, New York, N.Y. 10029, USA

H. FISCHBACH, Pathologisches Institut der Universität, Liebermeisterstraße 8, D-7400 Tübingen, Germany

E. GRISHMAN, Mount Sinai School of Medicine, Department of Pathology, Fifth Avenue and 100th Street, New York, N.Y. 10029, USA

E. HEILMANN, Medizinische Poliklinik der Westfälischen Wilhelms-Universität, Westring 3, D-4400 Münster, Germany

U. HELMCHEN, Pathologisches Institut der Universität, Liebermeisterstraße 8, D-7400 Tübingen, Germany

U. KNEISSLER, Pathologisches Institut der Universität, Liebermeisterstraße 8, D-7400 Tübingen, Germany

Y. KONDO, Department of Pathology, School of Medicine, Chiba University, 313 Inohanacho, 280 Chiba, Japan

H. LOEW, Medizinische Poliklinik der Westfälischen Wilhelms-Universität, Westring 3, D-4400 Münster, Germany

A. OKABAYASHI, Department of Pathology, School of Medicine, Chiba University, 313 Inohanacho, 280 Chiba, Japan

A. SAMIZADEH, Medizinische Poliklinik der Westfälischen Wilhelms-Universität, Westring 3, D-4400 Münster, Germany

H. SHIGEMATSU, Department of Pathology, School of Medicine, Chiba University, 313 Inohanacho, 280 Chiba, Japan

G. H. THOENES, I. Medizinische Klinik der Universität, Ziemssenstraße 1, D-8000 München 2, Germany

CH. WITTING, Pathologisches Institut der Universität. Westring 17, D-4400 Münster, Germany

Department of Pathology, School of Medicine, Chiba
University, Chiba, Japan

Cellular and Histopathologic Consequences of Immunologically Induced Experimental Glomerulonephritis

ATSUSHI OKABAYASHI, M.D., YOICHIRO KONDO, M.D., and
HIDEKAZU SHIGEMATSU, M.D.

With 14 Figures

Contents

I. Introduction 1

II. Immunologic Basis of Glomerular Injury 3

III. Morphologic Aspects of Immunologically Induced Glomerulonephritis 5
    1. Masugi Nephritis 5
      a) The First Phase of Masugi Nephritis 5
      b) The Second Phase of Masugi Nephritis 7
    2. Steblay Nephritis 12
    3. Acute Serum Sickness-Type Nephritis 14
      a) Active Serum Sickness Nephritis 14
      b) Passive Serum Sickness Nephritis 17
    4. Chronic Serum Sickness-Type Nephritis 18
    5. Heymann Nephritis 20
    6. Glomerulonephritis and Prolonged Antigenic Stimulation 21
    7. Glomerulonephritis Associated with Infection 21
      a) Glomerulonephritis in Aleutian Disease of Mink 21
      b) Glomerulonephritis in New Zealand Strain Mice 22
      c) Other Glomerulonephritis Correlated to Infectious Agents 23
    8. Miscellaneous Types of Glomerulonephritis of Possible Immune Origin . . . 24

IV. Some Pathogenic Considerations in Relation to Morphologic Manifestations 24
    1. Glomerular Alterations and Localization of Immune Reactants 24
    2. Phagocyte Accumulation and Proliferative Glomerular Changes 28
    3. Disorganizing Processes and Progressive Glomerulonephritis 30

V. Concluding Remarks 34

References 35

I. Introduction

It is now generally accepted that many, if not all, human cases of glomerulonephritis develop on the basis of immunologic mechanisms. Several key developments in experimental studies have contributed to our current understanding of the pathogenesis of glomerulonephritis.

The first historical step in the field of experimental glomerulonephritis was taken by Masugi about 40 years ago. Employing heterologous antikidney sera (nephrotoxic sera), he produced and thoroughly described a variety of glomerular diseases in animals compatible with acute, subacute, and chronic glomerulonephritis in humans (Masugi, 1933; Masugi, 1934). This experimental model (Masugi nephritis or nephrotoxic nephritis) is distinct from others because of its high reproducibility. Advances in methodology made it possible to analyze the underlying mechanisms responsible for the induction of Masugi nephritis (Kay, 1940; Hammer and Dixon, 1963; Fujimoto et al., 1964). It has been clarified that Masugi nephritis is basically a biphasic disease consisting of the first phase (initial or heterologous phase) and the second phase (secondary or autologous phase). In the first phase, nephrotoxic antibodies (NTAbs) are immediately localized along the glomerular basement membrance (GBM), with or without the immediate onset of glomerular lesions owing to the nature and amount of the NTAbs administered; the second phase occurs several days later following the formation of specific host antibodies that react with the antigen (NTAbs) fixed in the glomerulus resulting in either exacerbation or initiation of glomerular lesions (reviewed by: Unanue and Dixon, 1967b; McCluskey and Vassalli, 1969).

The next outstanding progress in this field was made through studies on experimental acute serum sickness produced by a single i.v. injection of a large amount of foreign serum (Rich and Gregory, 1943; Rich, 1947) or purified foreign serum antigen (Hawn and Janeway, 1947). Studying this "one-shot" serum sickness, special attention was directed to the host immune response in relation to the induction of serum sickness inflammations. The results obtained indicated that various tissue injuries, including proliferative glomerulonephritis, developed at the time of antigen–antibody interaction in the circulation (Germuth, 1953). Further investigation disclosed that the formation of antigen–antibody complexes (usually antigen excess, soluble complexes) and their tissue depositions were the major pathogenesis of acute serum sickness diseases (Dixon et al., 1958). The pathogenetic role of antigen–antibody complexes was again confirmed in experimental chronic serum sickness (Dixon et al., 1961). Probably considerable numbers of experimental or naturally occurring nephritis in animals may develop on the same immunologic basis as revealed in experimental serum sickness. It was also proposed that autoimmune disorders including lupus-like nephritis developed under the condition of prolonged antigenic stimulation, correlating with characteristic immune system alterations (Okabayashi, 1964).

Another important item of information comes from the observation that renal glomeruli can be damaged by autologous antikidney antibodies produced by repeated immunization with heterologous or homologous kidney antigens. At present, two well established models are available as examples (Heymann et al., 1959; Steblay, 1962).

In this review, we will describe pathologic processes in these glomerular diseases with some emphasis on their ultrastructural features.

II. Immunologic Basis of Glomerular Injury

In immunologically induced glomerulonephritis, there can be at least three possible patterns of immunologic processes taking place in renal glomeruli, particularly around the GBM as shown in Fig. 1.

In the first type the GBM *per se* acts as an antigen that is capable of reacting with either heterologous or autologous anti-GBM antibodies in the circulation. A typical example is the first phase of rat Masugi nephritis in which rabbit NTAbs combine with rat GBM in a characteristic continuous, linear fashion as revealed by the fluorescent antibody method (ORTEGA and MELLORS, 1956; ANDRES et al., 1962; SEEGAL et al., 1962). The antigen (rat GBM)–antibody interaction and the concurrent participation of complement (C3) usually result in the immediate onset of glomerulonephritis (UNANUE and DIXON, 1964). A similar mechanism may also be operative in other glomerular diseases produced after injection of heterologous antitissue sera that contain cross-reacting antibodies against the GBM (SEEGAL et al., 1963; CHASE et al., 1972). Another example is sheep nephritis caused by repeated injections of heterologous GBM antigen incorporated in Freund's complete adjuvant (STEBLAY, 1962). By the immunization, autologous anti-GBM antibodies are formed in the sheep and are then deposited in the glomerulus with a resultant induction of severe glomerulonephritis.

The second type is mediated by the interaction between an antigen previously localized on the GBM and a specific host antibody in the circulation, as seen in the second phase of Masugi nephritis. In this situation the NTAbs behave as an antigen. Therefore, a significant difference exists between the first and the second phase with regard to the sequence of immunologic events, although the importance of the NTAbs is critical for both occasions. Since the NTAbs have been localized diffusely along the GBM, the host antibody also distributes in a similar continuous linear fashion in immuno-fluorescence (ORTEGA and MELLORS, 1956). It is tempting to assume that some other antigens, which have no specific affinities to the glomerular constituents, are first deposited on the GBM and then interact with circulating antibodies. However, in no instances has this possibility been clearly proved.

The third type results from glomerular depositions of antigen–antibody complexes initially formed in the circulation. A well known model of this glomerulonephritis is seen in experimental acute serum sickness induced in rabbits by i.v. administration of a large amount of antigen, e.g. bovine serum albumin (BSA). Glomerular localizations of antigen–antibody complexes and complement (C3) are demonstrated by immunofluorescence (DIXON et al., 1958; FISH et al., 1966). The distribution pattern of the complexes is distinctly different from that seen in Masugi nephritis and is characterized by granular fluorescence scattered discontinuously on the capillary wall. The incidence of acute serum sickness nephritis is less frequent than Masugi nephritis since neither antigen nor antibody possesses any affinities to the glomerular constituents.

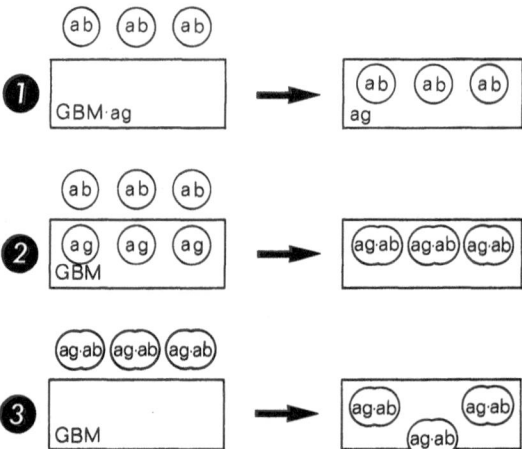

Fig. 1. Three possible immunologic processes occurring around the glomerular basement membrane (GBM). (1) Interaction between endogenous GBM antigens (ag) and circulating heterologous or autologous anti-GBM antibodies. (2) Interaction between antigens previously fixed on the GBM (ag) and circulating antibodies (ab). (3) Deposition of circulating antigen–antibody complexes (ag·ab) which have no specific affinities to the glomerular constituent

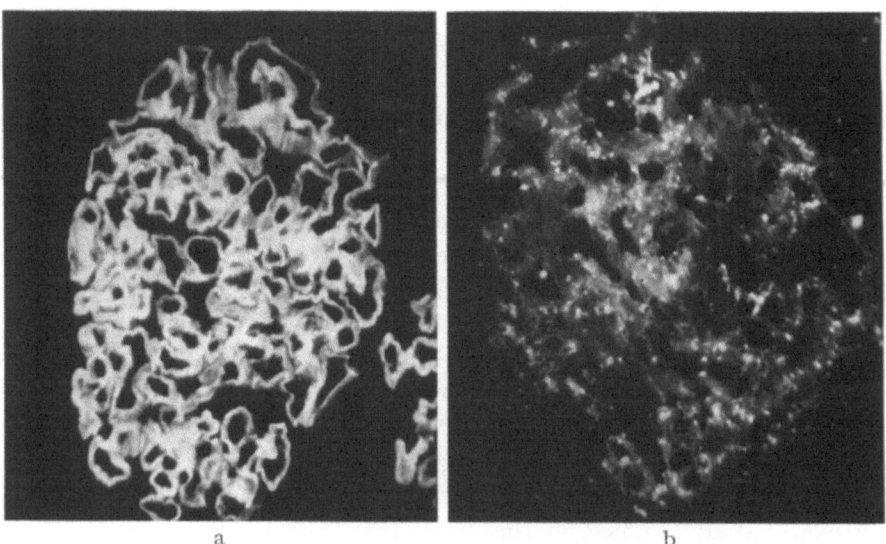

a   b

Fig. 2. (a) A fluorescent micrograph of a rat glomerulus in the first phase of Masugi nephritis. Characteristic linear localization of nephrotoxic rabbit IgG. × 500. (Courtesy of Dr. H. Tomioka.) (b) A fluorescent micrograph of a rabbit glomerulus in acute serum sickness nephritis. Discrete, finely granular fluorescence demonstrating deposition of rabbit IgG along the capillary walls and in the mesangium. × 540. (Courtesy of Dr. M. Sano)

Such a mechanism as shown in serum sickness nephritis would account for the pathogenesis of a number of acute as well as chronic experimental glomerulonephritis cases and various substances, e.g. foreign proteins, infectious agents, or endogenous cell and tissue components might serve as antigenic constituents of the nephritogenic immune complexes.

III. Morphologic Aspects of Immunologically Induced Glomerulonephritis

Although there have been many excellent publications dealing with pathologic features of immunologically induced glomerulonephritis, the references cited here will be limited to those concerned with the ultrastructural pathology and possible pathogenesis.

1. Masugi Nephritis

NTAbs are prepared in an animal by immunization with the kidney from a different species of animal. Masugi nephritis is elicited by a passive administration of the NTAbs into the donor animal of the kidney antigen and is divided into two phases. In general, definite glomerular changes are seen both in the first and the second phase when mammalian NTAbs are employed, whereas fowl NTAbs are not nephritogenic during the first phase. It has been demonstrated that the major nephritogenic antigen is included in the GBM (KRAKOWER and GREENSPON, 1951; CRUICKSHANK and HILL, 1953).

a) The First Phase of Masugi Nephritis

Pathologic processes during the first phase have been extensively analyzed in rat Masugi nephritis produced by injection with rabbit NTAbs (PIEL et al., 1955; MILLER and BOHLE, 1957; CHURG et al., 1960; FELDMAN et al., 1963; FUJIMOTO et al., 1964; COCHRANE et al., 1965). The rabbit NTAbs are fixed to the GBM immediately after injection and persist for at least several months (ORTEGA and MELLORS, 1956; SEEGAL et al., 1962). Localization is visualized by immunofluorescence in a uniform, linear pattern. Fixation of rat or guinea pig complement is also seen in a similar fashion (BURKHOLDER, 1961; VOGT and KOCHEM, 1961; UNANUE and DIXON, 1964). Glomerular changes shortly after injection of the NTAbs are recognizable only by electron microscopy, consisting of a slight loosening of the mesangium and circumscribed subendothelial accumulation of electron lucent material accompanying the detachment of the endothelial lining. More definitive changes are observed after several hours. There is a variable thickening of the GBM and local depositions of wispy, poorly delineated substances within or at the luminal side of the GBM (FELDMAN, 1963). Attenuated portions of the endothelium are often desquamated from the GBM so that the GBM is exposed directly to the capillary lumen. Simultaneously, accumulations of polymorphonuclear leukocytes (PMNs) are seen in the capillary tufts. An intraluminal aggregation of platelets and fibrin can also be seen in varying degrees depending upon the

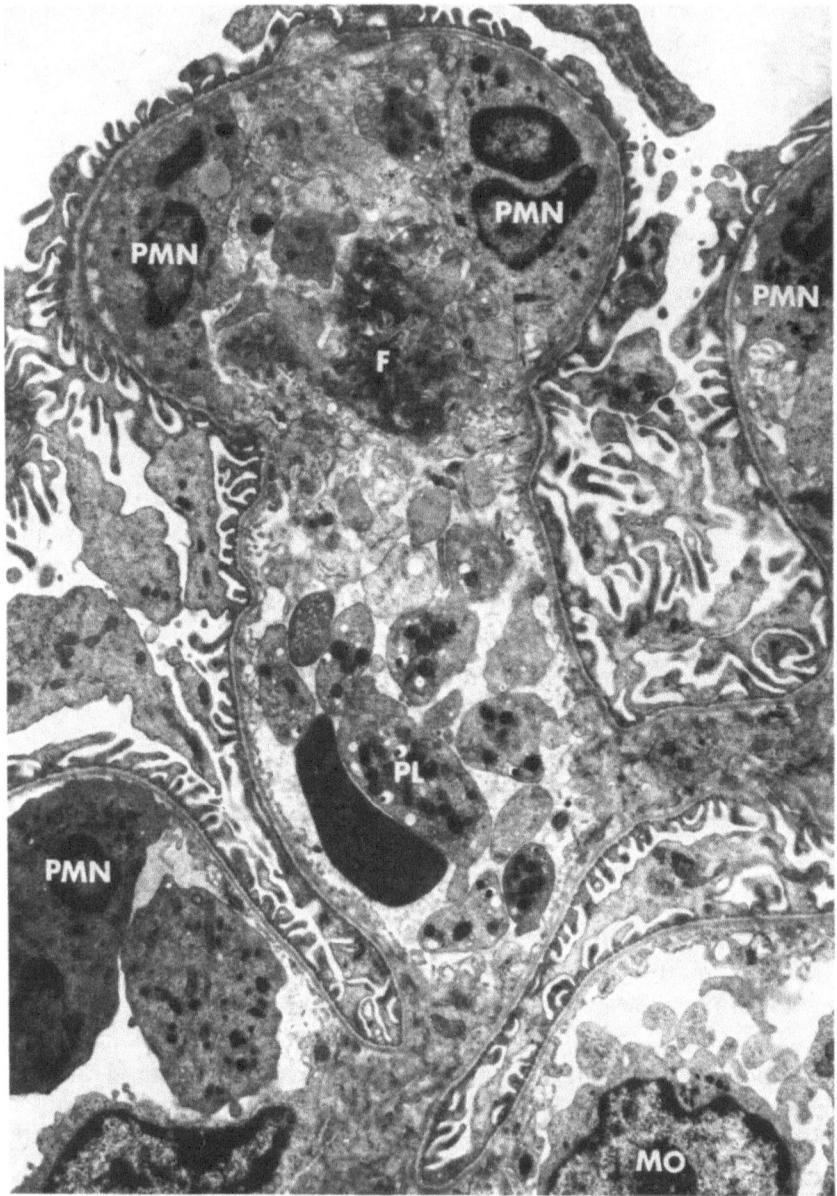

Fig. 3. Glomerular lesions of rat Masugi nephritis 2 hrs after injection with nephrotoxic rabbit IgG. The capillary lumens are occluded by leukocytes (PMN), fibrin (F), platelets (PL), and a monocyte (MO). PMNs show direct contact with basement membranes. ×5600. [H. Shigematsu, Virchows Arch. Abt. B **5**, 187 (1970)]

severity of the glomerular injury. Migrant PMNs exhibit direct contact with the denuded GBM or appear to be replacing the endothelium (Cochrane *et al.*, 1965; Shigematsu, 1970). Increased GBM permeability is suggested by the foot process fusion of podocytes. At 24 hours and thereafter PMNs disappear from the capillary tufts but the lumen is again crowded with monocytes. Some monocytes are found to be closely attached to the GBM (SHIGEMATSU, 1970). These monocytes exhibit prominent phagocytic activities for fibrin or cell fragments and change into large macrophages or epithelioid cells. The monocytic accumulation is transient and the patency of the lumen is well restored within 72 hours. The denuded GBM is again covered by the endothelium. In this reparatory process, the participation of endothelial cells is reflected by increased numbers of cytoplasmic ribosomes and occasional mitotic figures. It has been confirmed in rats tolerant to rabbit IgG (FELDMAN et al., 1963) that the first phase is transient and that the original glomerular architecture is restored within a few weeks.

On the other hand, marked thrombotic changes can be induced by the administration of a large dose of rabbit NTAbs (UNANUE et al., 1968). Under this condition, the migrant cell accumulation is not prominent and the glomerular capillary lumens are diffusely occluded by fibrin or fibrinoid material. Such exaggerated thrombotic lesions terminate in diffuse necrosis of the renal parenchyma and rapid uremic death of the diseased animals.

It has been suggested that the first phase of rat Masugi nephritis depends largely upon the participation of serum complement (HAMMER and DIXON, 1963; BAXTER and SMALL, 1963) and of PMNs mediated by the complement fixation (COCHRANE et al., 1965). In fact, glomerular changes are significantly modified in an experimental system in which there is little or no participation of complement. In rat Masugi nephritis produced by nephrotoxic guinea pig IgG_1 which did not fix complement *in vitro* at all but did so a little *in vivo*, endothelial exfoliation and fibrin deposition were detectable, but accumulation of PMNs was minimal (KOBAYASHI et al., 1973 a). $F(ab')_2$ fragments obtained from the nephrotoxic IgG_1 only caused endothelial exfoliation (KOBAYASHI et al., 1973 b). Moreover, it was reported that in congenitally complement deficient mice, NTAbs caused only a very mild glomerular disease in which leukocytic infiltration and proliferative change did not take place (UNANUE et al., 1967 b).

b) The Second Phase of Masugi Nephritis

The second phase develops several days after injection of NTAbs and is consistent with the appearance of autologous antibody (KAY, 1940). The autologous antibody specifically reacts with antigen (NTAb) fixed previously on the GBM so that its distribution is basically identical to that of antigen (ORTEGA and MELLORS, 1956; SEEGAL et al., 1963). Thus, in this phase, the host antibody is visualized by immunofluorescence as a continuous linear pattern. Simultaneously, complement is also fixed in the glomeruli in a similar fashion (UNANUE and DIXON, 1964). The pathologic changes in the second phase might be greatly modified by a number of factors such as animal species, the nature and amounts of NTAbs injected, and the intensity of host immune responses. In rat Masugi nephritis the kidney damage in the second phase is usually progressive, undergoing a chronic glomerular disease probably due to the continuing production of host antibody and its fixation to antigen (rabbit NTAb). This is in sharp contrast to the transient glomerular injury in the first phase as was proved in rats that were tolerant to rabbit IgG (Hammer and Dixon, 1963; Feldman et al., 1963).

Ultrastructurally, the predominant change in the second phase is the appearance of dense granular subendothelial deposits intimately applied to the GBM (Feldman, 1963; Feldman et al., 1963). Endothelial cells are swollen and mesangial cells increase in numbers (Suzuki et al., 1963). In a more chronic stage the mesangium is conspicuously widened due to an increase of the cellular elements as well as the basement membrane-like material or ground substance containing collagen fibers (Suzuki et al., 1963). The GBM is progressively thickened, apparently by incorporation of the subendothelial deposits (Feldman, 1963). The basement membrane-like material then appears in the lumen, irregularly separating the intracapillary cells. These processes may terminate in the virtual obliteration of the capillary tufts with destruction of the glomerular architecture.

An attempt has been made to clarify glomerular events limited to the second phase by using a weak rabbit NTAb that is not capable of inducing the first phase (Shigematsu and Kobayashi, 1971). The results obtained so far again confirm that the major change in the secondary phase is the GBM thickening with dense deposits. There were mild proliferative changes caused by intraluminal or subendothelial accumulation of migrant monocytes. The deposits were mostly observed at the subendothelial aspect of the GBM but some were also present at the outer aspect. With fluorescent microscopy, the subepithelial deposits were discernible as a granule located at the outer surface of linear fluorescence.

As compared to rat Masugi nephritis, a more severe, proliferative glomerular injury is seen in rabbit Masugi nephritis. It seems that this rabbit glomerulo-nephritis can serve as an excellent model for analyzing the nature of proliferative glomerular changes. Therefore, its pathologic features will be described below in some detail.

The second phase can be induced in rabbits without the preceding first phase by injection with an appropriate amount of duck NTAbs. The glomerulo-nephritis becomes manifest after a latent period of several days, and, within a month, a resolution occurs if the glomeruli have not been severely damaged. The GBM shows swelling and thickening, and appears somewhat porous because of its decreased density (Sakaguchi et al., 1957). Electron dense or opaque deposits are present at the subendothelial side of the GBM. The mesangial matrix is edematous and becomes inhomogeneous. These changes are often associated with the detachment of the endothelium from the GBM (Sakaguchi et al., 1957; Kondo and Shigematsu, 1972).

The second step of the process is characterized by marked glomerular hypercellularity. Obviously both endothelial cells and mesangial cells contribute in varying degrees to the proliferative glomerular change (SAKAGUCHI *et al.*, 1957; FUJIMOTO *et al.*, 1964). These fixed cells are swollen, proliferated, and their organelles are either enlarged or increased in number. However, with regard to the origin of increased mononuclear cells in the affected glomeruli, the progressive accumulation of migrant monocytes is more important (KONDO and SHIGEMATSU, 1972). Of particular note is that these monocytes show a remarkable tendency to contact intimately with the GBM. Their phagocytic activities are also prominent. Furthermore, a series of transformations of monocytes into macrophages, epithelioid cells, and occasional multinucleated giant cells is seen. Infiltration of PMNs is variable. Platelets, fibrin, or other thrombotic materials are seen occasionally in the lumen. As mentioned above, the proliferation of the fixed glomerular cells is important, yet it is not a major factor contributing to the hypercellularity. Therefore, the disappearance of migrant monocytes is principally followed by a resolution of the glomerular changes without severe structural alterations (KONDO and SHIGEMATSU, 1972). However, a thickening of the mesangium may persist for several months.

In contrast, rapidly progressive glomerulonephritis with a marked structural distortion is seen in rabbits receiving a larger amount of duck NTAbs (KONDO *et al.*, 1972). It seems that such a disorganizing glomerulonephritis is initiated by a conspicuous loosening of the mesangial matrix and the GBM. The mesangium is widened due to extensive edematous swelling or lysis of the matrix and hypertrophy as well as a proliferation of mesangial cells. There are local proliferations of endothelial cells and an enhanced accumulation of monocytic cells which are located in the capillary lumen, subendothelial space, and loosened mesangium. The tufts are frequently occluded by fibrin or fibrinoid substances and PMNs. The significance of mesangiolysis is a loss of the supporting element of the glomerular tuft structure which is then followed by an accentuation of lobular appearance in a mild case and, in an advanced stage, ballooning or globular transformation of the tufts. In fact, in a severely affected glomerulus, neither the mesangium nor the capillary lumen can be discerned, and the tufts are transformed into a dilated sack filled with numerous monocytes, proliferated glomerular cells (mostly mesangial cells), thrombotic material, and PMNs. Under these conditions, the GBM becomes progressively thinner and extended, eventually resulting in local or diffuse rupture. Owing to the GBM rupture a massive influx of monocytes or other blood elements occurs in Bowman's space. Although both visceral and parietal epithelial cells are involved in the process and damaged, their reactive overgrowth soon becomes evident. The extracapillary inflammation thus leads to formation of the crescent composed of monocytic cells and proliferated epithelial cells (KONDO *et al.*, 1972).

Little is known about mediators involved in the initiation and/or the persistence of the second phase, despite these remarkable histologic findings. It is unlikely from the morphologic aspect that PMNs again play a significant role as they do in the first phase of rat Masugi nephritis. The participation of complement is not *sine qua non*, although the disease process might be

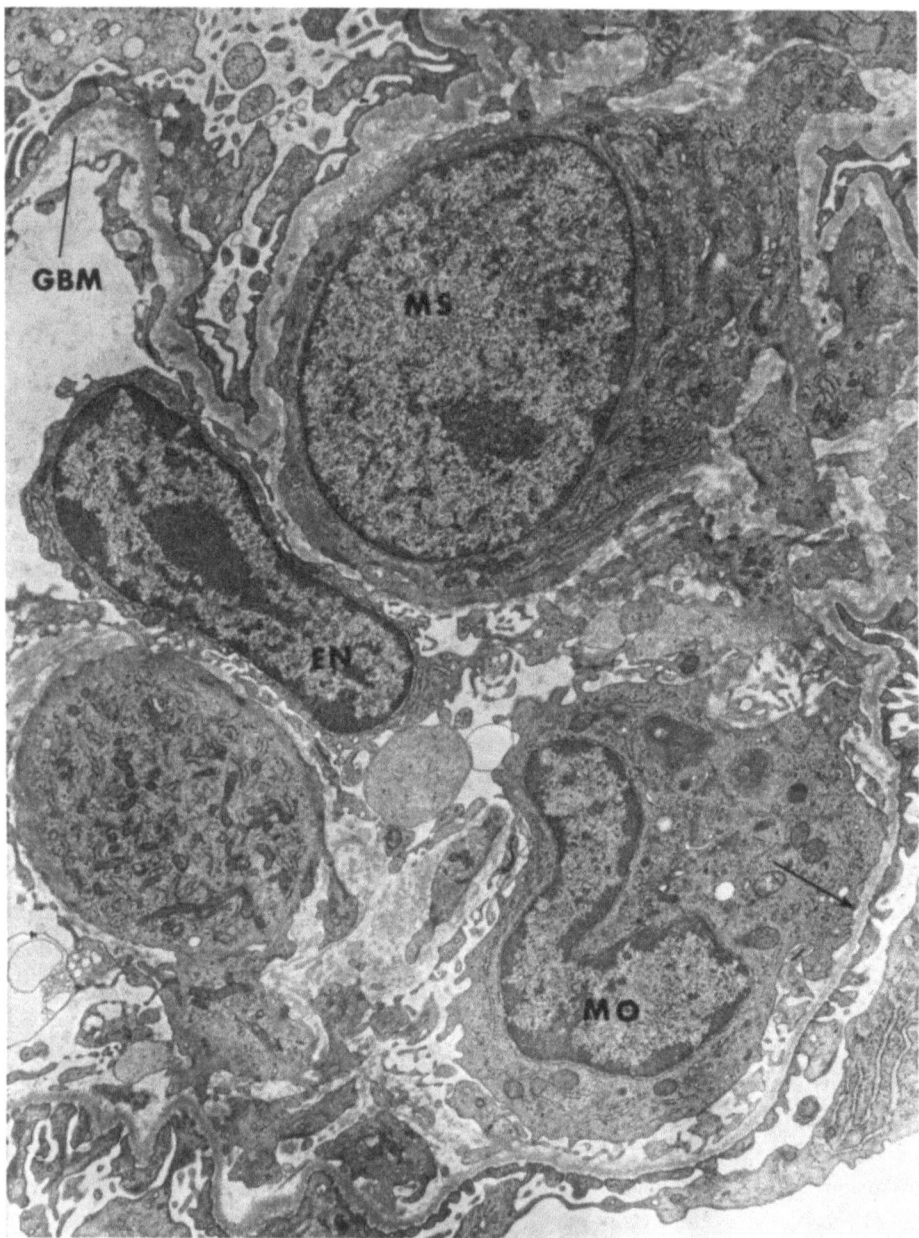

Fig. 4. An early glomerular change of rabbit Masugi nephritis induced by injection
with nephrotoxic duck antibody (second phase). Marked swelling of mesangial cells
(MS), a monocyte (MO) exhibiting localized contacts with basement membrane (arrow),
and subendothelial mottling of basement membrane (GBM) are seen. EN: endothelial
cell. ×8600

modified in complement deficient animals (UNANUE *et al.*, 1967b). Of the
many possible mediators accounting for the pathogenesis, the most outstanding
is the coagulation process. There is evidence that coagulation apparently

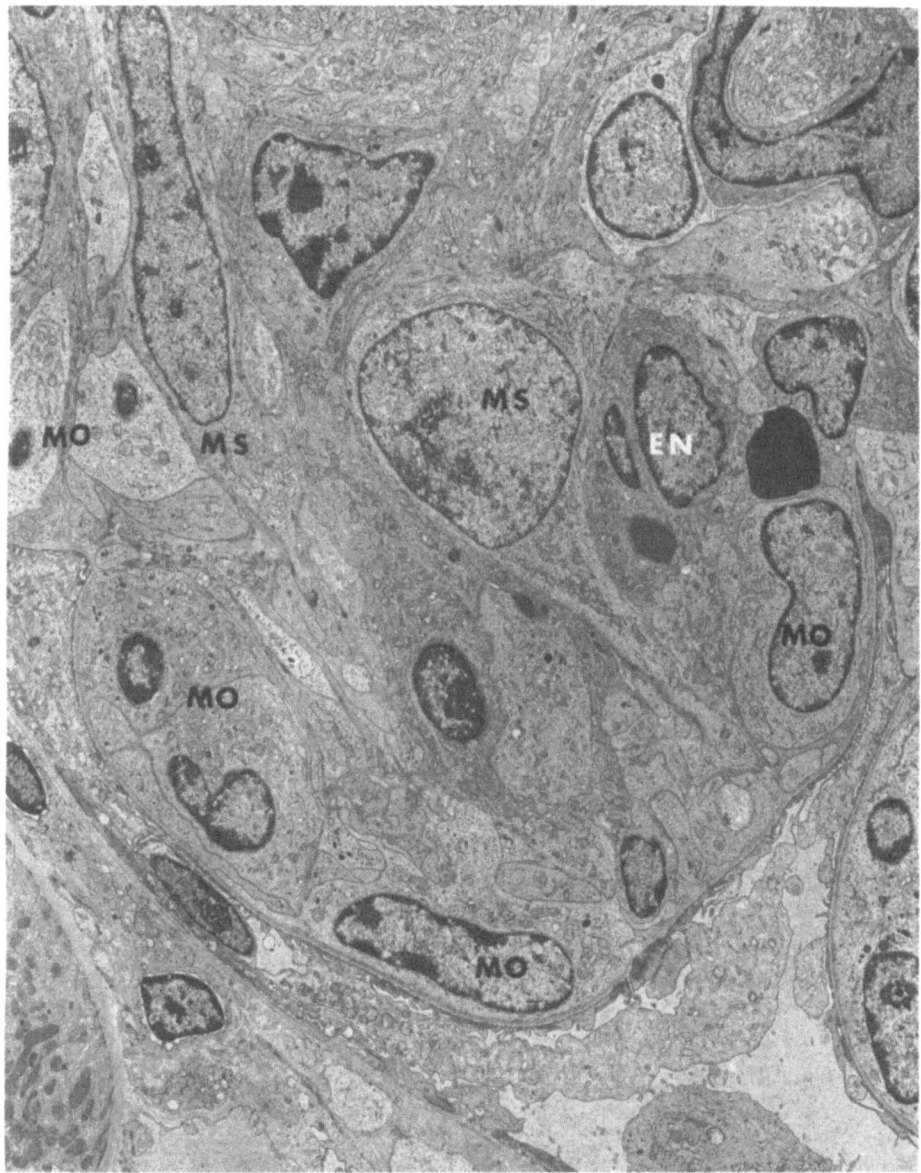

Fig. 5. Rabbit Masugi nephritis induced by injection with nephrotoxic duck antibody (second phase). Note a balloon-like distortion of a tuft filled with numerous monocytic cells (MO) and some swollen mesangial cells (MS), and endothelial cells (EN). ×4100

contributes to glomerular lesions in rabbit Masugi nephritis induced by a potent sheep NTAb (VASALLI and McCLUSKEY, 1964). About 5 days after injection of this sheep NTAb, a definite proliferation of endothelial and mesangial cells (intracapillary cells) developed, often associated with deposits of material with staining properties of fibrin. Fibrin and fibrinoid material were also seen in Bowman's space where they were invaded by proliferating epithelial cells (crescent formation). In contrast, it was found that these changes could be prevented strikingly, if the animals were treated with anti-coagulant (warfarin).

Ultrastructural analysis of Masugi nephritis has been performed in other animal species. In dogs injected with rabbit or sheep NTAb, the first phase was characterized by a "quellung" and occasional longitudinal splitting of the GBM, whereas in the second phase there was proliferation of intracapillary cells with a deposition of electron dense material between the endothelium and the GBM, and between the proliferated intracapillary cells (MOVAT et al., 1961). In the monkey, a proliferative glomerulonephritis appeared 6–10 days after injection of rabbit NTAb. Progressive basement membrane irregularities including thickening, splitting, and focal defects were observed, together with proliferations of endothelial, mesangial, and epithelial cells (BATTIFORA and MARKOWITZ, 1969).

2. Steblay Nephritis

Autologous antibodies with a nephritogenic property (autologous anti-GBM antibody) could be produced in some species of animals through immunization with homologous or heterologous GBM antigens. The sheep is particularly susceptible and fulminant glomerulonephritis is manifested within several months by repeated injections of human or other heterologous GBM antigens in Freund's complete adjuvant (STEBLAY, 1962). The antibody is localized linearly along the GBM as seen in immunofluorescence, and is capable of inducing glomerular injuries passively in the same species of animals, thereby indicating the autoimmune nature of the disease (LERNER and DIXON, 1966). Antibodies eluted from the GBM of nephritic sheep react, in vitro, with sheep GBM. They also react with lamb GBM in vivo, fix C3, and induce immediate glomerular injury (STEBLAY and RUDOFSKY, 1968). In the sheep or goat the glomerular lesions resulting in progressive renal failure are of a generalized crescentic type. Before the formation of fulminant crescents, characteristic GBM alterations are noted by electron microscopy (GERMUTH et al., 1972b; OHNUKI, 1975). The GBM shows irregular thickening and increased density, becomes tortuous, and terminates in its rupture. Such serious GBM damage is accompanied by a massive exudation of blood elements into Bowman's space. It seems that crescentic epithelial proliferation involving both visceral and parietal epithelium is partly stimulated by increased GBM permeability (proteinuria) but more intensely by the influx of red cells, PMNs, monocytes, and fibrin in the extracapillary space through the GBM break. Between the proliferated epithelial cells, basement membrane-like material may soon appear and the cell clusters undergo fibroepithelial crescents (STEBLAY, 1962). In contrast, intracapillary changes are not remarkable and no dense deposits have been detected so far (MUEHRCKE et al., 1967). Various glomerular alterations were also elicited in other animal species by similar procedures

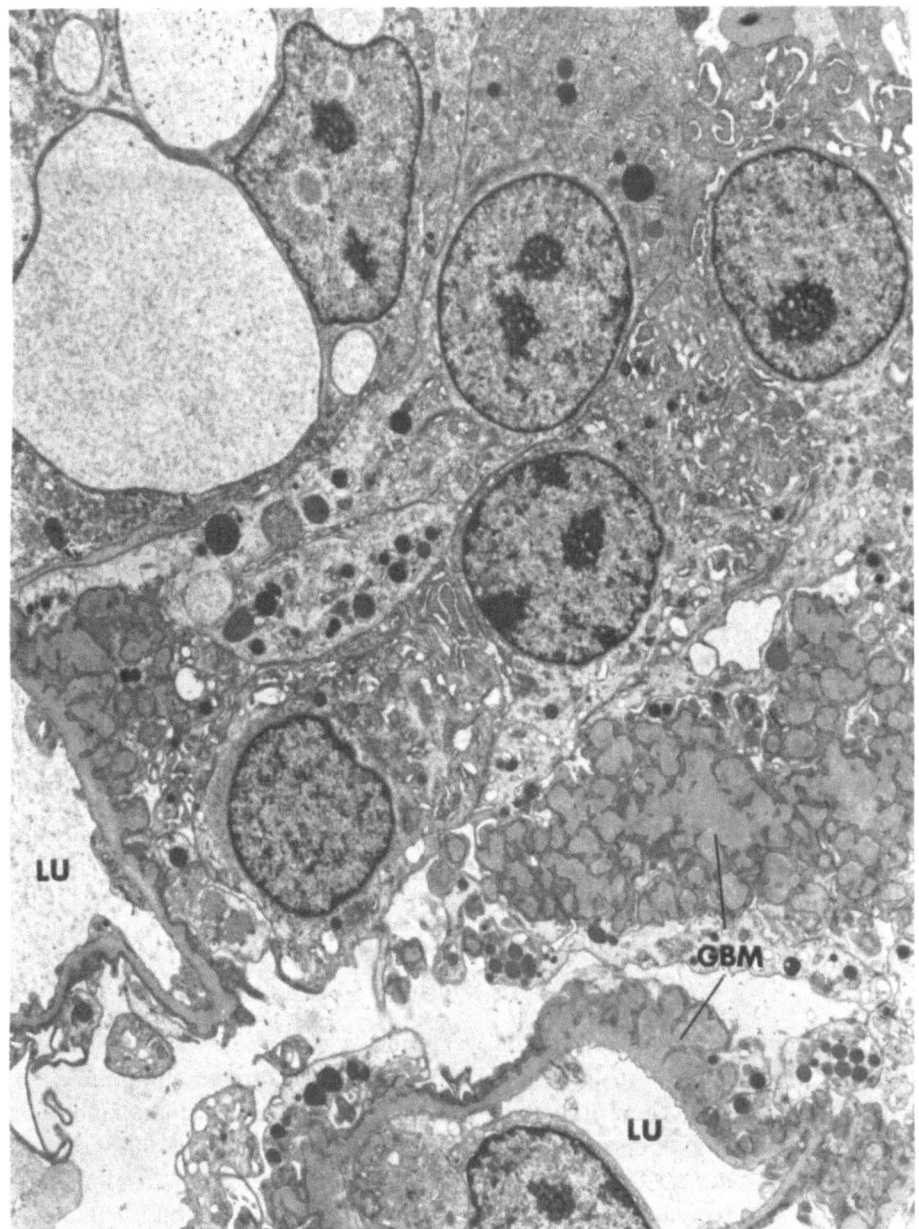

Fig. 6. A glomerular portion from a goat immunized with human glomerular basement membrane in Freund's adjuvant (a precrescentic stage of Steblay nephritis). Marked proliferation of podocytes and basement membrane irregularities (GBM) are seen. There are no peculiar abnormalities in the lumen (LU). ×5800. [T. OHNUKI, Acta path. jap. **25**, 319 (1975)]

and mechanisms (STEBLAY, 1963; PARONETTO and KOFFLER, 1967; UNANUE and DIXON, 1967a; UNANUE *et al.*, 1967a; COUSER *et al.*, 1973). The incidence of the glomerulonephritis could be increased by using enzymatically purified

GBM glycoprotein antigen (Shibata *et al.*, 1971). It is of interest that a very purified GBM antigen was no longer effective in stimulating animals to form anti-GBM antibodies, but was, for reasons unknown, still capable of producing glomerular lesions (Shibata *et al.*, 1972).

3. Acute Serum Sickness-Type Nephritis

In experimental acute serum sickness, a variety of tissue lesions including necrotizing angiitis and proliferative glomerulonephritis may develop in the rabbit some days after a single i.v. injection of a large dose of antigen ("one-shot" serum sickness) or within a few days after a second injection ("accelerated" serum sickness) (*see* McCluskey, 1965). It has been shown that the injected antigen (BSA) is eliminated from the circulation in three phases consisting of: (1) an equilibration of the antigen between the intravascular and extravascular fluid spaces, (2) non-immune catabolism by the host, and (3) a rapid elimination resulting from the formation of antigen–antibody complexes (Germuth, 1953; Dixon *et al.*, 1958). The onset of the tissue lesions is recognized during the immune phase of antigen elimination and they tend to disappear at the time when free antibody appears in the circulation. Indeed, it has been confirmed that soluble antigen–antibody complexes formed in the circulation in an antigen excess environment are capable of inducing the inflammation in serum sickness subsequent to their deposition at the tissue sites (Dixon *et al.*, 1958).

The pathogenic role of the complexes shown in this "active serum sickness" can be more directly evidenced in "passive serum sickness" which develops after i.v. injection of soluble antigen–antibody complexes prepared *in vitro* (McCluskey and Benacerraf, 1959).

a) Active Serum Sickness Nephritis

The glomerular disease occurs between one or two weeks after the antigen administration, consistent with the immune phase of antigen elimination. By immunofluorescence, the antigen, host antibody (IgG), and complement are detectable as scattered, discrete granules located along the glomerular capillary walls (Dixon *et al.*, 1958; Fish *et al.*, 1966). A common feature of glomerular alterations is an increased cellularity in which PMN accumulation is sometimes remarkable but at other times minimal. There is a marked proliferation and swelling of endothelial cells, often to such a degree that the lumens are completely occluded (Feldman, 1958; Feldman, 1964). Mesangial cells also contribute to the hypercellularity (Robertson and More, 1961; Arakawa and Kimmelstiel, 1970), and are related to the formation of the mesangial matrix or basement membrane-like material. It seems, however, that the hypercellularity is more often characterized by a massive influx of migrant monocytes (Kobayashi and Shigematsu, 1975). The monocytes (macrophages) and PMNs are present in the lumen and mesangium or subendothelial space.

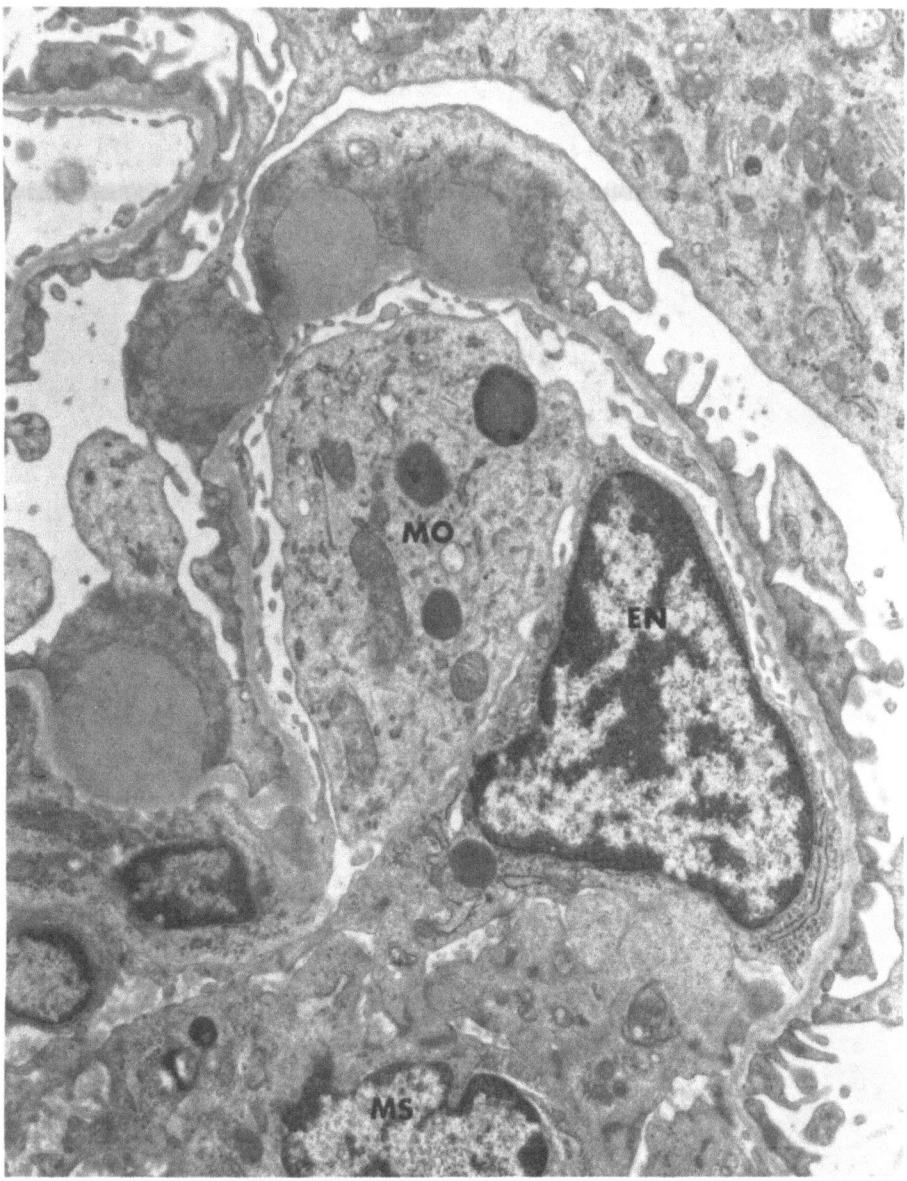

Fig. 7. "One-shot" serum sickness nephritis of a rabbit produced by i.v. injection with large dose of bovine serum albumin (healing stage). Large subepithelial deposits are seen. A capillary lumen is still occluded by a phagocyte (MO) and a swollen endothelial cell (EN). MS: mesangial cell. × 12000

Thrombotic, necrotizing changes are seen focally in severely involved glomeruli. Epithelial foot processes are fused in varying degrees. During the active stage, the GBM appears for the most part to be intact (FELDMAN, 1958; UNANUE et al., 1968), although detailed observation may disclose the presence of small subepithelial deposits (FELDMAN, 1958; ARAKAWA and KIMMELSTIEL, 1970).

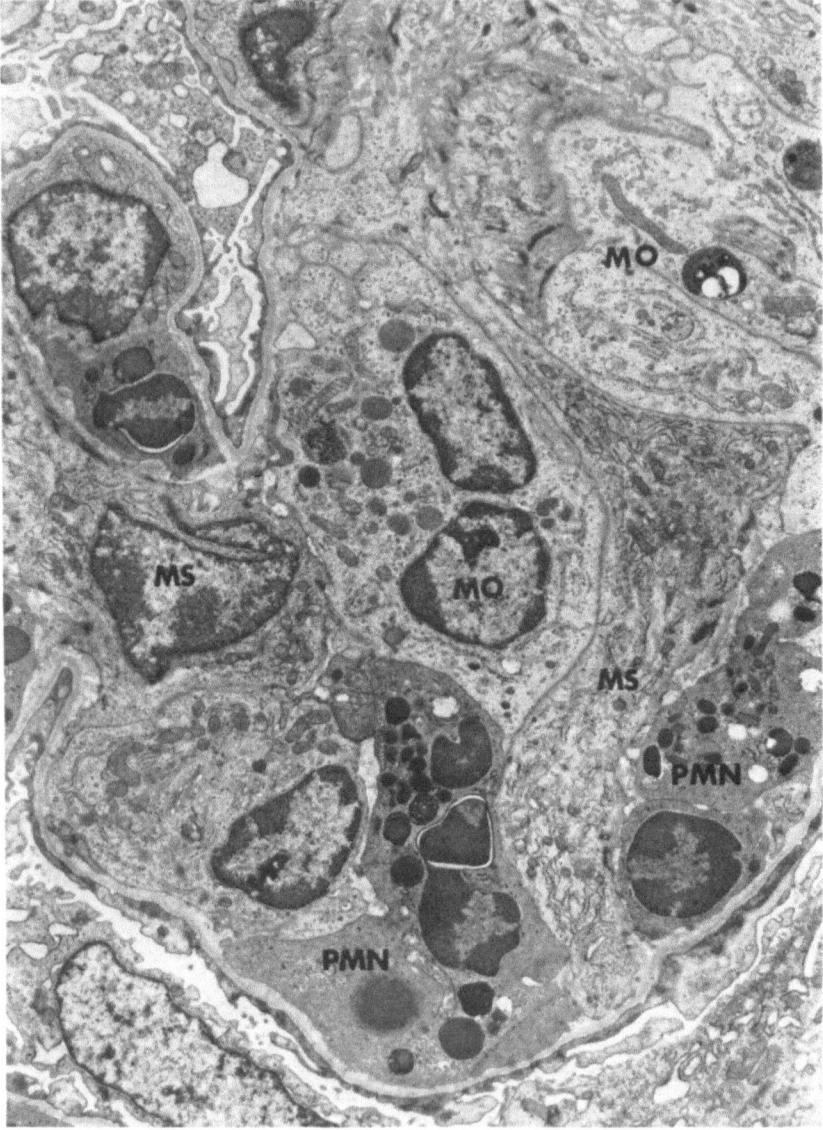

Fig. 8. Florid serum sickness nephritis of a rabbit produced by two injections of large dose of bovine serum albumin. Note disintegration of the mesangium and loss of normal capillary structure. The tuft is filled with mesangial cells (MS), monocytes (MO), and leukocytes (PMN). Some of PMNs are located directly on basement membrane. ×6400

Characteristic large subepithelial deposits, compatible with humps in human acute poststreptococcal glomerulonephritis (KIMMELSTIEL et al., 1962), are found after the antigen elimination when the inflammatory process is subsiding and a reparatory process is taking place in the affected glomeruli (FISH et al., 1966). Presumably the deposits are not causatively related to the glomerular inflammation (ARAKAWA and KIMMELSTIEL, 1970). The glomerular changes

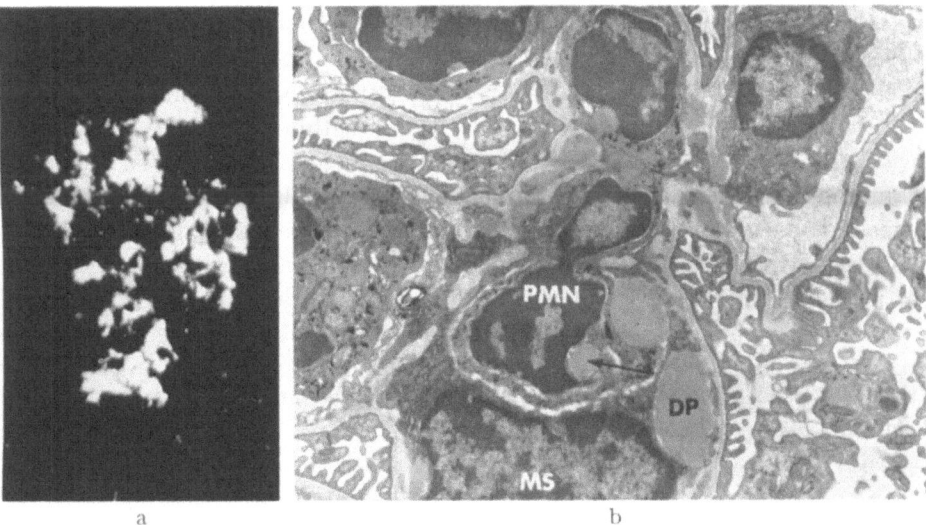

Fig. 9. Passive serum sickness nephritis of a mouse produced by i.v. injections of antigen (DNP-BSA)–antibody complex prepared *in vitro*. (a) A fluorescent micrograph of a glomerulus showing large aggregates of mouse IgG in the lumens and mesangium. × 360. (Courtesy of Dr. T. KOYAMA.) (b) Large dense deposits are seen in the mesangium (DP). Some deposits (arrow) are engulfed by an infiltrating leukocyte (PMN). MS: mesangial cell. × 7 800

are fairly well resolved within a few weeks, leaving focal sclerosing and collapsed areas. Vanishing processes of the subepithelial deposits have not yet been clarified.

Several procedures have been known to enhance the serum sickness disease, e.g. exaggerated glomerular lesions are evoked by an additional injection of the same dose of antigen into the rabbit just before the appearance of free antibody in the circulation (KOBAYASHI and SHIGEMATSU, 1975). The glomerular disease thus developed is characterized by prominent edema or lysis of the mesangium. The disorganized tufts are occluded by proliferated glomerular cells as well as migrant phagocytes, and proteinaceous substances. A crescent formation may also be seen whenever the GBM is severely damaged. It is interesting that subepithelial deposits are rarely encountered. After the inflammation has diminished, a sclerosing process takes place which rapidly terminates in collapse and scarring of the involved tufts. It should be emphasized that the ultrastructural pathology of this florid serum sickness nephritis strikingly resembles that just described in rabbit Masugi nephritis.

The deposition of immune complexes and the following tissue injury might be considerably modified by factors which will be discussed later.

b) Passive Serum Sickness Nephritis

Acute proliferative glomerulonephritis can be easily produced in mice or rats by a single or repeated injections of preformed antigen–antibody complexes (MCCLUSKEY and BENACERRAF, 1959; BENACERRAF et al., 1960; MCCLUSKEY et al., 1960; MILLER et al., 1960; OKUMURA et al., 1971). Fluorescent microscopy shows that both antigen and antibody are deposited in the glomerular mesangium, on the capillary wall, and within the lumen (MCCLUSKEY et al., 1962; MELLORS and BRZOSKO, 1962; OKUMURA et al., 1971). In mouse glomerulonephritis, deposits of large dense material in the mesangium are most prominent and accumulations of monocytes (macrophages) and PMNs (OKUMURA et al., 1971) are conspicuous. The deposits are sometimes detectable in the subendothelial space or within the GBM but there are no subepithelial deposits. The mesangium is infiltrated by these migrant phagocytes which contain numerous dense phagosomes, suggesting their role in the removal of the deposits. In contrast, the swollen endothelial and mesangial cells exhibit little phagocytic activity toward the deposits.

Both active and passive serum sickness nephritis may develop on a common immunologic basis; however, there are considerable differences between the two as to the site of deposits and the inflammatory tissue responses. This discrepancy is partly explained by the difference of the animal species used and the property of immune complexes deposited.

4. Chronic Serum Sickness-Type Nephritis

Animals receiving repeated injections of protein antigens may develop chronic glomerulonephritis. In rabbits that received daily i.v. injections of variable amounts of BSA or other antigens, it has been observed that the incidence of chronic glomerulonephritis is independent of the kind and absolute amount of antigen injected and is only seen in those animals responding with antibody barely sufficient to neutralize the antigen (DIXON et al., 1961). Histologically, glomerular lesions can be divided into two major types: proliferative or inflammatory glomerulonephritis, and degenerative glomerulonephritis. In immunofluorescence both are usually characterized by granular, often confluent, beaded deposits of antigen and host IgG distributed diffusely on the capillary walls (DIXON et al., 1961). Similar results have also been obtained in the animals immunized repeatedly with sufficient amounts of antigens via different parenteral routes (MOPPERT and FRESEN, 1967; KURIYAMA, 1973). Immunoelectron microscopy has revealed the sites of the deposition in great detail (ANDRES et al., 1963).

Lobulation of glomerular tufts, proliferation and swelling of endothelial cells, and subepithelial dense deposits with GBM thickening occur in the proliferative type. The mesangium is enlarged due to the increase in cellular and intercellular elements (FELDMAN, 1964). These changes lead to a progressive alteration of glomerular architecture resulting in collapse and scarred obsolescence of the glomeruli.

In addition to this rather common proliferative glomerulonephritis, a few rabbits show a different proliferative change confined to the mesangium (DIXON et al., 1961; GERMUTH et al., 1972a; KURIYAMA, 1973). By fluorescent

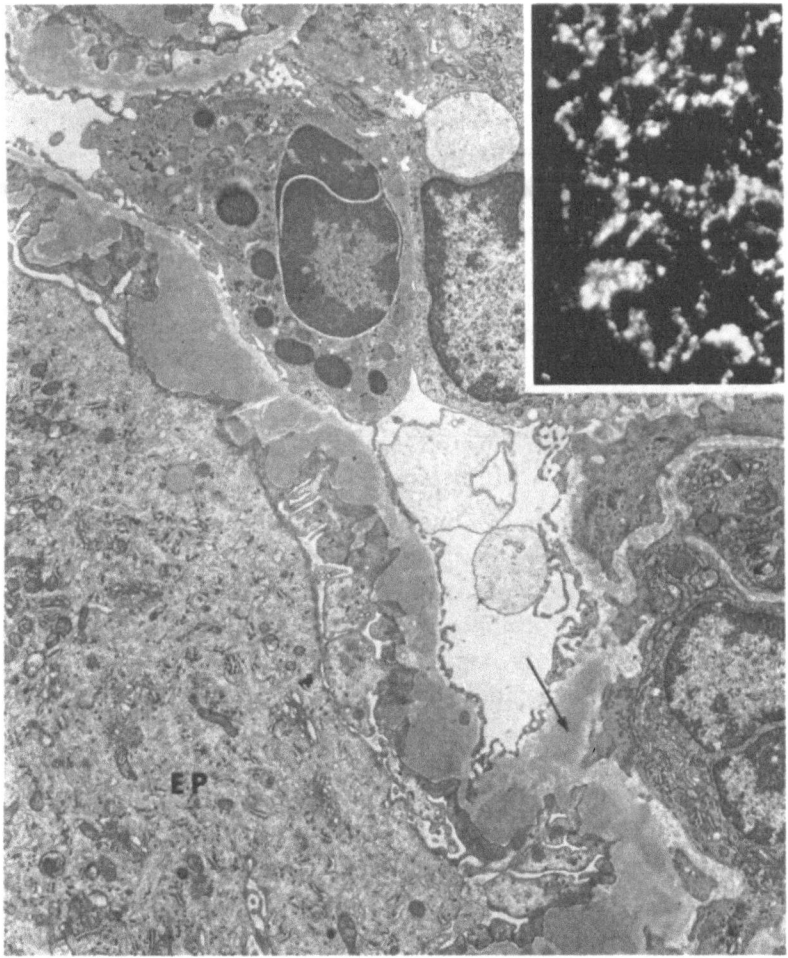

Fig. 10. Membranous nephropathy developed in a rabbit following repeated i.m. injections of egg albumin. Marked basement membrane thickening associated with numerous subepithelial deposits. Dense deposits are also present in the mesangium (arrow). Swelling of a podocyte (EP) and diffuse foot process fusions are seen. ×6500. (Courtesy of Dr. K. KURIYAMA.) Inset: A fluorescent micrograph of rabbit membranous nephropathy. Beaded deposits of rabbit IgG along capillary walls are evident. ×540. (Courtesy of Dr. N. SHINOHARA)

and electron microscopy, immune deposits are seen to occur mostly in the mesangium. The increased mesangial cells are occasionally located in the space between the endothelium and the GBM entirely along a capillary loop (KURIYAMA, 1973), exhibiting a feature which has been referred to as circumferential mesangial interposition (ARAKAWA and KIMMELSTIEL, 1969).

Degenerative glomerulonephritis is principally characterized by the presence of numerous dense deposits at the outer aspect of the GBM (DIXON et al., 1961). The deposition is frequently associated with GBM thickening but without significant proliferative changes. These features, together with the clinical manifestation of the nephrotic syndrome, closely resemble those of membranous nephropathy (membranous glomerulonephritis) in humans. Presumably the complexes are initially deposited at the subendothelial space as a flocculent, ill-defined mass. These deposits might be able to penetrate the GBM under conditions of increased GBM permeability and then aggregate at the subepithelial site, thus forming a typical dense deposit (KURIYAMA, 1973).

The subepithelial deposits are surrounded by newly formed basement membrane-like material so that GBM thickening gradually becomes manifest. The deposits enclosed within the GBM substance probably disintegrate; however, they would still persist after cessation of antigen injection over a period of many months (FELDMAN, 1963).

5. Heymann Nephritis

Some strains of rats, after receiving repeated i.p. injections of homologous renal tissue in complete Freund's adjuvant, develop a progressive glomerular disease with the nephrotic syndrome (HEYMANN et al., 1959). The glomerular disease resembles chronic serum sickness nephritis in many respects, namely granular localization of host immunoglobulin and C3 (OKUDA et al., 1965; DIXON et al., 1965) and a membranous thickening of the capillary wall without notable proliferative changes. The GBM thickening apparently results from subepithelial depositions of electron-dense material (BLOZIS et al., 1962; FELDMAN, 1963; ALOUSI et al., 1969; LAGUENS and SEEGAL, 1969; SUGISAKI et al., 1973). The deposits are rare, if present, and the GBM thickness is normal at the prenephrotic stage (ALOUSI et al., 1969). The deposits are finely granular and irregular in shape. They become larger and greater in number with time and are gradually surrounded or enclosed by newly formed GBM substances. Although the mesangium is more or less accentuated and the mesangial cells extend their cytoplasmic processes peripherally or into the lumen, changes in the luminal side of the tufts are not remarkable in most instances.

These features suggest that the glomerular disease is evoked by the deposition of immune complexes. This has been supported and further extended by several important observations. Firstly, the nephritogenic antigen has been identified as a renal tubular epithelium-specific antigen which is derived primarily from the brush border of proximal tubules of the rat kidney (EDGINGTON et al., 1968). Secondly, the renal tubular antigen has been demonstrated in the diseased glomerulus along with host immunoglobulin and C3 (GLASSOCK et al., 1968). Thirdly, circulating antibodies directed against the renal tubular epithelium have been detected in the nephrotic rat. In addition, immunoglobulin eluted from the diseased kidney reacts specifically with the luminal portion of the proximal tubular epithelium (GRUPE and KAPLAN, 1969). These results strongly indicate that this disease results from the glomerular deposition of peculiar immune complexes consisting of the renal tubular antigen(s) and the corresponding antibodies.

6. Glomerulonephritis and Prolonged Antigenic Stimulation

Alterations of immune responses should also be considered with respect to the pathogenesis of chronic serum sickness diseases since a wasting of immune system activities occurs in the later stage of prolonged antigenic stimulation. On the basis of such an alteration of the antibody forming tissues, a number of unusual antibodies appear in animals, including autoantibodies directed against blood cells and nuclear antigen (OKABAYASHI, 1964). In this situation inflammatory processes, e.g. glomerulonephritis, often exhibit a degenerative conversion (OKABAYASHI, 1970). In addition, some animals show wire-loop glomerular lesions along with a positive tissue, as well as *in vitro*, LE phenomenon, and other hallmarks of systemic lupus erythematosus (OKABAYASHI, 1964). Similar lupus-like nephritis has also been noted in C57BL mice bearing antinuclear antibodies during the course of prolonged antigenic stimulation (OKUMURA, 1973). In the diseased glomeruli, granular or lumpy deposits of mouse IgG are seen in the mesangium and on the capillary walls, whereas the antigen injected is not detectable. With the electron microscope, dense deposits are seen at the inner aspect of the GBM and within the mesangium where the deposits exhibit a peculiar organized structure resembling that which has been described in human lupus nephritis (GRISHMAN *et al.*, 1967).

7. Glomerulonephritis Associated with Infection

a) Glomerulonephritis in Aleutian Disease of Mink

A population of mink with a changed skin color (Aleutian mink; homozygous recessive for the Aleutian gene, aa) has been known to be affected by a fatal glomerular disease, in addition to systemic angiitis, massive infiltration of lymphocytes or plasma cells in various tissues, and hyperglobulinemia (reviewed by: NORTON, 1970; COCHRANE and KOFFLER, 1973). The mink disease apparently occurs associated with a spontaneous or experimental infection of virus (Aleutian disease virus). In renal glomeruli, slight to marked depositions of IgG and complement are seen by immunofluorescence in keeping with the severity of the disease. The fluorescence is granular or lumpy and is localized within the mesangium and along the capillary walls (HENSON *et al.*, 1969; PORTER *et al.*, 1969). Traces of virus antigen are found in a few cases (PORTER *et al.*, 1969). Broad eosinophilic thickening of the capillary walls with a wire-loop appearance, widening of the mesangium, and proliferation of glomerular cells are present. By electron microscopy, abundant dense deposits are seen in the subendothelial space, mesangium, and to a lesser extent at the subepithelial aspect of the GBM (HENSON *et al.*, 1967; KINDIG *et al.*, 1967; McKAY *et al.*, 1967; HENSON *et al.*, 1968; PAN *et al.*, 1970b). The deposits are also present within the cytoplasm of the endothelial and mesangial cells (HENSON *et al.*, 1968; PAN *et al.*, 1970b). The mesangial cells increase in numbers and extend their cytoplasmic processes everywhere. Infiltration of PMNs and other inflammatory cells is also seen in the lumen or mesangium, and these cells sometimes attach themselves to the deposits. Thrombotic changes are seen in varying degrees. Several months after the infection, degenerative glomerular lesions become evident (Pan et al., 1970a; Pan et al., 1970b). Almost all capillary loops are obliterated by massive depositions of eosinophilic sub- stances, and glomerular cells undergo degeneration or necrosis. A frequent complication of degenerative glomeruli is adhesion of the tufts to Bowman's capsule with or without crescent formation.

The pathogenesis of the glomerulonephritis in Aleutian mink disease is not exactly known. It has been reported that a large protein complex (22s–25s) is present and, in fact, virus antigen–antibody complexes circulate in infected mink (Porter et al., 1965; Porter et al., 1967). It is therefore reasonable to conclude that the disease is intimately related to the formation of viral antigen–antibody complexes and subsequent deposition in glomerular capil- laries (Porter et al., 1969). The importance of intravascular coagulation as a causative factor for the inflammation has also been suggested (McKay et al., 1967; Henson et al., 1967).

b) Glomerulonephritis in New Zealand Strain Mice

Various tissue and blood abnormalities appear spontaneously in the New Zealand (NZ) strain of mice, including glomerulonephritis, vasculitis, immuno- proliferative diseases, and autoantibodies against red blood cells and nuclear antigens (Mellors, 1966; Howie and Helyer, 1968). The mouse disease has therefore been referred to as a representative model of naturally occurring autoimmune disease. Frequency of renal involvement along with positive LE cell phenomenon is strikingly increased by hybridization between mice with black (NZB) and white (NZW) skin color, and the glomerular alterations are compatible with those of systemic lupus erythematosus in man (Helyer and Howie, 1963). Female (NZB × NZW)F$_1$ mice are more severely affected than males. Fluorescent microscopy reveals progressive granular or lumpy deposits of immunoglobulins along the capillary walls and within the mes- angium (Aarons, 1964; Mellors, 1965; Nairn et al., 1966) accompanied by inflammatory exudation of albumin and fibrinogen (McGiven and Hicks, 1967). There might be a broad histologic resemblance between the NZB and NZB × NZW mouse glomerulonephritis (Hicks and Burnet, 1966). At the early stage, when light and fluorescent microscopy do not show any changes, local deposits of dense materials can be detectable by electron microscopy, scattered sparsely on the GBM (McGiven and Lynraven, 1968). The deposits become more extensive with age and are seen on both sides of the GBM (Channing et al., 1965; Mellors, 1965; Dubois et al., 1966; Hicks and Burnet, 1966), and most abundantly at the subendothelial aspect, thereby resembling wire-loop lesions. The deposits are of such an extent as to entirely occlude the capillary lumens. The lumens are also obliterated by increased intracapillary cells. The mesangium is enlarged by an accumulation of dense deposits and by cellular proliferation. Although basement membrane-like material appears between the increased intracapillary cells, the GBM proper does not seem to be greatly altered (CHANNING et al., 1965). Fibrin is visible within the capillary tufts and sometimes in Bowman's space, accompanying crescentic epithelial proliferation. From the results of fluorescent and electron-microscopic studies, it is highly probable that the deposits are composed of a mixture of immune complexes and fibrinoid material. The disease process is progressive and results finally in the obliteration of the affected capillary loops.

In studying the pathogenesis of NZ-mouse disease, special attention has been directed to infection of wild type Gross leukemia virus (GLV). It was found that the NZ mice carried GLV throughout life and produced natural antibody against GLV antigens (MELLORS et al., 1969). The glomerulonephritis of $(NZB \times NZW)F_1$ hybrid mice became prevalent as the GLV antigens underwent immune elimination from the circulation and the antigens together with bound immunoglobulins were deposited in the diseased glomeruli (MELLORS et al., 1971). It is therefore proposed that the formation of natural antibody against GLV antigens and the subsequent glomerular deposition of the viral antigen–antibody complexes play a role in the pathogenesis of the glomerulonephritis. On the other hand, it was revealed that acid eluates from nephritic kidney contained antibodies against nuclear components and that glomerular changes could be exacerbated by immunization with nuclear antigens (LAMBERT and DIXON, 1968). Moreover, quantitative immunologic studies have disclosed that elutable IgG is directed largely to nucleoprotein and partly to GLV antigens (DIXON et al., 1971). These results imply that nuclear antigen–antinuclear antibody complexes are the principal immuno-reactant relevant to the pathogenesis and GLV antigen–antibody complexes are involved to a lesser extent. The source of nuclear antigens to which the mice respond is unknown.

c) Other Glomerulonephritis Correlated to Infectious Agents

Viral infections are the most common pathogenic mechanism of murine glomerular diseases. In some of the animals infected with a virus, e.g. lympho-cytic choriomeningitis virus, it was found that the viral antigen–antibody complexes were circulating in the blood and the complexes were deposited in the glomeruli in a granular fashion (OLDSTONE and DIXON, 1971). Glomerulo-nephritis associated with viral infection was also seen in chronic hog cholera, which was characterized by PMN accumulation and increasing deposition of dense material at the mesangial side of the GBM, in keeping with positive fluorescence for pig immunoglobulin (CHEVILLE et al., 1970). Direct viral damage to glomerular cells and deposition of viral antigen–antibody complexes were thought to be causative mechanisms.

Frequent glomerular abnormalities have been noted in animals with *Plasmodium* or *Schistosoma* infections. Mice infected with *P. berghei* developed slight to moderate proliferative glomerulonephritis with scattered electron-dense deposits in the mesangium and GBM (BOONPUCKNAVIG et al., 1972;

Suzuki, 1974). With the fluorescent microscope, malarial antigen, host immunoglobulin (exclusively IgM), and complement were detected in the glomeruli. In monkeys infected with S. mansoni, the affected glomeruli contained
host antibody but not schistosomal antigens (Brito et al., 1971). The parasitic
antigen was demonstrated in monkey glomerulonephritis produced by
S. japonicum infection, together with various immunoglobulins including IgE
and complement (Tada et al., 1975). The glomerulonephritis was possibly
modified by concurrent hepatic damage.

8. Miscellaneous Types of Glomerulonephritis of Possible Immune Origin

Spontaneously occurring glomerular diseases in various species of animals
are most likely of the immune complex variety, although this has not been
determined beyond doubt. Several inbred strains of mice were known to
uniformly exhibit glomerular alterations with age. These changes were characterized by progressive mesangial sclerosis with deposits of host antibody and
complement (Linder et al., 1972). Other species of animals, e.g. galagos
(Burkholder et al., 1971) or dogs (Murray et al., 1974), also showed spontaneous glomerulonephritis of a possible immune complex type. It has been
reported that glomerular lesions occur concomitantly with transplantation
immunity. A mild membranous glomerular change was frequently noted in
chronic allogeneic disease in mice (Lewis et al., 1968). Glomeruli were usually
involved in renal allograft rejection in rats (Lindquist et al., 1968) or dogs
(Horowitz et al., 1965; Kondo et al., 1974).

IV. Some Pathogenic Considerations in Relation to Morphologic Manifestations

Many conditions should be considered in studying the pathology of immunologically induced glomerulonephritis. Although available concepts have
recently accumulated to account for its pathogenesis and morphologic manifestations, many problems remain to be resolved. Since a detailed introduction of these is beyond the scope of the present review, a brief discussion
will be made here as to how and to what extent immunologic processes and
mediators involved are concerned with some characteristic glomerular alterations.

1. Glomerular Alterations and Localization of Immune Reactants

As mentioned before, it may well be that renal glomeruli are damaged
by antibodies directed against the glomerular constituents, most likely GBM,
or by depositions of nonglomerular antigen–antibody complexes.

In the first phase of rat Masugi nephritis, a representative model of the
antiGBM-type glomerulonephritis, rabbit NTAbs and complement (C3) are

specifically localized on the GBM entirely along the capillary loops (UNANUE and DIXON, 1964). The localization pattern has also been confirmed and further extended by immunoelectron microscopy (ANDRES et al., 1962; ARHELGER et al., 1963; VOGT et al., 1968; MASUGI, 1969; DRUET et al., 1972; HOEDEMAEKER et al., 1972), indicating that the GBM is a crucial site of the antigen–antibody interaction. This may lead one to assume that a diffuse alteration takes place all along the GBN; however, electron microscopy has failed to show any diffuse, uniform GBM changes. Only localized foci of subendothelial mottling or wispy deposits and variable thickening of the GBM were of note (FELDMAN, 1963). In contrast to indefinite GBM alterations, intraluminal changes are remarkable, consisting of PMN accumulation, thrombocyte aggregation, deposits of fibrin, and swelling and slight proliferation of glomerular cells. It has been suggested that many of these changes are relevant to the participation of the complement system (HAMMER and DIXON, 1963). The complement fixation was followed by an accumulation of PMNs and thus glomerulonephritis developed (COCHRANE et al., 1965). Either complement or PMN depletion (COCHRANE et al., 1965) and enzymatic digestions of the NTAbs (BAXTER and SMALL, 1963) were effective in preventing the onset of definite glomerular lesions except for endothelial detachment from the GBM (KOBAYASHI et al., 1973 b). It is questionable whether the first phase is completely complement dependent since duck NTAbs, which do not fix mammalian complement and possess a unique biological property distinct from rabbit NTAbs (FUJIMOTO et al., 1964), could elicit an immediate glomerular injury after the injection (STAVITSKY et al., 1956; HASSON et al., 1957; HAMMER and DIXON, 1963). This implies that in addition to the complement and PMN systems, other unknown mediators might be operative in the first phase.

In the second phase of Masugi nephritis, the NTAb, autologous antibody, and complement are seen to be localized along the GBM in immunofluorescence (UNANUE and DIXON, 1964). Here again, GBM alterations are not diffuse but rather focal and are recognizable in electron microscopy as ill-defined subendothelial deposits (FELDMAN, 1963) or occasionally as dense subepithelial deposits (SHIGEMATSU and KOBAYASHI, 1971). As compared to the first phase, proliferative or other glomerular changes are more severe and often self-perpetuating. They are largely dependent upon the host immune responses and could be intensified by passive administration of specific homologous antibody (VASSALLI and MCCLUSKEY, 1964) or additional antigenic stimulation (SHIGEMATSU and KOBAYASHI, 1973). The mediators involved in this phase have been poorly established. The role of PMNs and complement is not quite the same as in the first phase. It is interesting that intravascular coagulation is important in producing proliferative changes in the second phase of rabbit Masugi nephritis. The administration of an anticoagulant agent resulted not only in the prevention of deposits of fibrin but also in proliferative intra- and extracapillary changes (VASSALLI and MCCLUSKEY, 1964). It appears that the clotting process results from the effect of the antigen–antibody interaction on platelets (ROBBINS and STETSON, 1959; SIQUEIRA and NELSON, 1961;

BETTEX-GALLAND *et al.*, 1963). The importance of the clotting mechanism has also been evidenced by the experiment in which a variety of glomerular abnormalities are brought about by injecting several drugs which accelerate intravascular coagulation (VASSALLI *et al.*, 1963).

Discrete, granular distribution of antigen, antibody, and complement is a characteristic fluorescent finding in classic "one-shot" serum sickness nephritis in rabbits (DIXON *et al.*, 1958; FISH *et al.*, 1966). Frequently the antigen is difficult to detect, probably due to the covering of antigenic determinants by the host antibodies (WILSON and DIXON, 1970). Circulating antigen–antibody complexes are not always deposited in the tissue sites but appreciable portions are thought to be removed by the reticuloendothelial cells (BENACER-RAF *et al.*, 1959). It was shown that platelet depletion as well as the ad-ministration of antagonists of vasoactive amines similarly prevented the deposition and the onset of glomerular lesions (KNIKER and COCHRANE, 1968). A possible role of IgE antibody was also proposed in connection with the deposition (COCHRANE, 1971). Although arterial lesions in acute serum sickness was PMN and complement dependent, glomerulonephritis developed in the absence of PMNs (KNIKER and COCHRANE, 1965) and C3 or other components of complement (HENSON and COCHRANE, 1971). Thus mediation of glomerular injury subsequent to the deposition of immune complexes is not yet clearly understood. Whatever the mediators, the deposition is followed by proliferative changes of the glomeruli. The most prominent changes are swelling and proliferation of glomerular cells (FELDMAN, 1958; ARAKAWA and KIMMEL-STIEL, 1970). In the active stage of the disease, GBM alterations are not remarkable and the complexes are hardly visible by electron microscopy in terms of dense deposits (FELDMAN, 1958; FISH *et al.*, 1966). Typical sub-epithelial deposits are usually found late after antigen elimination when the glomerular inflammation tends to heal. In fact, there is no correlation between the inflammation and the subepithelial deposits (ARAKAWA and KIMMELSTIEL, 1970). It was speculated that the circulating complexes were nephritogenic while those deposited in the subepithelial space were no longer phlogogenic in spite of continued interaction with antibody and complement (WILSON and DIXON, 1970). Thus the glomerulonephritis in one-shot serum sickness is transient.

The frequency of glomerular deposition, sites of deposits, and pathologic features are greatly influenced by the size of the complexes. Very large com-plexes are effectively removed by the reticuloendothelial cells prior to the tissue deposition. The deposition with a resultant tissue injury was found almost exclusively in animals forming somewhat larger complexes, greater than 19s in size (COCHRANE and HAWKINS, 1968), while those smaller than 19s were rarely deposited. The importance of molecular size was again confirmed from the observation that typical proliferative glomerular changes occurred in rabbits forming BSA–antiBSA complexes with molecular weight ranging from $3-5 \times 10^5$ daltons, consistent with molecular ratios of Ag_2Ab and Ag_3Ab_2 (DREESMAN and GERMUTH, 1972). If still larger complexes were formed, the sequence of events might not be proliferative changes but intravascular coagulation in glomerular tufts (LEBER and McCLUSKEY, 1974).

In passive serum sickness nephritis in mice, preformed antigen–antibody complexes were mostly entrapped by the mesangium. The deposits were visible as a large aggregate in both immunofluorescence and electron microscopy (OKUMURA et al., 1971), in contrast to discrete peripheral distribution of the complexes in active serum sickness in rabbits. Aside from the difference in animal species and experimental procedures employed, one might assume that aggregation of the complexes more or less occurred in the capillary lumen in the mouse glomerulonephritis so that the complexes were not able to penetrate the GBM and were entrapped within the mesangium.

Renal glomeruli are most commonly involved in chronic serum sickness. It was proposed that slightly antigen-excess immune complexes were again nephritogenic (DIXON et al., 1961). Two different kinds of glomerular diseases have been produced in rabbits by repeated injections of an antigen: diffuse proliferative glomerulonephritis and membranous nephropathy (membranous glomerulonephritis). Both are characterized by abundant granular deposits of antigen–antibody-complement complexes in immunofluorescence and corresponding dense deposits distributed along the outer aspects of the GBM in electron microscopy (DIXON et al., 1961). Despite the close resemblance between the two types of glomerulonephritis in terms of immune deposits, the histologic manifestations differ greatly from each other. At present this could be interpreted in two ways, according to the size of the complexes or the property of the antibodies. Firstly, the proliferative glomerulonephritis developed only in rabbits possessing circulating complexes composed of highly avid antibody with molecular weight ranging from $5–7 \times 10^5$ daltons (GERMUTH et al., 1972a). Secondly, it has been suggested that the production of nonprecipitating antibodies favors the development of proliferative as well as membranous glomerular changes (PINCUS et al., 1968; CHRISTIAN, 1969). It is interesting that an animal with low molecular-weight complexes showed minimal inflammation, whereas others with circulating complexes heavier than 19s showed proliferative changes (PINCUS et al., 1968). Furthermore, it has been shown that the antibody formed in rabbit with membranous nephropathy is characterized by low avidity and low precipitating efficiency (KURIYAMA, 1973; NAKABAYASHI, 1974). Immune complexes composed of such nonprecipitating antibodies might be relatively small in size and circulate for much longer periods than larger complexes. If a circumstance exists in which such peculiar complexes are not abruptly but very gradually deposited in glomeruli, it is not unlikely that they penetrate the GBM and accumulate at the subepithelial space without definite inflammatory changes. The formation of nonprecipitating antibodies has been discussed in connection with valencies of antigenic determinants on the complex protein antigen (PINCUS et al., 1968; CHRISTIAN, 1969). It is also possible that the antibody is produced on the basis of altered immune responses developing in animals under conditions of prolonged antigenic stimulation (OKABAYASHI, 1972).

Membranous nephropathy is also produced in rats immunized with homologous kidney homogenates (Heymann nephritis). Subepithelial deposits found in this rat nephropathy are composed of renal tubular antigen–antibody complexes (EDGINGTON et al., 1968; GLASSOCK et al., 1968; GRUPE and KAPLAN, 1969). It has been supposed that the circulating immune complexes are formed in rats in an antibody excess state (LEBER and McCLUSKEY, 1974). As mentioned before, subepithelial deposits are not always phlogogenic; however, abundant subepithelial deposits can be correlated to the clinical manifestations of the nephrotic syndrome. Increased GBM permeability associated with the deposits has been demonstrated in Heymann nephritis by using several tracers (SCHNEEBERGER et al., 1974).

The localization pattern of immune complexes is significantly different in naturally occurring glomerulonephritis in the NZ-strain mouse and Aleutian mink than other chronic serum sickness-type glomerular diseases. As mentioned before, in the mouse and mink glomerulonephritis, subendothelial and mesangial deposits predominate more often than subepithelial deposits. Suggestive evidence accounting for this comes from the observation of chronic serum sickness in rabbits. It was stated that immune complexes of intermediate size of approximately 1×10^6 daltons or greater could not be deposited beyond the GBM and aggregated within the subendothelial and mesangial system (GERMUTH et al., 1972a). Although the exact nature of immune complexes circulating in nephritic mouse or mink is not yet fully determined, it may be assumed that the complexes are in most part much larger than those circulating in rabbits with membranous nephropathy. Obviously the immune deposits are causative of all of the glomerular changes in these two models of naturally occurring glomerulonephritis. The continual formation of the nephritogenic complexes under the condition of viral infection is attributed to the unusual immunologic background of these animals, possibly linked to as yet unknown genetic factors (reviewed by: NORTON, 1970; COCHRANE and KOFFLER, 1973).

2. Phagocyte Accumulation and Proliferative Glomerular Changes

Proliferative changes are frequently seen in experimental acute glomerulonephritis. The hypercellularity is generally caused by a proliferation of fixed glomerular cells (endothelial and mesangial cells) and a migration of blood phagocytes (PMNs and monocytes). With light microscopic observations in the past, the origin of increased mononuclear cells was ascribed to endothelial cells. Detailed examination with the aid of electron microscopy, however, has shown the importance of mesangial cells which almost always respond to nephritogenic stimuli and participate in glomerular inflammation.

In various forms of acute proliferative glomerulonephritis, many electron microscopic studies have described swelling and proliferation of endothelial cells. However, little is known about the mechanisms which provoke the endothelial reactions. That antigen, antibody, and complement complexes *per se* stimulate the endothelium to proliferate is unlikely since this has not been proved in the first phase of rat Masugi nephritis. The endothelial response might be related to some extent to reparative overgrowth against the preceding injury (SHIGEMATSU, 1970) or increased phagocytosis for fibrin or other clotting material (VASSALLI and McCLUSKEY, 1964). Proliferation and activation of mesangial cells could also be explained in similar ways.

Accumulation of PMNs is a common feature of many glomerular diseases. It was reported that antigen–antibody complexes were chemotactic for PMNs *in vitro* (BOYDEN, 1962) and that they did ingest the complexes in the inflammatory foci of Arthus type (COCHRANE *et al.*, 1959; URIUHARA and MOVAT, 1966). In passive serum sickness nephritis, antigen–antibody complexes were engulfed by PMNs (OKUMURA *et al.*, 1971). The role of PMNs has been thoroughly discussed in the first phase of rat Masugi nephritis in connection with complement (COCHRANE *et al.*, 1965); the PMNs exhibited intimate, broad contact with the GBM (COCHRANE *et al.*, 1965) and underwent degeneration following the formation of abundant phagocytic vacuoles (SHIGEMATSU, 1970). From these observations, it would appear that the PMNs accumulated in the glomeruli play a role in ingesting antigen, antibody, and complement complexes. Obviously the effective removal of the complexes is not successful in Masugi nephritis because of its peculiar situation in which the GBM, a solid glomerular structure, is included as the antigenic constituent. The degeneration of PMNs supposedly results in the release of injurious substances which are included in their primary or secondary lysosomes and in turn provokes increased GBM permeability and other glomerular abnormalities. There is supporting evidence for this, as follows: The urinalysis of a nephritic rat at a time when PMNs attacked the GBM disclosed the presence of large molecules such as IgG and GBM fragments (HAWKINS and COCHRANE, 1968). Some enzymes were liberated when PMNs attached themselves to noningestable complexes (HENSON, 1971). It was also demonstrated that GBM permeability was increased in the area where PMNs showed direct contact (GANG *et al.*, 1970). Animals injected with PMN lysates developed focal and local glomerular changes with slight proteinuria (MANALIGOD *et al.*, 1969). In other glomerular diseases, however, PMNs do not take an active role and glomerular changes do occur even in a state of PMN depletion. The relation between PMNs and tissue alterations other than rat Masugi nephritis still remains to be clarified.

Blood monocytes are another contributor to the hypercellularity in acute glomerulonephritis. Although the characteristic behavior of monocytes has been well documented both *in vitro* and *in vivo* experiments, little attention has been directed to their role in proliferative glomerulonephritis. It might be that previous electron microscopic studies were incapable of differentiating the monocytic cells from fixed glomerular cells due most probably to inadequate processing methods during the preparation of tissue specimens. It is now clearly evident that migrant monocytes are frequently the major increased cell line in a variety of proliferative glomerulonephritis (SHIGEMATSU, 1970; OKUMURA *et al.*, 1971; KONDO and SHIGEMATSU, 1972; KOBAYASHI and SHIGEMATSU, 1975). The monocytes presumably accumulate to remove various

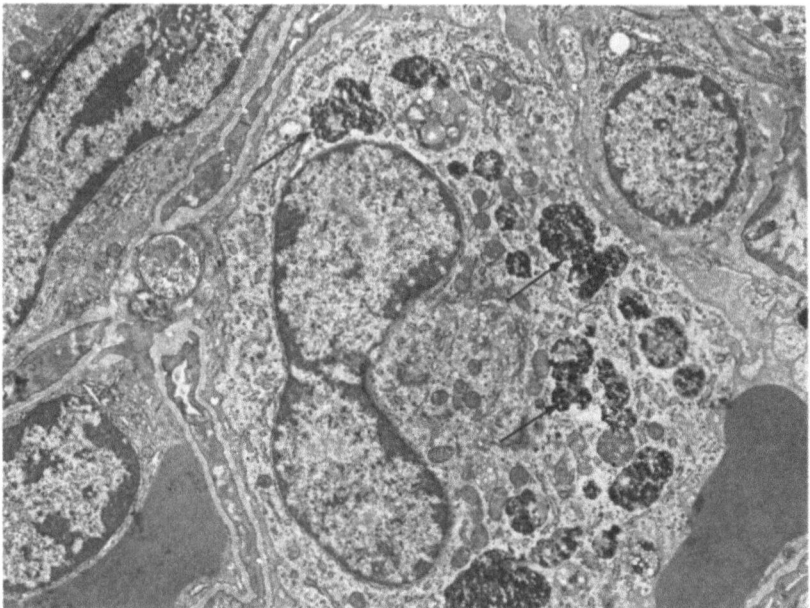

Fig. 11. A glomerular portion of a rabbit with acute serum sickness nephritis. Injected india-ink particles are selectively ingested by a migrant monocyte (arrows) and are not seen in fixed glomerular cells. ×6000. (Courtesy of Dr. M. SANO)

products provided by tissue damage, e.g. fibrin and cell or tissue fragments. They also ingested antigen–antibody complexes (OKUMURA et al., 1971). Through the phagocytic process, the monocytes were transformed into macrophages, epithelioid cells, and giant cells (SHIGEMATSU, 1970; KONDO and SHIGEMATSU, 1972). The location of the monocytic cells was extremely variable and they were found even in Bowman's space as a component of crescents (KONDO et al., 1972). It is likely that this peculiar behavior of the monocytic cells has not been well understood and they have even been erroneously referred to as endothelial or intracapillary cells.

The question arises as to whether the influx of monocytes is ascribed to an immune mechanism or whether they merely act as scavengers in the inflamed glomeruli. An attractive hypothesis is that they accumulate specifically for some relation to cellular immunity. The possibility has been suggested in some types of human glomerular diseases (BENDIXEN, 1968; ROCKLIN et al., 1970; ZABRISKIE et al., 1970; DARDENNE et al., 1972; MAHIEU et al., 1972; MALLICK et al., 1972). However, the mediators that trigger the monocytic response have not yet been characterized in any experimental glomerulonephritis.

3. Disorganizing Processes and Progressive Glomerulonephritis

Experimental acute glomerulonephritis is usually reversible. With the intensified nephritogenic stimuli, however, a rapidly progressive glomerular

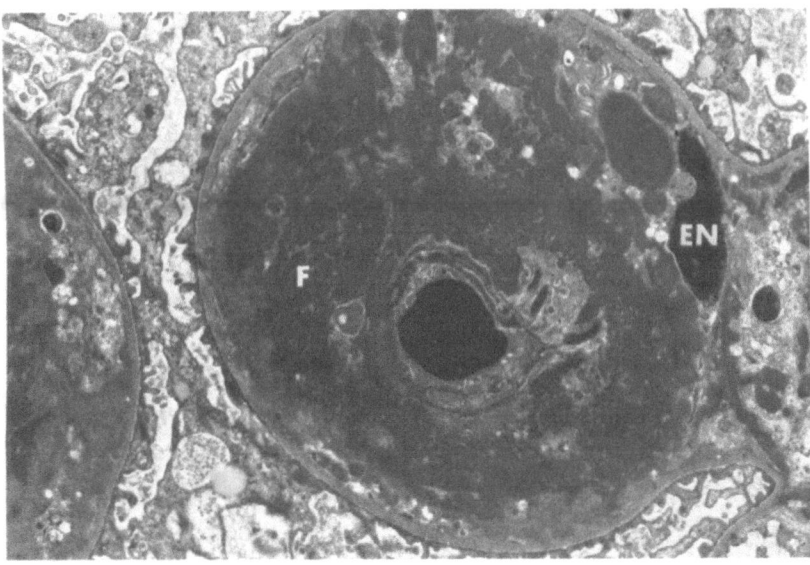

Fig. 12. Conspicuous intravascular coagulation seen in the first phase of rat Masugi nephritis. Capillary lumens are entirely obliterated by fibrin (F), fibrinoid material, and cell debris. Note necrosis of an endothelial cell (EN). ×4500

injury appears which is characterized by one or a combination of the changes described below.

Firstly, varying degrees of clotting lesions are almost always seen in progressive glomerulonephritis. The clotting process is activated by antigen–antibody interaction (LEE, 1963) on one hand and is enhanced by the lack of fibrinolytic activities on the other. It was speculated that fibrinolytic activity operated well in the presence of intact endothelial cells (WARREN, 1963; MYHRE-HENSEN, 1971; WAREN and KHAN, 1974), whereas it was lost by endothelial damage (BERGSTEIN et al., 1974). With the injection of a potent NTAb, massive intravascular coagulation was brought about in rats, diffusely obliterating the glomerular tufts (FUJIMOTO et al., 1964; SHIGEMATSU, 1970). The exaggerated coagulation did not cause cellular proliferation but promptly resulted in glomerular and cortical necrosis. Moderate deposits of fibrin or fibrinoid material were, however, thought to be responsible for the induction of crescentic glomerular changes (VASSALLI and McCLUSKEY, 1964). It is likely that a chronic glomerular disease becomes manifest when the clotting materials are not removed because of either impaired fibrinolytic activities or a lack of phagocytosis.

Secondly, the progressive glomerulonephritis is often characterized by marked disintegration of the mesangium, similar to that described in the glomerular injury in Habu snake poisoning, referred to as "mesangiolysis" (KITAMURA et al., 1957; SUZUKI et al., 1963). The lytic process involving the mesangium and GBM has been noted in immunologically induced glomerulo-

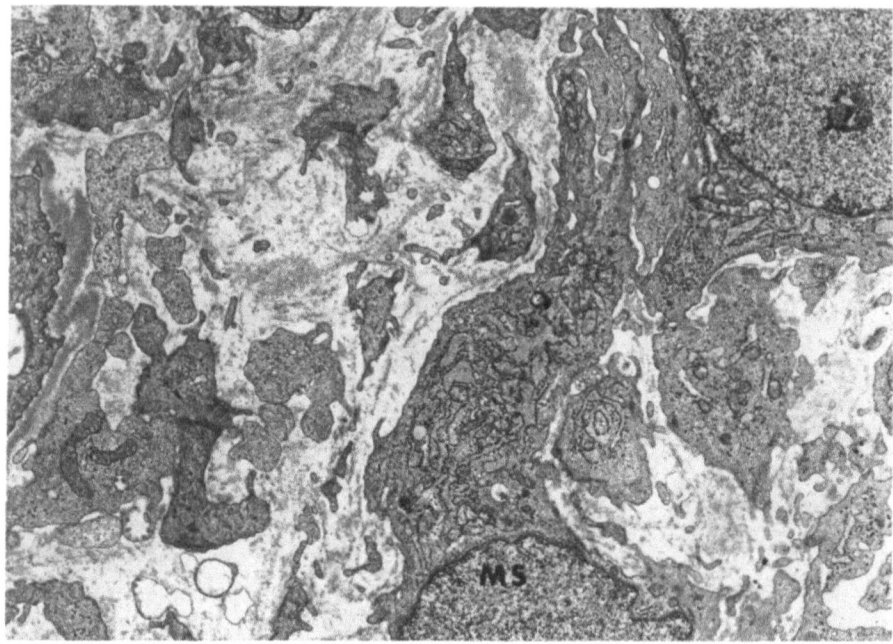

Fig. 13. Prominent edematous swelling or lysis of the mesangial matrix with an activation of mesangial cells (MS) in the second phase of rabbit Masugi nephritis. ×6400

nephritis as a fundamental pathologic phenomenon (OKABAYASHI, 1970). The change is most prominent in enhanced serum sickness nephritis (KOBAYASHI and SHIGEMATSU, 1975) and Masugi nephritis in rabbits (KONDO et al., 1972). The mesangiolysis was conceivably initiated by exaggerated edematous swelling of the matrix resulting from transudation of the blood liquid. The sequence of events was globular or balloon-like distortion of the tuft structure together with enhanced exudative and proliferative changes. The tufts then underwent an enmeshed or granulomatous disorganization, terminating in a rapid scarring of the glomeruli. The mesangiolysis in Habu snake poisoning was caused by edema, degeneration, and loss of the matrix that led to a conversion of the glomerulus into a blood-filled cystic cavity surrounded merely by the preserved GBM (KITAMURA et al., 1957; SUZUKI et al., 1963); there were no additional inflammatory changes, suggesting that the process was provoked by a rather simple toxic or enzymatic action on the mesangium. In immunologically induced glomerulonephritis, the mesangiolysis was followed by the extensive inflammatory reaction and cellular proliferation, indicating that the promoting mechanisms would be more complicated and unique. Unfortunately there is no further information at hand.

Thirdly, the formation of crescents is another characteristic of progressive glomerulonephritis. Ultrastructural observations have made it clear that the crescents occur on the basis of characteristic GBM changes. It was shown in

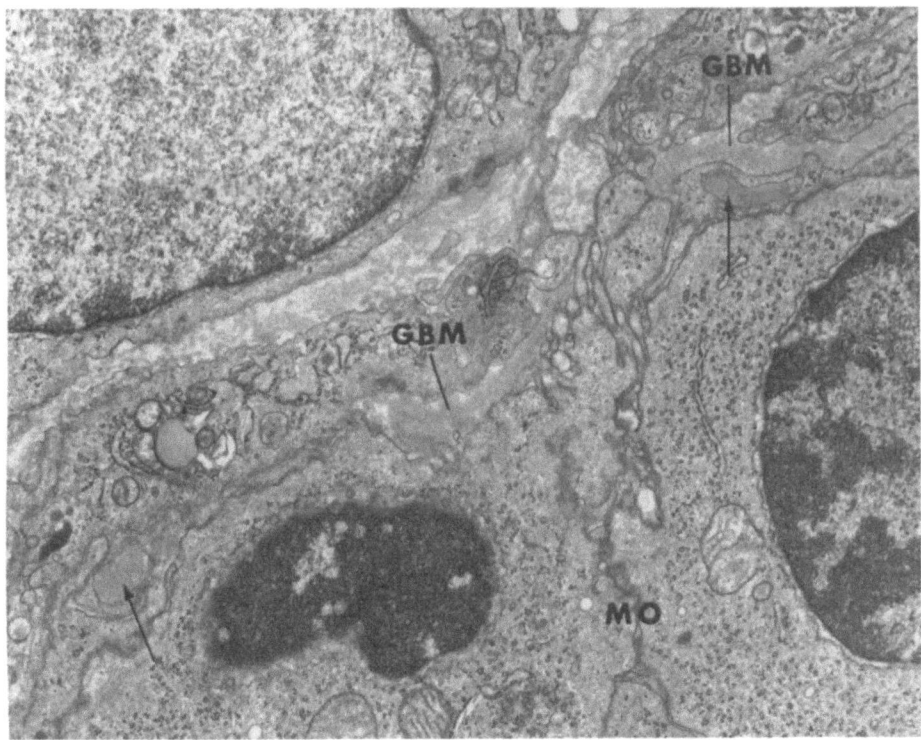

Fig. 14. Interruption of glomerular basement membrane (GBM) in the second phase of rabbit Masugi nephritis. Basement membrane fragments (arrows) are seen enclosed within the cytoplasm of unidentified cells. Two mononuclear cells (MO) are seen migrating into Bowman's space. ×12000

both serum sickness nephritis and Masugi nephritis that an intense intracapillary inflammation frequently affected the GBM to the extent of becoming attenuated and virtually interrrupted (KONDO et al., 1972; SHIGEMATSU and KOBAYASHI, 1973; KOBAYASHI and SHIGEMATSU, 1975). Once the GBM rupture developed, the inflammation extended into Bowman's space and the tufts or lobuli disappeared. The cell clusters obliterating Bowman's space were composed of epithelial cells and migrated inflammatory cells. A massive influx of fibrin and proteinaceous substances might stimulate the epithelial cells to proliferate. Simultaneously the periglomerular tissue was also included in the process. As a whole, the glomerulus was transformed into a granulomatous structure (KONDO et al., 1972). The disorganizing glomerulonephritis was apparently brought about subsequent to the intracapillary changes; there was no evidence to indicate that the crescents were produced by direct immunologic action on Bowman's epithelium. Lytic or necrotizing processes taking place in the tufts were probably responsible for the development of the GBM rupture. Enzymes included in PMNs may be mediators as has been suggested in other experiments (COCHRANE and AIKINS, 1966; JANOFF and ZELIGS, 1968).

V. Concluding Remarks

We are now able to produce a wide variety of glomerulonephritis experimentally in animals by immunologic procedures. It is entirely clear that experimental results have provided much information useful for elucidating important questions on human renal diseases. For example, nephrotoxic serum nephritis originally reported by MASUGI (1933, 1934) has long been regarded as an example of a highly artificial disease. Reasonable speculations, however, led to the attempt to produce autologous antiGBM-type glomerulonephritis, which was successfully carried out (STEBLAY, 1962). This in turn stimulated the search for the human counterpart. It has thus been demonstrated that there is indeed human glomerulonephritis of this type (LERNER et al., 1967). Extensive studies on experimental serum sickness have clarified the pathogenic importance of circulating antigen–antibody complexes for the development of acute, subacute, and chronic glomerulonephritis (DIXON et al., 1961), and have established the concept of immune complex disease. An appreciable proportion of human cases may be affected by the mechanism relating pathogenetically to immune complexes. Acute poststreptococcal glomerulonephritis is the most likely disease caused by deposits of immune complexes. Unfortunately, in many other situations, the possibility still remains obscure because of the difficulty in demonstrating antigen(s) or, conversely, in determining the specificity of antibody. Not infrequently, it is noticeable in experimental glomerulonephritis that changes developed are very similar, apart from differences in the underlying immune process, as was described in Section III. In general, the severity of lesions largely depends upon the amount of immune reactants localized in the glomeruli. The bulk of evidence also suggests that the variety in physicochemical as well as immunochemical properties of nephritogenic complexes would be reflected by different morphologic manifestations. In addition, the alteration of immune responses is another important factor in the pathogenesis of chronic glomerular diseases, especially those occurring in experimental autoimmune disorders. Also important are mediators involved in the antigen–antibody interaction by which cellular and tissue alterations are actually elicited. Several mediators have been proved to have a role in some experimental systems but not in others. In brief, only fragmentary information is available concerning possible mediators that may actually trigger multitudinous glomerular lesions. On the other hand, the continuance of a disease cannot necessarily be ascribed to the persistence of immune reactants. It is highly probable that if a significant architectural distortion of the glomerulus has once developed, there appears a self-perpetuating process undergoing hyaline scarring regardless of the presence of any nephritogenic stimuli. All of these considerations are, in turn, required for the study on human glomerular diseases.

From the morphologic aspect, the inflammatory process is not completely distinct from that which takes place in other vascular or connective tissues (JONES, 1951; JONES, 1953). Any acute phlogogenic stimuli would cause increased permeability, sticking of PMNs and mononuclear cells, and a proliferation of proper tissue cells, the changes being no more than the hallmarks of a common acute inflammation. The accumulation of migrant phagocytes is often remarkable but usually transient. This may well be the reason why a prompt resolution occurs in acute proliferative glomerulonephritis in man. With the intensified stimuli, extravasation of cellular and fluid elements of the blood would take place associated with lysis or destruction of the capillary structure involving the surrounding tissue and finally resulting in scarring. Be that as it may though, glomerulonephritis is a unique inflammation because of its pathogenesis in immune origin and of the specific anatomic and physiologic condition of the glomerulus. In a deeper insight into the pathobiological implications of Masugi and other immunologically induced glomerulonephritides described above, a clue may possibly be furnished solving problems of the pathology of the immune response.

References

AARONS, I.: Renal immunofluorescence in NZB/NZW mice. Nature **203**, 1080–1081 (1964)

ALOUSI, M. A., POST, R. S., HEYMANN, W.: Experimental autoimmune nephrosis in rats. Amer. J. Path. **54**, 47–71 (1969)

ANDRES, G. A., MORGAN, C., HSU, K. C., RIFKIND, R. A., SEEGAL, B. C.: Electron microscopic studies of experimental nephritis with ferritin-conjugated antibody. The basement membranes and cisternae of visceral epithelial cells in nephritic rat glomeruli. J. Exp. Med. **115**, 929–936 (1962)

ANDRES, G. A., SEEGAL, B. C., HSU, K. C., ROTHENBERG, M. S., CHAPEAU, M. L.: Electron microscopic studies of experimental nephritis with ferritin-conjugated antibody. Localization of antigen-antibody complexes in rabbit glomeruli following repeated injections of bovine serum albumin. J. Exp. Med. **117**, 691–704 (1963)

ARAKAWA, M., KIMMELSTIEL, P.: Circumferential mesangial interposition. Lab. Invest. **21**, 276–284 (1969)

ARAKAWA, M., KIMMELSTIEL, P.: The glomerulonephritis of acute serum sickness. A study using light and electron microscopy. Amer. J. Clin. Path. **54**, 60–70 (1970)

ARHELGER, R. B., GRONVAL, J. A., CARR, O. B., BRUNSON, J. G.: Electron microscopic localization of nephrotoxic serum in rabbit glomeruli with ferritin-conjugated antibody. Lab. Invest. **12**, 33–37 (1963)

BATTIFORA, H. A., MARKOWITZ, A. S.: Nephrotoxic nephritis in monkeys. Sequential light, immunofluorescence, and electron microscopic studies. Amer. J. Path. **55**, 267–281 (1969)

BAXTER, J. H., SMALL, P. A.: Antibody to rat kidney: In vivo effects of univalent and divalent fragments. Science **140**, 1406–1407 (1963)

BENACERRAF, B., POTTER, J. L., McCLUSKEY, R. T., MILLER, F.: The pathologic effects of intravenously administered soluble antigen-antibody complexes. II. Acute glomerulonephritis in rats. J. Exp. Med. **111**, 195–200 (1960)

BENACERRAF, B., SEBESTYEN, M., COOPER, N. S.: The clearance of antigen-antibody complexes from the blood by the reticuloendothelial system. J. Immunol. **82**, 131–137 (1959)

BENDIXEN, G.: Organ-specific inhibition of the in vitro migration of leucocytes in human glomerulonephritis. Acta Med. Scand. **184**, 99–103 (1968)

BERGSTEIN, J. M., HOYER, J. R., MICHAEL, A. F.: Glomerular fibrinolytic activity following endotoxin induced glomerular fibrin deposition in the pregnant rat. Amer. J. Path. **75**, 195–202 (1974)

BETTEX-GALLAND, M., LUSCHER, E. F., SIMON, G., VASSALLI, P.: Induction of viscous metamorphosis in human platelets by means other than thrombin. Nature **200**, 1109–1110 (1963)

BLOZIS, G. G., SPARGO, B., ROWLEY, D. A.: Glomerular basement membrane changes with the nephrotic syndrome produced in the rat by homologous kidney and Hemophilus pertussis vaccine. Amer. J. Path. **40**, 153–165 (1962)

BOONPUCKNAVIG, S., BOONPUCKNAVIG, V., BHAMARAPRAVATI, N.: Immunopathological studies of plasmodium berghei-infected mice. Arch. Path. **94**, 322–330 (1972)

BOYDEN, S.: The chemotactic effect of mixture of antibody and antigen on polymorphonuclear leucocytes. J. Exp. Med. **115**, 453–466 (1962)

BRITO, T. DE, GUNJI, J., CAMARGO, M. E., CERAVOLO, A., SILVA, L. C. DA: Glomerular lesions in experimental infections of Schistosoma mansoni in Cebus apella monkeys. Bull. WHO, **45**, 419–422 (1971)

BURKHOLDER, P. M.: Complement fixation in diseased tissues. I. Fixation of guinea pig complement in sections of kidney from human with membranous glomerulonephritis and rats injected with anti-rat kidney serum. J. Exp. Med. **114**, 605–616 (1961)

BURKHOLDER, P. M., BERGERSON, J. A., SHERWOOD, B. F., HACKEL, D. B.: A histopathologic survey of *Galago* in captivity. Virchows Arch. Abt. A **354**, 80–98 (1971)

CHANNING, A. A., KASUGA, T., HOROWITZ, R. E., DUBOIS, E. L., DEMOPOULOS, H. B.: An ultrastructural study of spontaneous lupus nephritis in the NZB/BL-NZW mouse. Amer. J. Path. **47**, 677–694 (1965)

CHASE, W. H., PAINE, L. D., LAMOUREUX, G., TAYLOR, H. E.: Ultrastructural study of the glomerulonephritis produced by antilymphocyte globulin in monkeys. Lab. Invest. **27**, 393–399 (1972)

CHEVILLE, N. F., MENGELING, W. L., ZINOBER, M. R.: Ultrastructural and immunofluorescent studies of glomerulonephritis in chronic hog cholera. Lab. Invest. **22**, 458–469 (1970)

CHRISTIAN, C. L.: Immune complex disease. New Engl. J. Med. **280**, 878–884 (1969)

CHURG, J., GRISHMAN, E., MAUTNER, W.: Nephrotoxic serum nephritis in the rat. Electron and light microscopic studies. Amer. J. Path. **37**, 729–749 (1960)

COCHRANE, C. G.: Mechanisms involved in the deposition of immune complexes in tissues. J. Exp. Med. **134**, 75s–89s (1971)

COCHRANE, C. G., AIKINS, B. S.: Polymorphonuclear leukocytes in immunologic reactions. The destruction of vascular basement membrane in vivo and in vitro. J. Exp. Med. **124**, 733–752 (1966)

COCHRANE, C. G., HAWKINS, D.: Studies on circulating immune complexes. III. Factors governing the ability of circulating complexes to localize in blood vessels. J. Exp. Med. **127**, 137–154 (1968)

COCHRANE, C. G., KOFFLER, D.: Immune complex disease in experimental animals and man. In Adv. Immunol, Vol. 16, Eds.: E. J. DIXON and H. G. KUNKEL, p. 185–264. New York and London: Academic Press 1973

COCHRANE, C. G., UNANUE, E. R., DIXON, F. J.: A role of polymorphonuclear leukocytes and complement in nephrotoxic nephritis. J. Exp. Med. **122**, 99–116 (1965)

COCHRANE, C. G., WEIGLE, W. O., DIXON, F. J.: The role of polymorphonuclear leukocytes in the initiation and cessation of the Arthus vasculitis. J. Exp. Med. **110**, 481–494 (1959)

COUSER, W. G., STILMANT, M., LEWIS, E. J.: Experimental glomerulonephritis in the guinea pig. I Glomerular lesions associated with antiglomerular basement membrane antibody deposits. Lab. Invest. **29**, 236–243 (1973)

CRUICKSHANK, B., HILL, A. G. S.: The histochemical identification of a connective-tissue antigen in the rat. J. Path. Bact. **66**, 283–289 (1953)

DARDENNE, M., ZABRISKIE, J., BACH, J. F.: Streptococcal sensitivity in chronic glomerulonephritis. Lancet **1**, 126–128 (1972)

DIXON, F. J., FELDMAN, J. D., VAZQUEZ, J. J.: Experimental glomerulonephritis. The pathogenesis of a laboratory model resembling the spectrum of human glomerulonephritis. J. Exp. Med. **113**, 899–920 (1961)

DIXON, F. J., OLDSTONE, M. B. A., TONETTI, G.: Pathogenesis of immune complex glomerulonephritis of New Zealand mice. J. Exp. Med. **134**, 65s–71s (1971).

DIXON, F. J., UNANUE, E. R., WATSON, J. I.: Immunopathology of the kidney. In: IVth Intern. Symp. Immunopath. Eds.: P. GRABAR and P. A. MIESCHER, p. 363–373. Basel/Stuttgart: Schwabe 1965

DIXON, F. J., VAZQUEZ, J. J., WEIGLE, W. O., COCHRANE, C. G.: Pathogenesis of serum sickness. Arch. Path. **65**, 18–28 (1958)

DREESMAN, G. R., GERMUTH, F. G.: Immune complex disease. IV. The nature of the circulating complexes associated with glomerulonephritis in the acute BSA-rabbit system. Johns Hopkins Med. J. **130**, 335–343 (1972)

DRUET, P., BARIETY, J., BELLON, B., LALIBERTE, F.: Nephrotoxic serum nephritis in the rat. Ultrastructural localization of nephrotoxic rabbit antibodies using peroxidase-labeled conjugates. Lab. Invest. **27**, 157–164 (1972)

DUBOIS, E. L., HOROWITZ, R. E., DEMOPOULOS, H. B., TEPLITZ, R.: NZB/NZW mice as a model of systemic lupus erythematosus. J. A. M. A. **195**, 285–289 (1966)

EDGINGTON, T. S., GLASSOCK, R. J., DIXON, F. J.: Autologous immune complex nephritis induced with renal tubular antigen. I. Identification and isolation of the pathogenetic antigen. J. Exp. Med. **127**, 555–572 (1968)

FELDMAN, J. D.: Electron microscopy of serum sickness nephritis. J. Exp. Med. **108**, 957–962 (1958)

FELDMAN, J. D.: Pathogenesis of ultrastructural glomerular changes induced by immunological means. In IIIrd Intern. Symp. Immunopath. Eds.: P. GRABAR and P. A. MIESCHER, p. 263–281. Basel/Stuttgart: Schwabe 1963

FELDMAN, J. D.: Ultrastructure of immunologic processes. In: Adv. Immunol. Vol. 4. Eds.: F. J. DIXON and J. H. HUMPHREY, p. 175–248. New York and London: Academic Press 1964

FELDMAN, J. D., HAMMER, D. K., DIXON, F. J.: Experimental glomerulonephritis. III. Pathogenesis of glomerular ultrastructural lesions in nephrotoxic serum nephritis. Lab. Invest. **12**, 748–763 (1963)

FISH, A. J., MICHAEL, A. F., VERNIER, R. L., GOOD, R. A.: Acute serum sickness nephritis in the rabbit. An immune deposit disease. Amer. J. Path. **49**, 997–1022 (1966)

FUJIMOTO, T., OKADA, M., KONDO, Y., TADA, T.: The nature of Masugi nephritis. Histo- and immunopathological studies. Acta path. jap. **14**, 275–310 (1964)

GANG, N. F., TRACHTENBERG, E., ALLERHAND, J., KALANT, N., MAUTNER, W.: Nephrotoxic serum nephritis. III. Correlation of proteinuria, excretion of the glomerular basement membrane-like protein, and changes in the ultrastructure of the glomerular basement membrane as visualized with lanthanum. Lab. Invest. **23**, 436–441 (1970)

GERMUTH, F. G.: A comparative histologic and immunologic study in rabbits of induced hypersensitivity of the serum sickness type. J. Exp. Med. **97**, 257–282 (1953)

GERMUTH, F. G., CHOI, I., TAYLOR, J. J., RODRIGUEZ, E.: Antibasement membrane disease. I. The glomerular lesions of Goodpasture's disease and experimental disease in sheep. Johns Hopkins Med. J. **131**, 367–384 (1972b)

GERMUTH, F. G., SENTERFIT, L. B., DREESMAN, G. R.: Immune complex disease. V. The nature of the circulating complexes associated with glomerular alterations in the chronic BSA-rabbit system. Johns Hopkins Med. J. **130**, 344–357 (1972a)

GLASSOCK, R. J., EDGINGTON, T. S., WATSON, J. I., DIXON, F. J.: Autologous immune complex nephritis. II. The pathogenetic mechanism. J. Exp. Med. **127**, 573–588 (1968)

GRISHMAN, E., PORUSH, J. C., ROSEN, S. M., CHURG, J.: Lupus nephritis with organized deposits in the kidneys. Lab. Invest. **16**, 717–725 (1967)

GRUPE, W. E., KAPLAN, M. H.: Demonstration of an antibody to proximal tubular antigen in the pathogenesis of experimental autoimmune nephrosis in rats. J. Lab. Clin. Med. **74**, 400–409 (1969)

HAMMER, D. K., DIXON, F. J.: Experimental glomerulonephritis. II. Immunologic events in the pathogenesis of nephrotoxic serum nephritis in the rat. J. Exp. Med. **117**, 1019–1034 (1963)

HASSON, M. W., BEVANS, M., SEEGAL, B. G.: Immediate or delayed nephritis in rats produced by duck anti-rat-kidney sera. Arch. Path. **64**, 192–204 (1957)

HAWKINS, D., COCHRANE, C. G.: Glomerular basement membrane damage in immunological glomerulonephritis. Immunology **14**, 665–681 (1968)

HAWN, C. V. Z., JANEWAY, C. A.: Histological and serological sequences in experimental hypersensitivity. J. Exp. Med. **85**, 571–590 (1947)

HELYER, B. J., HOWIE, J. B.: Renal disease associated with positive lupus erythematosus tests in a cross-bred strain of mice. Nature **197**, 197–197 (1963)

HENSON, P. M.: Interaction of cells with immune complexes: Adherence, release of constituents and tissue injury. J. Exp. Med. **134**, 114s–135s (1971)

Henson, P. M., Cochrane, C. G.: Acute immune complex disease in rabbits. The role of complement and of a leukocyte-dependent release of vasoactive amines from platelets. J. Exp. Med. **133**, 554–571 (1971)

Henson, J. B., Gorham, J. R., Padgett, G. A., Wash, P., Davis, W. C.: Pathogenesis of the glomerular lesions in Aleutian disease of mink. Immunofluorescent studies. Arch. Path. **87**, 21–28 (1969)

Henson, J. B., Gorham, J. R., Tanaka, Y.: Renal glomerular ultrastructure in mink affected by Aleutian disease. Lab. Invest. **17**, 123–139 (1967)

Henson, J. B., Gorham, J. R., Tanaka, Y., Padgett, G. A.: The sequential development of ultrastructural lesions in the glomeruli of mink with experimental Aleutian disease. Lab. Invest. **19**, 153–162 (1968)

Heymann, W., Hackel, D. B., Harwood, S., Wilson, S. G. F., Hunter, J. L. P.: Production of nephrotic syndrome in rats by Freund's adjuvant and rat kidney suspensions. Proc. Soc. Exp. Biol. Med. **100**, 660–664 (1959)

Hicks, J. D., Burnet, F. M.: Renal lesions in the "auto-immune" mouse strains NZB and F1 NZB×NZW. J. Path. Bact. **91**, 467–477 (1966)

Hoedemaeker, P. J., Feenstra, K., Nijkeuter, A., Arends, A.: Ultrastructural localization of heterologous nephrotoxic antibody in the glomerular basement membrane of the rat. Lab. Invest. **26**, 610–613 (1972)

Horowitz, R. E., Burrows, L., Paronetto, F., Dreiling, D., Kark, A. E.: Immunologic observations on homografts. II. The canine kidney. Transplantation **3**, 318–325 (1965)

Howie, J. B., Helyer, B. J.: The immunology and pathology of NZB mice. In: Adv. Immunol. Vol. 9. Eds.: F. J. Dixon and H. G. Kunkel, p. 215–266. New York and London: Academic Press 1968

Janoff, A., Zeligs, J. D.: Vascular injury and lysis of vascular basement membrane in vitro by neutral protease of human leukocytes. Science **161**, 702–704 (1968)

Jones, D. B.: Inflammation and repair of the glomerulus. Amer. J. Path. **27**, 991–1009 (1951)

Jones, D. B.: Glomerulonephritis. Amer. J. Path. **29**, 33–51 (1953)

Kay, C. F.: The mechanism by which experimental nephritis is produced in rabbits injected with nephrotoxic duck serum. J. Exp. Med. **72**, 559–572 (1940)

Kimmelstiel, P., Kim, O. J., Beres, J.: Studies on renal biopsy specimens with the aid of the electron microscope. II. Glomerulonephritis and glomerulonephrosis. Amer. J. Clin. Path. **38**, 280–296 (1962)

Kinding, D., Spargo, B., Kirsten, W. H.: Glomerular response in Aleutian disease of mink. Lab. Invest. **16**, 436–443 (1967)

Kitamura, W., Hashiguchi, T., Hamada, R., Ooyama, M.: Pathological study on the snake poisoning. Nichibyokaishi **46**, 355–355 (1957)

Kniker, W. T., Cochrane, C. G.: Pathogenic factor in vascular lesions of experimental serum sickness. J. Exp. Med. **122**, 83–98 (1965)

Kniker, W. T., Cochrane, C. G.: The localization of circulating immune complexes in experimental serum sickness. The role of vasoactive amines and hydrodynamic forces. J. Exp. Med. **127**, 119–136 (1968)

Kobayashi, Y., Shigematsu, H.: Accelerated serum sickness. In preparation, 1975

Kobayashi, Y., Shigematsu, H., Tada, T.: Nephritogenic properties of nephrotoxic guinea pig antibodies. I. Glomerulonephritis induced by guinea pig IgG_1 antibody in rats. Virchows Arch. Abt. B **14**, 259–271 (1973a)

Kobayashi, Y., Shigematsu, H., Tada, T.: Nephritogenic properties of nephrotoxic guinea pig antibodies. II. Glomerular lesions induced by $F(ab')_2$ fragments of nephrotoxic IgG_1 antibody in rats. Virchows Arch. Abt. B **15**, 35–44 (1973b)

Kondo, Y., Okamura, T., Nishijima, H., Okumura, K., Suzuki, N., Iwasaki, Y.: Glomerular changes in acute renal allograft rejection in the dog. Virchows Arch. Abt. B **17**, 63–78 (1974)

Kondo, Y., Shigematsu, H.: Cellular aspects of rabbit Masugi nephritis. I. Cell kinetics in recoverable glomerulonephritis. Virchows Arch. Abt. B **10**, 40–50 (1972)

Kondo, Y., Shigematsu, H., Kobayashi, Y.: Cellular aspects of rabbit Masugi nephritis. II. Progressive glomerular injuries with crescent formation. Lab. Invest. **27**, 620–631 (1972)

KRAKOWER, C. A., GREENSPON, S. A.: Localization of the nephrotoxic antigen within the isolated renal glomerulus. Arch. Path. **51**, 629–639 (1951)

KURIYAMA, T.: Chronic glomerulonephritis induced by prolonged immunization in the rabbit. Lab. Invest. **28**, 224–235 (1973)

LAGUENS, R., SEGAL, A.: Experimental autologous immune complex nephritis: An electron microscope and immunohistochemical study. Exp. Mol. Path. **11**, 89–98 (1969)

LAMBERT, P. H., DIXON, F. J.: Pathogenesis of the glomerulonephritis of NZB/W mice. J. Exp. Med. **127**, 507–522 (1968)

LEBER, P. D., McCLUSKEY, R. T.: Immune complex diseases. In: The Inflammatory Process, 2nd ed. Vol. III. Eds.: B. W. ZWEIFACH, L. GRANT, and R. T. McCLUSKEY, p. 401–441. New York and London: Academic Press 1974

LEE, L.: Antigen-antibody reaction in the pathogenesis of bilateral renal cortical necrosis. J. Exp. Med. **117**, 365–376 (1963)

LERNER, R. A., DIXON, F. J.: Transfer of ovine experimental allergic glomerulonephritis (EAG) with serum. J. Exp. Med. **124**, 431–442 (1966)

LERNER, R. A., GLASSOCK, R. J., DIXON, F. J.: The role of anti-glomerular basement membrane antibody in the pathogenesis of human glomerulonephritis. J. Exp. Med. **126**, 989–1004 (1967)

LEWIS, R. M., ARMSTRONG, M. Y. K., ANDRÉ-SCHWARTZ, F., MUFTUOGLU, A., BELDOTTI, L., SCHWARTZ, R. S.: Chronic allogeneic disease. I. Development of glomerulonephritis. J. Exp. Med. **128**, 653–679 (1968)

LINDER, E., PASTERNACK, M., EDGINGTON, T. S.: Pathology and immunology of age associated disease of mice and evidence for an autologous immune complex pathogenesis of the associated renal disease. Clin. Immunol. Immunopath. **1**, 104–121 (1972)

LINDQUIST, R. R., GUTTMANN, R. D., MERRILL, J. P.: Renal transplantation in the inbred rat. II. An immunohistochemical study of acute allograft rejection. Amer. J. Path. **52**, 531–545 (1968)

MAHIEU, P., DARDENNE, M., BACH, J. F.: Detection of humoral and cell-mediated immunity to kidney basement membranes in human diseases. Amer. J. Med. **53**, 185–192 (1972)

MALLICK, N. P., WILLIAMS, R. J., McFARLANE, H., ORR, W. McN., TALYLOR, G., WILLIAMS, G.: Cell-mediated immunity in nephrotic syndrome. Lancet 1, 507–509 (1972)

MANALIGOD, J. R., KRAKOWER, C. A., GREENSPON, S. A.: Glomerular changes induced by extrarenal foci of inflammation and by polymorphonuclear cell lysates. Amer. J. Path. **56**, 533–551 (1969)

MASUGI, M.: Über das Wesen der spezifischen Veränderungen der Niere und der Leber durch das Nephrotoxin bzw. das Hepatotoxin. Zugleich ein Beitrag zur Pathogenese der Glomerulonephritis und der eklamptischen Lebererkrankung. Beitr. Path. Anat. **91**, 82–112 (1933)

MASUGI, M.: Über die experimentelle Glomerulonephritis durch das spezifische Antinierenserum. Ein Beitrag zur Pathogenese der diffusen Glomerulonephritis. Beitr. Path. Anat. **92**, 429–466 (1934)

MASUGI, Y.: Immunoelectron microscopic studies on local vascular changes after immunological tissue injuries—especially on the mechanism of nephrotoxic nephritis. Acta path. jap. **19**, 265–281 (1969)

McCLUSKEY, R. T.: Experimental serum sickness. In: Inflammatory Process. Eds.: B. W. ZWEIFACH, L. GAND, and R. T. McCLUSKEY, p. 649–683. New York and London: Academic Press 1965

McCLUSKEY, R. T., BENACERRAF, B.: Localization of colloidal substances in vascular endothelium. A mechanism of tissue damage. II. Experimental serum sickness with acute glomerulonephritis induced passively in mice by antigen-antibody complexes in antigen excess. Amer. J. Path. **35**, 275–283 (1959)

McCLUSKEY, R. T., BENACERRAF, B., MILLER, F.: Passive acute glomerulonephritis induced by antigen-antibody complexes solubilized in hapten excess. Proc. Soc. Exp. Biol. Med. **111**, 764–768 (1962)

McCLUSKEY, R. T., BENACERRAF, B., POTTER, J. L., MILLER, F.: The pathologic effects of intravenously administered soluble antigen-antibody complexes. I. Passive serum sickness in mice. J. Exp. Med. **111**, 181–194 (1960)

McCLUSKEY, R. T., VASSALLI, P.: Experimental glomerular diseases. In: The Kidney: Morphology, Biochemistry, Physiology, Vol. II. Eds.: C. ROUILLER and A. F. MULLER, p. 83–198. New York and London: Academic Press 1969

McGIVEN, A. R., HICKS, J. D.: The development of renal lesions in NZB/NZW mice. Immunohistological studies. Brit. J. Exp. Path. **48**, 302–304 (1967)

McGIVEN, A. R., LYNRAVEN, G. S.: Glomerular lesions in NZB/NZW mice. Electron microscopic study of development. Arch. Path. **85**, 250–261 (1968)

McKAY, D. G., PHILIPS, L. L., KAPLAN, H., HENSON, J. B.: Chronic intravascular coagulation in Aleutian disease of mink. Amer. J. Path. **50**, 899–912 (1967)

MELLORS, R. C.: Autoimmune disease in NZB/BL mice. I. Pathology and pathogenesis of a model system of spontaneous glomerulonephritis. J. Exp. Med. **122**, 25–40 (1965)

MELLORS, R. C.: Autoimmune and immunoproliferative diseases of NZB/Bl mice and hybrids. In: Intern. Rev. Exp. Path. Vol. 5. Eds.: G. W. RICHTER, and M. A. EPSTEIN, p. 217–252. New York and London: Academic Press 1966

MELLORS, R. C., AOKI, T., HUEBNER, R. T.: Further implication of murine leukemia-like virus in the disorders of NZB mice. J. Exp. Med. **133**, 1045–1062 (1969)

MELLORS, R. C., BRZOSKO, W. J.: Studies in molecular pathology. I. Localization and pathogenic role of heterologous immune complexes. J. Exp. Med. **115**, 891–902 (1962)

MELLORS, R. C., SHIRAI, T., AOKI, T., HUEBNER, R. J., KRAWCZYNSKI, K.: Wild-type gross leukemic virus and the pathogenesis of the glomerulonephritis of New Zealand mice. J. Exp. Med. **133**, 113–132 (1971)

MILLER, F., BENACERRAF, B., McCLUSKEY, R. T., POTTER, J. L.: Production of acute glomerulonephritis in mice with soluble antigen-antibody complexes prepared from homologous antibody. Proc. Soc. Exp. Biol. Med. **104**, 706–709 (1960)

MILLER, F., BOHLE, A.: Elektronenmikroskopische Untersuchungen am Glomerulum bei der Masugi-Nephritis der Ratte. Virchows Arch. Path. Anat. **330**, 483–497 (1957)

MOPPERT, J., FRESEN, K. O.: Experimentelle Glomerulonephritis und Glomerulonephrose bei der Maus nach wiederholten Ovalbumin-Injektionen. Eine licht-fluorescenz- und elektronen-optische Untersuchung. Virchows Arch. Path. Anat. **342**, 304–318 (1967)

MOVAT, H. Z., McGREGOR, D. D., STEINER, J. W.: Studies of nephrotoxic nephritis. II. The fine structure of the glomerulus in acute nephrotoxic nephritis of dogs. Amer. J. Clin. Path. **36**, 306–321 (1961)

MUEHRCKE, R. C., RUDOFSKY, U., STEBLAY, R. W.: Studies on autoimmune nephritis in sheep and rats. III. The pattern and significance of the ultrastructural changes in the glomerular lesions. Fed. Proc. **26**, 743–743 (1967)

MURRAY, M., PATH, M. R. C., WRIGHT, N. G.: A morphologic study of canine glomerulonephritis. Lab. Invest. **30**, 213–221 (1974)

MYHRE-JENSEN, O.: Localization of fibrinolytic activity in the kidney and urinary tract of rats and rabbits. Lab. Invest. **25**, 403–411 (1971)

NAIRN, R. C., McGIVEN, A. R., IRONSIDE, P. N. J., NORINS, L. C.: Plasma proteins in the glomerular lesions of NZB/NZW mice. Brit. J. Exp. Path. **47**, 99–103 (1966)

NAKABAYASHI, M.: Immunochemical properties of rabbit antibodies in membranous glomerulonephritis. Acta path. jap. **24**, 63–77 (1974)

NORTON, W. L.: Aleutian mink and New Zealand mice: Models of viral induced connective tissue disease. In: Rheumatology, Vol. 3. Ed.: J. ROTSTEIM, p. 194–223. Basel, Munich, and New York: Karger 1970

OHNUKI, T.: Crescentic glomerulonephritis induced by homologous or heterologous glomerular basement membrane antigen in the goat. Acta path. jap. **25**, 319–331 (1975)

OKABAYASHI, A.: Induction of a disease resembling systemic lupus erythematosus in later stage of prolonged sensitization in rabbits. Acta path. jap. **14**, 345–371 (1964)

OKABAYASHI, A.: Nephritides and dysimmunization. With special reference to the significance of lytic process in immunologically induced experimental glomerulonephritis. Jap. J. Nephrol. **12**, 1–17 (1970)

OKABAYASHI, A.: Hematologic- and immunologic-central organs in a systemic lupus erythematosus-like disease of the rabbit experimentally induced in the later stage of prolonged sensitization. Acta heam. jap. **35**, 83–100 (1972)

OKUDA, R., KAPLAN, M. H., CUPPAGE, F. E., HEYMANN, W.: Deposition of autologous gamma globulin in kidneys of rats with nephrotic renal disease of various etiologies. J. Lab. Clin. Med. **66**, 204–215 (1965)

OKUMURA, K.: Induction of a disease resembling systemic lupus erythematosus in C57BL/6J mice by prolonged immunization with egg albumin. Acta path. jap. **23**, 695–704 (1973)

OKUMURA, K., KONDO, Y., TADA, T.: Studies on passive serum sickness. I. The glomerular fine structure of serum sickness nephritis induced by preformed antigen-antibody complexes in the mouse. Lab. Invest. **24**, 383–391 (1971)

OLDSTONE, M. B. A., DIXON, F. J.: Immune complex disease in chronic viral infections. J. Exp. Med. **134**, 32s–40s (1971)

ORTEGA, L. G., MELLORS, R. C.: Analytical pathology. IV. The role of localized antibodies in the pathogenesis of nephrotoxic nephritis in the rat. J. Exp. Med. **104**, 151–170 (1956)

PAN, I. C., TSAI, K. S., GRINYER, I., KARSTAD, L.: Glomerulonephritis in Aleutian disease of mink: Ultrastructural studies. J. Path. **102**, 33–40 (1970b)

PAN, I. C., TSAI, K. S., KARSTAD, L.: Glomerulonephritis in Aleutian disease of mink: Histological and immunofluorescence studies. J. Path. **101**, 119–127 (1970a)

PARONETTO, F., KOFFLER, D.: Autoimmune proliferative glomerulonephritis in monkeys. Amer. J. Path. **50**, 887–894 (1967)

PIEL, C. F., DONG, L., MODERN, F. W. S., GOODMAN, J. R., MOORE, R.: The glomerulus in experimental renal disease in rats as observed by light and electron microscopy. J. Exp. Med. **102**, 573–580 (1955)

PINCUS, T., HABERKERN, R., CHRISTIAN, C. L.: Experimental chronic glomerulonephritis. J. Exp. Med. **127**, 819–832 (1968)

PORTER, D. D., DIXON, F. J., LARSEN, A. E.: Metabolism and function of gamma globulin in Aleutian disease of mink. J. Exp. Med. **121**, 889–900 (1965)

PORTER, D. D., LARSEN, A. E.: Aleutian disease of mink: Infectious virus-antibody complexes in the serum. Proc. Soc. Exp. Biol. Med. **125**, 680–682 (1967)

PORTER, D. D., LARSEN, A. E., PORTER, H. G.: The pathogenesis of Aleutian disease of mink. I. In vivo viral replication and the host antibody response to viral antigen. J. Exp. Med. **130**, 575–593 (1969)

RICH, A. R.: Hypersensitivity in diseases; With especial reference to periarteritis nodosa, rheumatic fever, disseminated lupus erythematosus and rheumatoid arthritis. Harvey Lect. **42** (1946–47), 106–147 (1947)

RICH, A. R., GREGORY, J. E.: The experimental demonstration that periarteritis nodosa is a manifestation of hypersensitivity. Bull. Johns Hopkins Hosp. **72**, 65–82 (1943)

ROBBINS, J., STETSON, C. A.: An effect of antigen-antibody interaction on blood coagulation. J. Exp. Med. **109**, 1–8 (1959)

ROBERTSON, D. M., MORE, R. H.: Structure of glomerular axial region in normal and nephritic rabbits. Arch. Path. **72**, 331–342 (1961)

ROCKLIN, R. E., LEWIS, E. J., DAVID, J. R.: In vitro evidence for cellular hypersensitivity to glomerular-basement-membrane antigens in human glomerulonephritis. New Engl. J. Med. **283**, 497–501 (1970)

SAKAGUCHI, H., SUZUKI, Y., YAMAGUCHI, T.: Electron microscopic study of Masugi nephritis. I. Glomerular change. Acta path. jap. **7**, 53–66 (1957)

SCHNEEBERGER, E. E., LEBER, P. D., KARNOVSKY, M. J., McCLUSKEY, R. T.: Altered functional properties of the renal glomerulus in autologous immune complex nephritis. An ultrastructural tracer study. J. Exp. Med. **139**, 1283–1302 (1974)

SEEGAL, B. C., HSU, K. C., ANDRES, G. A.: Specific nephrotoxic nephritis: Old facts and present concept. In IIIrd Intern. Symp. Immunopath. Eds.: P. GRABAR and P. A. MIESCHER, p. 208–219. Basel/Stuttgart: Schwabe 1963

SEEGAL, B. C., HSU, K. C., ROTHENBERG, M. S., CHAPEU, M. L.: Studies of the mechanism of experimental nephritis with fluorescein-labeled antibody. II. Localization and persistence of injected rabbit or duck anti-rat-kidney serum during the course of nephritis in rats. Amer. J. Path. **41**, 183–203 (1962)

SHIBATA, S., NAGASAWA, T., MIYAKAWA, Y., NARUSE, T.: Nephritogenic glycoprotein. I. Proliferative glomerulonephritis induced in rats by a single injection of the soluble glycoprotein isolated from homologous glomerular basement membrane. J. Immunol. **106**, 1284–1294 (1971)

SHIBATA, S., SAKAGUCHI, H., NAGASAWA, T., NARUSE, T.: Nephritogenic glycoprotein. II. Experimental production of membranous glomerulonephritis in rats by a single injection of homologous renal glycopeptide. Lab. Invest. **27**, 457–465 (1972)

Shigematsu, H.: Glomerular events during the initial phase of rat Masugi nephritis. Virchows Arch. Abt. B 5, 187–200 (1970)

Shigematsu, H., Kobayashi, Y.: The development and fate of the immune deposits in the glomerulus during the secondary phase of rat Masugi nephritis. Virchows Arch. Abt. B 8, 83–95 (1971)

Shigematsu, H., Kobayashi, Y.: The distortion and disorganization of the glomerulus in progressive Masugi nephritis in the rat. Virchows Arch. Abt. B 14, 313–328 (1973)

Siqueira, M., Nelson, R. A.: Platelet agglutination by immune complexes and its possible role in hypersensitivity. J. Immunol. 86, 516–525 (1961)

Stavitsky, A. B., Heymann, W., Hackel, D. B.: Relation of complement fixation to renal disease in rat injected with duck antikidney serum. J. Lab. Clin. Med. 47, 349–356 (1956)

Steblay, R. W.: Glomerulonephritis induced in sheep by injections of heterologous glomerular basement membrane and Freund's complete abjuvant. J. Exp. Med. 116, 253–272 (1962)

Steblay, R. W.: Glomerulonephritis induced in monkeys by injections of heterologous glomerular basement membrane and Freund's adjuvant. Nature 197, 1173–1176 (1963)

Steblay, R. W., Rudofsky, U.: In vitro and in vivo properties of autoantibodies eluted from kidneys of sheep with autoimmune glomerulonephritis. Nature 218, 1269–1271 (1968)

Sugisaki, T., Klassen, J., Andres, G. A., Milgrom, F., McCluskey, R. T.: Passive transfer of Heymann nephritis with serum. Kidney Intern. 3, 66–73 (1973)

Suzuki, M.: Plasmodium berghei: Experimental rodent model for malarial renal immunopathology. Exp. Parasitol. 35, 187–195 (1974)

Suzuki, Y., Churg, J., Grishman, E., Mautner, W., Dachs, S.: The mesangium of the renal glomerulus. Electron microscopic studies of pathologic alterations. Amer. J. Path. 43, 555–578 (1963)

Tada, T., Kondo, Y., Okumura, K., Sano, M., Yokokawa, M.: Immunopathological studies on the nephritis induced by experimental infection with Schistosoma japonicum in Maccaca monkeys. Exp. Parasitol. (1975, in press)

Unanue, E. R., Dixon, F. J.: Experimental glomerulonephritis. IV. Participation of complement in nephrotoxic nephritis. J. Exp. Med. 119, 965–982 (1964)

Unanue, E. R., Dixon, F. J.: Experimental allergic glomerulonephritis induced in the rabbit with heterologous renal antigens. J. Exp. Med. 125, 149–162 (1967a)

Unanue, E. R., Dixon, F. J.: Experimental glomerulonephritis: Immunological events and pathogenetic mechanisms. In: Adv. Immunol., Vol. 6. Eds.: F. J. Dixon and J. H. Humphrey, p. 1–90. New York and London: Academic Press 1967b

Unanue, E. R., Dixon, F. J., Feldman, J. D.: Experimental allergic glomerulonephritis induced in the rabbit with homologous renal antigens. J. Exp. Med. 125, 163–176 (1967a)

Unanue, E. R., Dixon, F. J., Feldman, J. D.: Experimental immunologic diseases of the kidney. In: Textbook of Immunopathology, Vol. I. Eds.: P. A. Miescher and H. J. Müller-Eberhard, p. 164–178. New York and London: Grune & Stratton 1968

Unanue, E. R., Mardiney, M. R., Dixon, F. J.: Nephrotoxic serum nephritis in complement intact and deficient mice. J. Immunol. 98, 609–617 (1967b)

Uriuhara, T., Movat, H. Z.: The role of PMN-leukocyte lysosomes in tissue injury, inflammation and hypersensitivity. I. The vascular changes and the role of PMN-leukocytes in the reversed passive Arthus reaction. Exp. Mol. Path. 5, 539–558 (1966)

Vassalli, P., McCluskey, R. T.: The pathogenic role of the coagulation process in rabbit Masugi nephritis. Amer. J. Path. 45, 653–677 (1964)

Vassalli, P., Simon, G., Rouiller, C.: Electron microscopic study of glomerular lesions resulting from intravascular fibrin formation. Amer. J. Path. 43, 579–617 (1963)

Vogt, A., Bockhorn, H., Kozima, K., Sasaki, M.: Electron microscopic localization of the nephrotoxic antibody in the glomeruli of the rat after intravenous application of purified nephritogenic antibody-ferritin conjugates. J. Exp. Med. 127, 867–878 (1968)

Vogt, A., Kochem, H. G.: Immediate and delayed nephrotoxic nephritis in rats. The role of complement fixation. Amer. J. Path. 39, 379–392 (1961)

WARREN, B. A.: Fibrinolytic properties of vascular endothelium. Brit. J. Exp. Path. **444**, 365–372 (1963)

WARREN, B. A., KHAN, S.: The ultrastructure of the lysis of fibrin by endothelium in vitro. Brit. J. Exp. Path. **55**, 138–148 (1974)

WILSON, C. B., DIXON, F. J.: Antigen quantitation in experimental immune complex glomerulonephritis. I. Acute serum sickness. J. Immunol. **105**, 279–290 (1970)

ZABRISKIE, J. B., LEWSHENIA, R., MÖLLER, G., WEHLE, B., FALK, R. E.: Lymphocytic responses to streptococcal antigens in glomerulonephritic patients. Science **169**, 1105–1108 (1970)

Pathologisches Institut der Universität Münster/W.
(Director: Prof. Dr. E. Grundmann)

The Terminology of Glomerulonephritis
A Review

Christian Witting

With 3 Figures

The history of renal diseases can be traced back to Hippocrates and Avicenna who, in their time, saw and etiologic correlation between general dropsy and renal disease. The era of modern scientific nephrology began in 1827 when Richard Bright, an English clinician, published his first book *Diseased Kidney in Dropsy*, in which a causal relationship was established between general dropsy and certain anatomic changes in the kidney. From that time, these three parallel symptoms—dropsy, albuminuria, and anatomic changes in the kidney—were called "Bright's disease." Bright had defined renal changes exclusively on the basis of macroscopic symptoms, with some very cautious suggestions about pathogenesis. During the following years Bright's observations were discussed in England by Copland (1832–1858), Prout (1823) and Graves (1831), in France by Rayer (1840) and Solon (1838), in Germany until 1852 by Henle (1846), Rokitansky (1861), Reinhard (1850), Frerichs (1851) and, last but not least, by Virchow (1852). Most of these publications used the term "nephritis" for renal diseases. The special name of "glomerulonephritis" appeared first in Klebs's *Handbuch der Pathologischen Anatomie*, published in 1876. He wrote, in Vol. I: "One can designate glomerulonephritis as a form of interstitial nephritis in which the interstitial tissue of the glomeruli is involved exclusively."

An early classification of hematogenous, nonpurulent renal inflammations- a popular definition in the following years- was presented in 1899 by Senator:

1. Acute Nephritis

   a) Parenchymatous nephritis
   b) Diffuse nephritis

2. Chronic Diffuse Nephritis without Induration

(chronic parenchymatous nephritis)

3. Chronic Indurative Nephritis (Nephrocirrhosis)

   a) Secondary induration
   b) Primary indurative nephritis
   c) Arteriosclerotic indurations

This classification included the terms "acute" and "chronic," to describe the potential clinical course of the disease. Together with "subchronic" and "subacute", these terms, though much disputed, characterized the classification of glomerulonephritis over the next six decades. Similar criteria were adopted by LÖHLEIN in 1910, although he made no explicit mention of them. His classification runs as follows:

1. Glomerulonephritis of Several Days' Duration

LÖHLEIN's paradigm of this type of glomerulonephritis was scarlet fever nephritis in addition to some less frequent infections. In this disease he found the glomeruli severely enlarged, the capsule nearly or completely filled, the loops broad and long, and the prognosis uncertain.

2. Glomerulonephritis of Several Weeks' or Months Duration

In this type the predominant etiologic role is played by streptococcal infections with the subsequent influence of bacterial toxins on the kidneys. LÖHLEIN distinguished a more rapid from a milder type, calling the former "subacute glomerulonephritis." Frequent epithelial "crescents" are a striking histologic feature, and death occur after a course of about 4 weeks. In the mild type, on the other hand, large glomeruli possess coarse loops full of cellular elements. Epithelial crescents are found in only a few glomeruli or in none of them.

3. Chronic Glomerulonephritis

In this manifestation, all glomeruli are changed severely, epithelial crescents may be found occasionally, or even glomeruli that have been completely obliterated. The characteristic pattern of this type is its progress over many years. The disease may set in after acute nephritis following scarlet fever or tonsillitis.

LÖHLEIN proposed the following classification of hematogenous renal affections: Focal manifestations were separated from diffuse ones, and in the diffuse type, forms without severe involvement of glomeruli were distinguished from those with predominant glomerular involvement.

LÖHLEIN's definition was supported by VOLHARD and FAHR in 1914, who saw nephritis in opposition to nephrosis, defining nephritis as a disease state in which the inflammation is clearly manifest. The histologic picture is dominated by proliferative changes in vascular connective tissue. The authors differentiated interstitial nephritis from glomerulonephritis according to the location of proliferations in either interstitial or glomerular parts.

In addition to distinguishing between focal and diffuse changes, VOLHARD and FAHR adopted the terms acute, subchronic, and chronic to define the most striking differences:

1. Acute Glomerulonephritis

In this form microscopic changes are not so characteristic. Loops are elongated and broadened, occasionally distended, and blood is found, as a rule, within the capsule and in the tubules. The predominant feature is a significant increase of cells in each glomerulus. VOLHARD and FAHR see the distention of loops as a sign of florid inflammation, while the absence of this phenomenon is taken as a sign of decreasing inflammation. Acute glomerulo-nephritis can be cured completely in the majority of cases. Sometimes it passes into the second stage.

2. Subchronic Glomerulonephritis

Microscopy reveals particular intensification of proliferative, exudative, and desquamative processes, and even regular and intense involvement of channel epithelia manifested as a degenerative process. VOLHARD and FAHR separated, moreover, an extracapillary from an intracapillary type: the extra-capillary type was characterized by proliferative and desquamative reactions in tuft epithelia, the intracapillary type by marked cell proliferation inside the glomerular loops, as a result of which all the tufts become noticeably enlarged. In this stage regression is more than doubtful or even improbable.

3. Chronic Glomerulonephritis

a) Without granulation

The kidney is not substantially smaller or more compact than normal. Histologically, the original glomerular loops are transformed into plaque-like hyaline lumps, and nucleosis is diminished. Some glomeruli are completely obliterated, most of them exsanguinated. Bleeding into Bowman's capsule is found in some parts. This "smooth" type of chronic glomerulonephritis is rather rare; it is based on regular and simultaneous obliteration of all glo-meruli.

b) With granulation

Besides a great number of more or less totally obliterated glomeruli, others show free and open loops filled with blood. Remarkable attempts at regeneration of parenchyma are considered to be responsible for the granular macroscopic appearance of the kidney surface. As a rule, vessels are severely altered in this third chronic stage of glomerulonephritis. In the intima, elastic and hyperplastic thickening is found together with regressive changes. The media is often hypertrophic. VOLHARD and FAHR expressed the opinion that a substantial cause of arteriosclerotic processes in the kidney should not be seen in rising blood pressure, but in local changes inside the kidney.

In 1918 VOLHARD changed his opinion about the classification criteria "acute," "subacute," and "chronic," declaring them inadequate for sub-dividing the various forms of glomerulonephritis. His new definitions were the following:

1. Nephrosis: parenchymatous (dropsical) nephritis without increased blood pressure

2. Focal Nephritis: hemorrhagic (nondropsical) nephritis without increased blood pressure

3. *Acute Diffuse Glomerulonephritis:* hemorrhagic (dropsical or nondropsical) nephritis with increased blood pressure

4. *Chronic Diffuse Glomerulonephritis:* parenchymatous (dropsical) nephritis with increased blood pressure

The clinical terms, acute, subacute or subchronic, and chronic, were supplemented during subsequent years by criteria deduced from morphologic and pathoanatomic changes in the kidney. Hypotheses about etiology and pathogenesis of certain renal alterations were also incorporated in some of the classifications. Russell (1930) distinguished ischemic nephritis from toxic nephritis. The histologic picture is dominated by hyaline sedimentation in the tubules, collagenous crescents, and sclerotic thickening of Bowman's capsule. Toxic nephritis is subdivided into:

a) Proliferative glomerulonephritis, at first characterized by proliferation of endothelial cells, in a later stage by additional hyaline necroses

b) Proliferative capsulitis, showing typical proliferation of endothelia in Bowman's capsule

c) Focal sclerosis, characterized by unstructured hyaline areas in the glomeruli associated with capsular adhesion; hence "adhesive glomerulitis"

Bell in 1938 retained the classifications of acute, subacute, and chronic glomerulonephritis. Based upon etiologic and morphologic criteria, acute glomerulonephritis is subdivided in the following groups:

1. Acute Proliferative Glomerulonephritis

Characterized by numerical increase of capillary endothelial cells, thickening of basement membranes, accumulation of leukocytes, partial or total obstruction of capillaries, and extracapillary epithelial crescents.

2. Thrombosis of Glomerular Capillaries

No proliferations or exudations. This type occurs in sepsis without endocarditis.

3. Exudative Type

Characterized by abundance of leukocytes in the glomerular capillaries; this type is found in staphylococcal infections.

4. Thrombosis of Afferent Arterioles

Etiology can be traced to either pneumonia, pneumococcal peritonitis, or congenital syphilis.

5. Embolism Type with Uremia

Characterized by proliferative processes either strictly focal or diffuse. Endocarditis can be associated with this type.

6. Hemorrhagic Type with Obstruction of Tubules

Characterized by pronounced hematuria, frequent after infection of various kinds.

7. Acute Lipid Nephrosis

BELL identified a morphologic criterium of subacute glomerulonephritis in the general obstruction of all the glomeruli, without hyalinization but with tubular atrophy. In contrast to this, chronic glomerulonephritis shows 10% of glomeruli in hyalinization, capillary membranes are not thickened, capillaries are not narrowed. BELL mentions further an azotemic subtype of chronic glomerulonephritis.

ELLIS (1942) published his definition of two different types of glomerulonephritis in 1942; it was cited and discussed frequently in the following years:

Type I: The clinical characteristic is an acute onset after a previous infection accompanied by hematuria. Complete healing is possible, but transition to a rapidly progressing pattern is also possible. A third course was reported as transition into a persistent form with albuminuria, or development of hypertension and uremia. In histology, proliferation of the cellular component of the glomeruli is found together with leukocytes and erythrocytes inside Bowman's capsule and tubules. Fibrinoid necroses of arterioles and epithelial crescents are later symptoms, especially in the rapidly progressing type. If the disease continues over several years there are interstitial fibrosis and diminishing of glomeruli, enlarged glomeruli with increased cell population, decreased number of loops in frequent adhesion to the capsule. Moreover, pericapsular fibroses and a deterioration of interlobular arteries are defined as endarteritic changes.

Type II: The characteristics are generalized edema and severe albuminuria, but minimal hematuria. Complete healing is very rare; continuous progress with persisting edemas and intercurrent infections, is most common. The disease continues over many years and is often complicated by hypertension. ELLIS did not describe any histologic precursor stages of this type. In the small number of cases collected in his report, histologic changes were closely coordinated with those of nephrosis: some few focal necroses of glomeruli, adhesions to the capsule, and fatty degeneration of tubular epithelia. After prolonged course of the disease proliferative glomerulitis is found with lobular accentuation, followed by focal deposits of hyaline substances that can be found, in typical cases, in the stroma between capillaries. Changes are seen in the basement membranes of capillaries, but membrane thickening without proliferation or lobulation is also observed. This pattern of change is generally diffuse; histology reveals mainly a progress of glomerular hyalinization in the loops.

In contrast to VOLHARD, who had more or less rejected the terms acute, subacute, and chronic, FAHR maintained these classification criteria in a new publication in 1944. He saw diffuse glomerulonephritis as a paradigm of allergic inflammation provoked by streptococcal or pneumococcal infections. FAHR clearly refuted primary ischemia as a cause of glomerulonephritis, as had been postulated by VOLHARD. FAHR's classification was established as follows:

1. Acute Glomerulonephritis

Macroscopic changes are neither characteristic nor uniform in general. Microscopy reveals inflammatory hyperemia followed by exudation and proliferation of glomeruli, proliferation of glomerular endothelia and diffuse capillariitis in glomerular loops. Tubular changes are of minor importance.

2. Subacute or Subchronic Glomerulonephritis

The macroscopic picture is either the enlarged white kidney, or the large "colored" one. In microscopy, FAHR separated an intracapillary from an extracapillary type: in the former, changes are restricted to the interior of the loops, in the latter, they are manifested as a proliferative or desquamative process at the capsular endothelium. According to FAHR, the course of the former is more rapid and severe.

3. Chronic Glomerulonephritis

FAHR maintained the distinction between the smooth and the granulated cirrhotic kidney. The microscopic picture is dominated by striking intra-capillary changes in the glomeruli. Clinicians will distinguish further in this type, a stage of compensation from a stage of decompensation.

Moreover, FAHR opposed the focal glomerulonephritis to the more diffuse changes mentioned above; in focal glomerulonephritis he distinguished three forms of toxic, bacterial, or embolic origin.

This classification was adopted by BECHER in 1947.

The method of percutaneous renal biopsies was introduced in 1951 by IVERSEN and BRUN, who inaugurated a new era in kidney research. While the definition and identification of pathologicoanatomic changes had previously been restricted to autopsy findings, the methodical performance of renal biopsies now permitted more and more continuous observation of the early stages and of progress in renal disease.

Some authors still cling to the clinic-oriented prognostic definitions: JONES (1953) maintained the terms "acute, subacute and chronic" in his publication. BOHLE et al. (1969) attempted to combine the terms "peracute, acute, post-acute, and chronic" with morphologic criteria (Fig. 1).

HABIB (1961) was the first to abandon these terms completely. She confined her definitions strictly to morphologic criteria. She anticipated KINCAID-SMITH (1972), who wrote:

"At present a classification must be based on morphology. Clinical symptoms are too similar in association with a wide range of different glomerular lesions to permit more than a very simple and superficial classification. An etiological classification is desirable but we are ignorant about etiological factors in the vast majority of cases of glomerulonephritis. We are also at present unable to base a classification on pathogenetic mechanisms."

Accordingly, HABIB propose the following classification of glomerulo-nephritis accompanied by nephrotic syndromes:

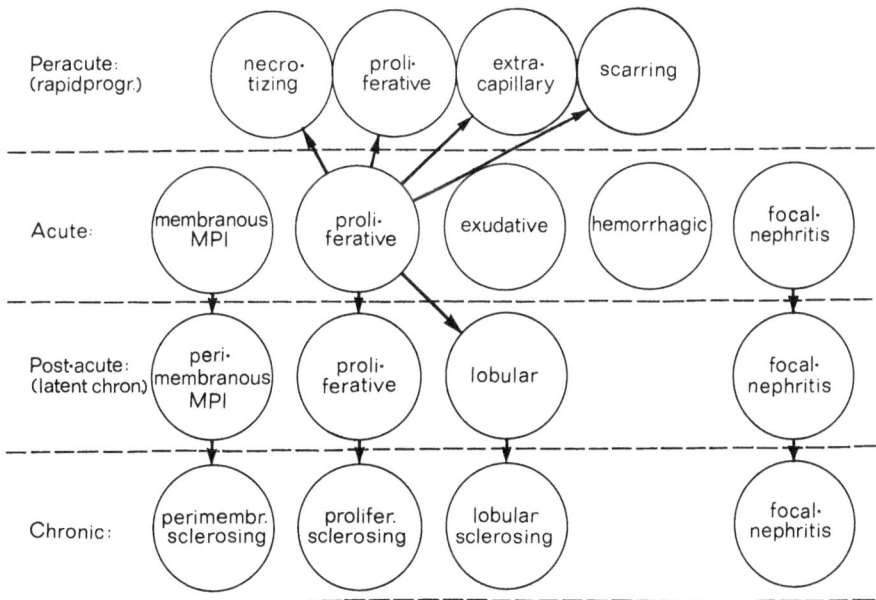

Fig. 1. Classification of acute and chronic forms of glomerulonephritis based on biopsy and autopsy findings (*MPI* = minimal proliferative intercapillary), BOHLE, 1969

1. Minimal Lesions

While light microscopy shows mainly regular glomerular structures, electron microscopy reveals, in particular, foot process fusion of epithelia and other signs of epithelial changes.

2. Thickening of Capillary Walls (Membranous Glomerulonephritis)

Silver impregnation is properly suited to reveal diffuse thickening of glomerular capillaries. In fact, these changes are often discernible only in electron microscopy, which is able to reveal subendothelial deposits in some places.

3. Extracapillary, Proliferative Glomerulitis

Characterized by the appearance of crescents and of occasional capillary adhesions.

4. Endocapillary Proliferative Glomerulitis

Diffuse endocapillary cell proliferations without thickening of capillary walls dominate, accompanied by occasional lobulations of the glomerular loops.

5. Endocapillary Proliferative Glomerulitis with Hyaline Nodules (Lobular Glomerulitis)

In addition to a distinctive narrowing, lobulation of capillaries is seen with endocapillary cell proliferation of varying grades.

6. This group comprises complex forms that do not fit into the preceding classifications

Kinoshita (1966) prefers morphologic criteria in general, although some clinical classification is maintained in view of prognosis:

1. Acute Glomerulonephritis

Histology reveals exudative changes, in particular mesangial proliferation of varying extent. Edema, hypertension, proteinuria, and hematuria dominate the clinical picture. About one-half of all patients are eventually cured, the other half is liable to turn into type 3.

2. Subacute Glomerulonephritis

Under morphologic aspects intramembranous or extramembranous proliferations are found with interstitial cellular changes. This type correlates to the "progressive form" described by Löhlein. It leads towards severe proteinuria and hematuria, to uremia and eventually to death in a few weeks or months.

3. "Elapsed" Acute Glomerulonephritis

This is a lighter type of pattern, similar to the changes in acute glomerulonephritis. Clinical symptoms continue for 6 or even 12 months, but essential alterations cannot be identified after those in renal functions. About one-half of the patients will be completely cured; in the others the disease may take a more chronic aspect—in particular that of the subchronic type.

4. Subchronic Glomerulonephritis

Truly irreversible glomerular changes are never or rarely found in this type. Kinoshita has subdivided it further into four groups according to the degree of intensity.

5. Chronic Glomerulonephritis

Characteristic features of this type are: irreversible changes in the glomeruli and pronounced interstitial fibrosis associated with fibrinoid degeneration of arterioles and of glomerular capillaries, and with epithelial crescents. The clinical picture is dominated by hypertension, proteinuria, and hematuria. The course is often slow, dragging over years, but ending in uremia and death.

6. Chronic Sclerosing Glomerulonephritis

Complete destruction of kidney parenchyma leads to irreversible changes in renal functions and finally to uremia.

In a similar manner Zollinger (1966) combined morphologic criteria with clinical and prognostic aspects. His classifications are:

1. Diffuse Acute Glomerulonephritis

    a) Acute diffuse glomerulonephritis
    b) Subacute diffuse glomerulonephritis
    c) Chronic diffuse glomerulonephritis

2. Glomerular Focal Nephritis

a) Embolic purulent focal glomerulitis
b) Thrombocapillariitis
c) Purely proliferative focal glomerulitis
d) Focal glomerulitis in lupus erythematodes
e) Focal glomerulitis in Wegener's granulomatosis

HEPTINSTALL (1966) was the first to attempt a synthesis of the outstanding classifications of glomerulonephritis published up to that point. Having enumerated and characterized different criteria of classification, he proposed his own table as an optimal compromise of all contemporary definitions—clinical, and pathologicoanatomic:

1. Acute glomerulonephritis
2. Rapid progressing glomerulonephritis
3. Chronic glomerulonephritis including the chronic lobular, and chronic idiopathic membranous types
4. Types of glomerulonephritis associated with nephrotic syndromes
5. Focal glomerulonephritis

EARLE (1970) proposed to "chronic glomerulonephritis" be subdivided morphologically as follows:

1. Diffuse proliferative glomerulonephritis
2. Diffuse membranous glomerulonephritis
3. Glomerulonephritis of mixed membranous-proliferative type (lobular, progressive, and hypocomplementemic)
4. Focal glomerulonephritis (membranous, proliferative, or mixed)
5. Glomerulonephritis associated with other diseases (amyloidosis, diabetes, periarteriitis or lupus erythematosus)
6. Family nephropathies

Acute glomerulonephritis is seen by EARLE as identical with acute proliferative poststreptococcal glomerulonephritis.

In 1970 HABIB presented her new classification of glomerular lesions based exclusively on morphologic criteria:

1.   Nephrosis (nephrotic syndrome with minimal glomerular changes)
2.   Specific glomerular lesions
2.1.   Glomerulonephritis in diabetes
2.2.   Glomerulonephritis in amyloidosis
2.3.   Thrombotic microangiopathy
2.4.   Lupus nephritis
3.   Unspecific glomerular changes
3.1.   Diffuse glomerulonephritis
3.1.1. Glomerulonephritis with extramembranous deposits
3.1.2. Proliferative glomerulonephritis
  a) Purely endocapillary type (with or without exudation)
  b) Membranoproliferative type
  c) Lobular type
  d) Endo- or extracapillary type + 3 subtypes
3.2.   Focal glomerulonephritis
3.2.1. Segmental and focal type

3.2.2. Segmental and focal hyalinosis
3.2.3. Glomerular, global and focal fibrosis
3.3.   Unclassifiable chronic glomerulonephrites

CHURG (1970) stet starts in the same fashion, from purely morphologic criteria; like HABIB, he separates diffuse from focal glomerulonephritis. But his subdivision of diffuse glomerulonephritis differentiates the proliferative from the exudative type, both sharply opposed to the rapidly progressing glomerulonephritis (the so-called malignant or extracapillary glomerulonephritis). In further contrast to HABIB, CHURG maintains the term "chronic glomerulonephritis," subdivided into the early subacute type, the sclerosing type, and end-stage glomerulonephritis. In the beginning, proliferative and sclerosing conditions seem to be in balance, but the later stages are dominated by sclerosing processes.

CHURG mentions several special types: lobular glomerulonephritis and membranoproliferative glomerulitis, suggesting "mesangio-capillary glomerulonephritis" as a more appropriate term for the latter.

CHURG's subdivision of focal glomerulonephritis also differs from that of HABIB in several essential points. CHURG enumerates the proliferative type, the proliferative necrotizing type, the sclerosing scarring type, and the segmental sclerosing type.

The classification of GLYDA (1971) is based equally on clinical prognostic and pathologicoanatomic principles. His gross classification contains four types with several subdivisions:

Type I

1.1. Acute proliferative glomerulonephritis
    Proliferation of mesangial and endothelial cells, narrowing of capillary lumina and of Bowman's capsule, ischemia of glomeruli
1.2. Acute exudative glomerulonephritis
    Sharp increase of leukocytes in glomeruli and in the stroma plus a somewhat lesser mesangial and endothelial proliferation
1.3. Subacute glomerulonephritis
    Epithelial proliferation in Bowman's capsule leading to formation of crescents, beginning adhesions
1.4. Rapid progressive glomerulonephritis
    Intense proliferation of epithelia in Bowman's capsule, crescent formation throughout glomeruli
1.5. Mesangial proliferative glomerulonephritis
    Proliferation of mesangial cells, increase of mesangial matrix; no changes in capillaries or in capsule epithelia, no adhesions
1.6. Chronic proliferative glomerulonephritis
    Evidence of a long = lasting inflammation, lobulation, increase of mesangium and endothelia
1.7. Chronic lobular glomerulonephritis
    Striking lobulation of glomeruli associated with proliferation of mesangium and endothelial cells
1.8. Chronic atrophic glomerulonephritis
    Fibrosis and hyalinization of glomeruli, fibrosing Bowman's capsule, partial hyalinization, lobulation and adhesions
1.9. Chronic mixed glomerulonephritis
    Mixture of forms 1.1 and 1.2

GLYDA's classification comprises further "big" type 2: membranous glomerulonephritis; type 3: "submicroscopic" glomerulonephritis; and type 4: focal glomerulonephritis with several subdivisions.

In 1972, CAMERON attempted to summarize all previous classification criteria in glomerulonephritis. Judging the terminology as rather confused and misleading, he traced the difficulties back to the actual interpretation of renal findings. The resulting classification resembles, more or less, that of HABIB:

1. Minimal Changes

This type is characterized by very small changes; fusion of epithelial foot processes is revealed only by electron microscopy.

2. Membranous (Epimembranous) Nephropathies

Deposits of IgG or C3 at basement membranes. These phenomena are demonstrated particularly in silver staining and/or electron microscopy.

3. Focal Glomerulosclerosis (Segmental Hyalinosis)

The type is identical with HABIB's segmental or focal hyalinosis.

4. Proliferative Glomerulonephritis

In parallel to the classification criteria of HABIB and CHURG, CAMERON distinguished 6 subtypes:

a) Active, diffuse endothelial form
b) Mesangial form
c) Proliferative glomerulonephritis with abundant epithelial crescents
d) Mesangiocapillary form
e) Focal form
f) Endothelial (endocapillary) form

The most comprehensive classification based exclusively on morphologic criteria was presented by KINCAID-SMITH (1972):

1. No Glomerular Lesions by light microscopy or minor or minimal lesions by light microscopy.

1.1. Normal on light microscopy, fluorescent microscopy, and electron microscopy
1.2. Glomeruli normal on light microscopy but showing foot process fusion on elecrone microscopy; findings typical in the so-called nil or minimal lesion nephrotic syndrtom or lipid nephrosis; immunofluorescence findings usually negative, response to steroids high
1.3. Minor lesions on light microscopy with diffuse mesangial IgA and IgG deposits; immunofluorescence findings essential to determine this category; electron microscopy shows also mesangial deposits; characteristic clinical symptom is hematuria, often associated with focal and segmental proliferative glomerulonephritis
1.4. Minor or doubtful proliferation on light microscopy; immunofluorescence staining often inconclusive
1.5. Minor or doubtful increase in mesangial matrix or thickening of basement membrane; immunofluorescence findings often negative; electron microscopy useful for clear decision

2. Diffuse Glomerular Lesions

2.1. Diffuse membranous glomerulonephritis; diffuse changes in all glomeruli; silver spikes on epithelial side of basement membrane, deposits of Ig between spikes; term "membranous glomerulonephritis" comprehends intramembranous as well as extramembranous changes; immunofluorescence is typical and characteristic; deposits of IgG, complement, at times also of fibrin and IgM along capillary walls; deposits can be demonstrated on electron microscopy

2.2. Diffuse proliferative glomerulonephritis

2.2.1. Diffuse endocapillary proliferative and exudative glomerulonephritis; increase in number of cells and in leukocytes; poststreptococcal form of glomerulonephritis. IgG, complement, and fibrin are revealed on immunofluorescence staining, sometimes also IgM and IgA; extramembranous deposits in shape of "humps"

2.2.2. Diffuse endocapillary glomerulonephritis

2.2.3. Diffuse mesangial proliferative glomerulonephritis; increase in mesangial matrix and mesangial cells

2.2.4. Diffuse proliferative glomerulonephritis with associated epithelial crescents; if over 80% of glomeruli show crescents, prognosis is bad; if more than 50% show crescents, prognosis is also invariably bad

2.2.5. Diffuse proliferative glomerulonephritis with focal and segmental mesangio-capillary (membranoproliferative) changes; group is small, probably a subgroup of 2.2.6

2.2.6. Diffuse mesangiocapillary (membranoproliferative) glomerulonephritis; includes both lobular and diffuse mesangiocapillary glomerulonephritis

2.2.7. Diffuse mesangiocapillary glomerulonephritis with dense deposits in basement membranes

2.3. Diffuse mesangial and/or basement membrane lesions without proliferation

3. Focal Glomerular Lesions

3.1. Segmental and focal proliferative glomerulonephritis

3.2. Segmental and focal hyalinosis

3.3. Segmental and focal fibrosis or sclerosis

THOENES (1972, 1973, 1974) also published a classification which combines the previous results of HABIB, CHURG, and KINCAID-SMITH with his own observations and deductions, and which, finally, presents a "Pathological System of Inflammatory Glomerulopathies" (see Fig. 2):

1. Diffuse Glomerulonephritides (Glomerulopathies)

1.1. Necrotizing glomerulonephritis (rapidly progressing)

1.2. Exudative, or exudative and proliferative glomerulonephritis (acute)

1.3. Proliferative glomerulonephritis

1.3.1. Intra- and extracapillary proliferative glomerulonephritis (rapidly progressing)

1.3.2. Mesangial (endocapillary) proliferative glomerulonephritis

1.3.3. Membranoproliferative and lobular glomerulonephritis

1.3.4. Proliferative sclerosing glomerulonephritis

1.4. (Peri)membranous glomerulonephritis

1.5. Minimal lesions

1.5.1. Minimal changes; nephrosis

1.5.2. Minimal glomerulitis

2. Focal and Segmental Glomerulonephritides (Glomerulopathies)

2.1. Proliferative form

2.1.1. Focal and segmental proliferative glomerulonephritis

2.1.2. Associated with certain basic diseases as one symptom among others, e.g. in: Schönlein-Henoch's purpura, disseminated lupus erythematosus, Goodpasture's syndrome, Wegener's granulomatosis

MORPHOLOGY

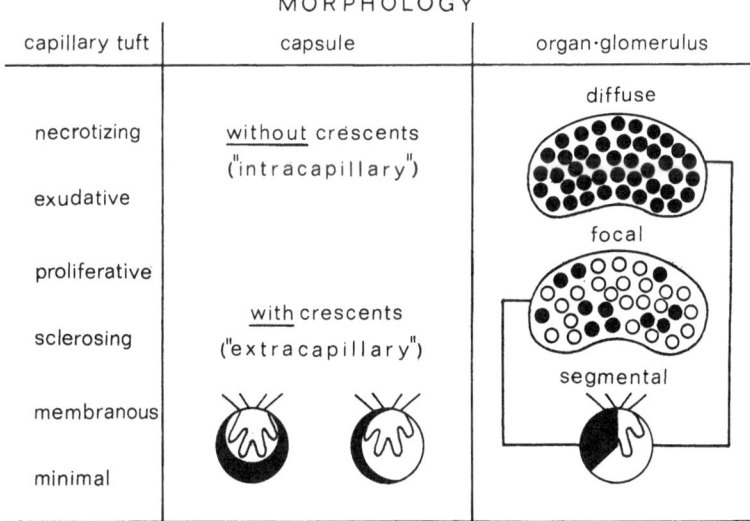

Fig. 2. Terms used for the classification of glomerulonephritis according to THOENES
(1972, 1973, 1974)

2.2.   Sclerosing form
2.2.1. Focal segmental sclerosing glomerulonephritis (focal sclerotic lesion, hyalinose
        segmentaire et focale)
2.2.2. Associated with some basic diseases, e.g. sarcoidosis

In 1974, ZOLLINGER modified his nomenclature by adopting morphologic
criteria (see Fig. 3):

1. Diffuse Glomerulonephritis

1.1.   Diffuse glomerulonephritis, streptococcal type
1.1.1. Exudative phase (formerly: acute)
1.1.2. Proliferative phase (subacute)
1.1.2.1. Mesangioproliferative diffuse glomerulonephritis; panmesangial mesangioprolif-
        erative glomerulonephritis; axial mesangioproliferative glomerulonephritis;
        special form: mesangioproliferative glomerulonephritis with IgA deposits;
        minimal mesangioproliferative glomerulonephritis
1.1.2.2. Extracapillary and mesangioproliferative glomerulonephritis
1.1.3. Sclerosing phase (chronic); subtypes as above
1.2.   Diffuse membranoproliferative glomerulonephritis (formerly: intracapillary-
        lobular glomerulonephritis)
1.3.   Diffuse epimembranous glomerulonephritis
1.4.   Glomerulonephritis shrinkage

2. Focal Glomerulonephritis

2.1. Purulent embolic form
2.2. Thrombocapillaritis (LÖHLEIN)

The new classification published by BOHLE in 1974 is also based on morphology. In many aspects his criteria are in accordance with those or HABIB,
but they differ on some points:

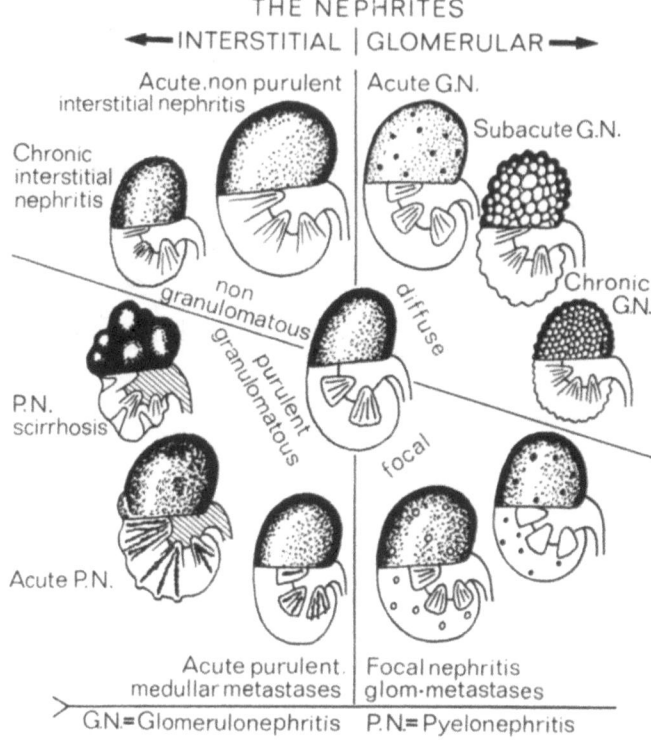

Fig. 3. Diagram of classification of interstitial and glomerular nephritis, ZOLLINGER, 1966

1. Endocapillary (acute) glomerulonephritis (poststreptococcal type)
2. Mesangioproliferative glomerulonephritis
   a) Without focal epithelial crescents
   b) With focal epithelial crescents

3. Intercapillary glomerulonephritis with minimal proliferation minus nephrotic syndrome (HABIB: minimal changes without nephrotic syndrome)

4. Intercapillary glomerulonephritis with minimal proliferation plus nephrotic syndrome (HABIB: Minimal changes with nephrotic syndrome)

5. Intercapillary glomerulonephritis with minimal proliferation and so-called focal sclerosis (HABIB: hyalinose segmentaire et focale, et fibrose glomérulaire globale et focale)

6. Peri-, extra-, epimembranous glomerulonephritis

7. Membranoproliferative glomerulonephritis
   a) Simple form
   b) Lobular variant

8. a) mesangioproliferative glomerulonephritis with diffuse epithelial crescents (HABIB: type III) (rapid progress)
   b) necrotizing glomerulonephritis (rapid progress)

8. Exudative glomerulonephritis
9. Genuine lobular glomerulonephritis
10. Glomerular focal nephritis (LÖHLEIN type)

One hundred and fifty years ago, Richard BRIGHT published his first report on the symptom complex that was subsequently named after him. Many clinicians and morphologists have concentrated their research on the various manifestations of glomerulonephritis or glomerulopathies; their different approaches have led to very varied classifications. Our review of these 150 years of research may be appropriately summarized in a quotation from THOENES's introduction to his classification system:

"Pathology of glomerulonephritis used to be a field that could be surveyed without difficulty: our knowledge was based on autopsy findings and their interpretation by light microscopy. Modified conditions have called for a fundamental revision of this approach:

1. Frequent renal biopsies in clinical diagnosis have enabled us to observe and define even the early stages of glomerular lesions.

2. Fresh biopsy samples of human kidneys can be subjected to modern methods of tissue examination: embedding in plastics, semi-thin sections, electron microscopy and, in particular, immunofluorescence microscopy.

3. Remarkable progress in experimental nephrologic immunology has made it possible to explain the basic mechanisms of immune reactions. The interpretation of experimental results has been fruitful in human pathology

A great variety of techniques and methods has yielded a wealth of information about glomerulonephritis in children and in adults. But we are still a long way from understanding them in every detail, and quite as far from managing their adequate classification.'

References

BECHER, E.: Nierenkrankheiten, Vol. II. Jena: Fischer 1947

BELL, E. T.: The pathology and pathogenesis of clinical acute nephritis. Amer. J. Pathol. **13**, 497–552 (1937)

BELL, E. T.: A clinical and pathological study of subacute and chronic glomerulo-nephritis, including lipoid nephrosis. Amer. J. Pathol. **14**, 691–741 (1938)

BOHLE, A.: In: Nierenkrankheiten, Physiologie, Pathophysiologie, Untersuchungs-methoden, Klinik, Therapie. Ed.: SARRE, H. Stuttgart: Thieme (in press)

BOHLE, A., BUCHBORN, E., EDEL, H. H., RENNER, E., WEHNER, H.: Zur pathologischen Anatomie und Klinik der Glomerulonephritis. Klin. Wschr. **47**, 733–759 (1969)

BRIGHT, R.: Cases and observations illustrating renal diseases accompanied with the secretion of albuminous urine. Guy's Hosp. Rep. **1**, 338 (1836)

CAMERON, J. S.: The natural history of glomerulonephritis. In: Renal Disease. Ed.: BLACK, D. Oxford and London: Blackwell 1972

CHURG, J.: Pathology of glomerulonephritis. Bull. N. Y. Acad. Sciences II **46**, 761–768 (1970)

COPLAND, J.: A Dictionary of Practical Medicine. London 1832–1858

EARLE, D. P.: Glomerulonephritis: Clinical aspects. Bull. N. Y. Acad. Sciences **46**, 749–760 (1970)

ELLIS, A.: Natural history of Bright's disease. Lancet I/1942, 1–7, 34–36, 72–76 (1942)

FAHR, TH.: In: Nierenkrankheiten, Vol. I. (Ed.: BECHER, E., ed.) Jena: Fischer 1944

FREY, W.: Die hämatogenen Nierenkrankheiten. In: Handbuch der Inneren Medizin, Vol. 8. W. FREY und F. SUTER: Nieren und ableitende Harnwege. Berlin-Göttingen-Heidelberg: Springer 1951

FRERICHS, TH.: Die Brightsche Nierenkrankheit und deren Behandlung. Braunschweig: 1851

GLYDA, J.: Attempt of morphological classification of primary glomerulonephritis on the basis of light microscopy examination of needle biopsy material. Polish Med. J. 11, 1640–1674 (1972)

GRAVES, R. J. G.: London Medical Gazette (1831)

HABIB, RENÉE: Classification anatomique des néphropathies glomérulaires. Päd. Fortbildungskurse 28, 3–47 (1970)

HABIB, RENÉE, MICHIELSEN, P., DE MONTERA, E., HINGLAIS, N., GALLE, P., HAMBURGER, J.: Clinical, microscopic and electron microscopic data in the nephrotic syndrome of unknown origin. In: Ciba Symposium on Renal Biopsy. (Eds.: WOLSTENHOLME, G. E. W., and CAMERON, M. P.). London: J. & A. Churchill Ltd. 1961

HENLE, J.: Handbuch der rationalen Pathologie. Braunschweig 1846

HEPTINSTALL, R. H.: Pathology of the Kidney. London: J. & A. Churchill 1966

IVERSEN, P., BRUN, C.: Aspiration biopsy of kidney. Amer. J. Med. 11, 324–330 (1951)

JONES, D. B.: Glomerulonephritis. Amer. J. Pathol. 29, 33–52 (1953)

KINCAID-SMITH, P., HOBBS, J. B.: Glomerulonephritis. A classification based on morphology with comments on the significance of vessel lesions. Med. J. Austral. 2, 1397–1403 (1972)

KINOSHITA, Y., YAMAD, A., FUJISAKI, S., HIRASAWA, Y., WATABE, Y., OSAWA, G., MIKAMI, A., TAKAHASHI, G., MORITA, T.: New classification of diffuse glomerulonephritis based on prognosis, especially new proposal of subchronic glomerulonephritis. Acta Medica et Biologica 14, 35–49 (1966)

KLEBS, E.: Handbuch der Pathologischen Anatomie, Bd. I/2. Berlin: A. Hirschwald 1876

LÖHLEIN, M.: Über die entzündlichen Veränderungen der Glomeruli der menschlichen Nieren und ihre Bedeutung für die Nephritis. Leipzig: S. Hirzel 1906

LÖHLEIN, M.: Über Nephritis nach dem heutigen Stande der pathologisch-anatomischen Forschung. In: Ergebnisse der Inneren Medizin und Kinderheilkunde 5, 411–458 (1910)

PROUT, W. P.: *Cited by* WAGNER

RAYER, P. F.: Traité des maladies des reins. Paris: 1837–1841

REINHARDT, B. E. H. R.: Zur Kenntnis der Bright'schen Krankheit. Charité Annalen 1, 185 (1850)

ROKITANSKY, K. V.: Lehrbuch der pathologischen Anatomie III. Wien 1861

RUSSELL, D. S.: A classification of Bright's disease. Brit. J. Urol. II, 219–232 (1930)

SENATOR, H. S.: Über chronische interstitielle Nephritis. Virchows Arch. 73, 1 (1878)

SOLON (MARTIN-SOLON, F.): *Cited by* WAGNER

THOENES, W.: Immunmorphologische Prinzipien und pathohistologische Systematik der Glomerulonephritis. In: Immunsuppression bei Nierenkrankheiten. Symposium Nürnberg. München: Dustri-Verlag 1972

THOENES, W.: Pathohistologische Systematik der Glomerulonephritis unter Berücksichtigung klinischer Aspekte. Nieren- u. Hochdr.krankh. 2, 199–208 (1973)

THOENES, W.: Pathomorphologische Prinzipien und Formen der Glomerulonephritis. Mschr. Kinderheilkunde 122, 728–740 (1974)

VIRCHOW, R.: Über parenchymatöse Entzündung. Virchows Arch. 4, 260 (1852)

VOLHARD, F.: Die doppelseitigen hämatogenen Nierenerkrankungen (Bright'sche Krankheit). In: Handbuch der Inneren Medizin. (Eds.: MOHR, L., and STAEHELIN, R.) III/2. Berlin: Springer 1918

VOLHARD, F., FAHR, TH.: Die Bright'sche Nierenkrankheit. Klinik, Pathologie und Atlas. Berlin: Springer 1914

WAGNER, E.: Der Morbus Brightii. In: Handbuch der speziellen Pathologie und Therapie. (Ed.: ZIEMSSEN, H. v.) IX/1. Leipzig: Vogel 1882

ZOLLINGER, H. U.: Niere und ableitende Harnwege. In: Spezielle pathologische Anatomie. (Eds.: DOERR, W., und UEHLINGER, E.), Bd. III. Berlin-Heidelberg-New York: Springer 1966

ZOLLINGER, H. U.: Harnorgane. In: Organpathologie. (Hrsg. : DOERR, W.), Bd. II/6, 1–62. Stuttgart: G. Thieme 1974

Medizinische Universitätsklinik, Immunbiologisches Labor
8 München 2, Ziemssenstr. 1, Germany

The Immunohistology of Glomerulonephritis — Distinctive Marks and Variability*

GUNTHER H. THOENES

With 10 Figures and 9 Plates

I. Introduction 61
II. Methodology 63
   1. Antisera 63
   2. Biopsy Treatment 64
   3. Fluorescence Microscopy and Photodocumentation 65
III. The Immunohistologic Manifestations of Clinically and/or Histologically Defined
   Forms of Glomerulonephritis 66
   1. Rapidly Progressing (Subacute Glomerulonephritis, Necrotizing, Extra-
      capillary, Crescentic) Glomerulonephritis 66
   2. Acute Glomerulonephritis (Postinfectious, Exudative, Endocapillary Prolif-
      erative, Mesangioproliferative, "Resolving") 67
   3. IgA Mesangioproliferative Glomerulonephritis (IgA-IgG Mesangial Nephro-
      pathy, Focal Proliferative Glomerulonephritis with IgA, Recurrent (Gross)
      Hematuria) 75
   4. Membranoproliferative Glomerulonephritis (Mesangiocapillary, Lobular,
      Dense-Deposit Disease, Mixed Membranous, Hypocomplementemic Persistent
      Glomerulonephritis) 78
   5. (Peri-) Membranous Glomerulonephritis (Idiopathic Membranous Glomerulo-
      nephropathy, Extramembranous Glomerulonephritis) 82
   6. Focal Segmental Sclerosing Glomerulonephritis (Glomerulopathy) (Focal
      Sclerosis, Focal and Segmental Hyalinosis, Global and Focal Fibrosis) . . . 86
IV. Glomerular Lesions in Systemic Diseases 90
   1. Systemic Lupus Erythematosus (SLE) 90
   2. Contrasting Examples of Renal Involvement in Systemic Disease: Schönlein-
      Henoch Nephritis (Anaphylactoid Purpura) 91
      Amyloidosis 91
V. Concluding Remarks 91
Acknowledgements 98
References 99

I. Introduction

The rediscovery of nephrotoxic antibodies (LINDEMANN, 1900) by MASUGI (1933) was a historical event. In spite of many unanswered questions the general concept of immunopathogenesis offers today the most likely possibility for providing a causal explanation for human glomerulonephritis. In fact there appears to be justification in most cases for assuming that pathohistologic

* Supported by Deutsche Forschungsgemeinschaft, SFB 37 (C5).

Fig. 1. A singular immune deposit along the basement membrane can be detected by immunofluorescence and with conventional magnification whereas with electron microscopy the single deposit can only be found after extensive search in many sections.
IgG, ×1 320

glomerular change is directly related to the respective immunopathogenic process (Germuth and Rodriguez, 1973).

Although *descriptive pathohistology* is the most effective method of providing a nosologic basis for glomerulonephritis, it must be supplemented by other methods such as electron microscopy, immunohistology, and immunochemistry because, especially by means of the latter, pathogenically static morphologic findings may be interpreted. Even when the premise of *immunopathogenesis* does not stand up to criticism (Hamburger *et al.*, 1973), immunohistology provides a possibility for describing the diagnosis of forms of glomerulonephritis that cannot be obtained by other means.

Immunofluorescence has become a relatively independent method and a standard procedure in the clinical-immunological laboratory. In no other organ are materializing immunologic processes reflected *in vivo* in such an extensive, regular, and differentiated manner as in the kidney. Almost 20 years after the first kidneys obtained by autopsy were examined by immunohistologic methods and after intensive experience on biopsy material, it appears imperative to summarize the "distinctive marks and the variability" of glomerulonephritis as seen by immunofluorescence.

This review will be limited almost exclusively to the description of human glomerulonephritis. The problem of *pathohistologic classification* of glomerulonephritis pertains to immunohistology only insofar as the morphologically described diseases will be part of the basis of description. The classifications of Churg and Duffy (1973) and W. Thoenes (1974) will serve as guidelines. The immunohistologic method has one definite advantage in the examination of kidney diseases. The strength of immunohistology (Fig. 1) is apparent in those cases where sensitivity to detail is wanting in conventional histology and where electron microscopy cannot provide a survey of the entire structure.

The detail—one single immune depot (Fig. 1)—may be located in an enlargement from an optical microscope with almost the same sensitivity as with the electron microscope. It is to be hoped that joint work combining all three methods will yield further knowledge on the pathogenesis of human glomerulonephritis.

II. Methodology

In 1950 COONS and KAPLAN introduced immunofluorescence as a method for examining tissue (COONS et al., 1941). At that time, however, at least three preconditions were missing which prevented wide application of immunofluorescence to the study of human glomerulonephritis. At about the same time, intensive work began on glomerulonephritis models *on the basis of animal experiments*, which later contributed to a differentialized understanding of the pathogenesis of human glomerulonephritis (DIXON et al., 1961). The production of antisera specific for a particular immunoglobulin was, for a long time to come, to depend upon individual research laboratories having the required immunochemical experience (LACHMANN et al., 1962). Intravital renal biopsy was first introduced in 1951. Autopsy material for histochemical examination is disadvantageous, because tissue preservation is poor. Moreover, in the final stages of glomerulonephritis, little information can be obtained about the development of the disease. Since the first immunohistologic contributions relating to glomerulonephritis—made by MELLORS and ORTEGA (1956), MELLORS et al. (1957), FREEDMAN et al. (1960), and FREEDMAN and MARKOWITZ (1962)—the technique has improved to such an extent that immunohistology has been used routinely since 1965 to 1967 (KOFFLER and PARONETTO, 1965; McCLUSKEY et al., 1966; BERGER et al., 1967). Not since the early 1970s have extensive case data, also examined on an immunohistologic basis, been available to larger nephrologic groups (BARIÉTY and DRUET, 1971). Standardization of immunofluorescent technique (NAIRN, 1964), necessary for routine application, has been sought since 1967 (HOLBOROW, 1970). A comprehensive paper on glomerulonephritis has recently been published by MERRILL (1974).

1. Antisera

The quality of fluorochrome-labeled antisera is essential for the use of immunofluorescence on tissues. Today, most investigators, including the author, use *commercial sera*. It is advisable to use products of two or three experienced manufacturers concomitantly. Preparations tested for good quality should be purchased in large quantities for long-term use, bottled in individual unthinned portions, and stored at $-80°C$. The *specificity* of the antibodies for the proteins to be identified should be self-evident and should be achieved by insoluble immunoabsorbents in order to avoid soluble immune complexes which remain in the serum. For labeling purposes, the IgG fraction is best. The *antibody contents* should amount to at least 150 μg antibody N/ml with a *protein concentration* of about 10 mg/ml. Fluorescein isothiocyanate is a common fluorochrome. The fluorescent preparation must be *free of unbound dye* and must not contain over- or underlabeled molecules (*optimum F/P ratio* between 1 and 4). Many commercial preparations are distributed in a lyophilic state. In our laboratory, we prefer those preparations which are sent in a *liquid cooled state and with conservation agents*, because there appears to be less danger to their stability. To increase stability, albumin is often added. This prevents subsequent determination of the F/P ratio. Only a few publications state whether the preparations are used in the original concentration or diluted. In the case of an optimum F/P ratio, the unspecific tissue fluorescence (background) should be so low that dilution is unnecessary. My experience is that diluted preparations lose some dyeing brillancy. We therefore use the preparations in an undiluted concentration with *minimum background dyeing*. This decision of course partly depends on how the tissue is prepared (see below).

The following proteins are currently important for the examination of renal biopsies: IgG, IgM, IgA, IgE, C_3, C_4, properdin, fibrinogen, and albumin and transferrin for control solutions. Proof of these proteins in the biopsy is generally best carried out by *direct immunofluorescence*. Our experience has shown that any gain in proof sensitivity by an indirect method is lost in tissue examination due to increased background dyeing. Furthermore, the same applies to *proof of the antigen*, i.e. direct fluorescent labeling of the anti-antigen antibodies achieves the least ambiguous results. It is particularly advantageous if human antibodies can be used. Streptococci antigens (Treser et al., 1969), hepatitis antigens (Combes et al., 1971), DNA (Koffler et al., 1967), and tubulus antigens (Naruse et al., 1973) are currently important antigen in practice.

2. Biopsy Treatment

The immunohistologic examination is made on the frozen preparation. In order to examine the biopsy by several methods (histology, electron microscopy, immunohistology) the material to be examined may be divided or the biopsy repeated. The latter approach is not usual in German clinics and biopsies are normally very thin. For this reason, we perform a double examination on the same tissue sample. This requires a very careful shock-freezing technique on the unfixed material so that the tissue has as few artefacts as possible (for electron microscopy, the tissue must be fixed directly and unfrozen.) In case of a sufficient amount of biopsy material, a part of it must be fixed directly also for conventional histology.

Due to the small size of the tissue samples, the biopsies are embedded in rabbit liver and are shock-frozen in liquid nitrogen. This method also permits careful transport in a frozen state (dry ice), the advantage being that nephrologic centers that have no immunopathologic department can obtain an immunohistologic assessment of renal biopsies. The frozen sections are produced routinely at a thickness of about 4 μ, on a cryostat microtome. The tissue is sectioned as economically as possible, thawed at room temperature, and fixed in formalin. The sections are thawed and dried by a stream of cool air on a microscope slide that has been cleaned with acid. Further treatment should be carried out immediately. Brief fixing in acetone is the next step in many laboratories. We do *not* do this because we believe that the rinsing process in a buffered NaCl solution, which follows in any case, is more effective without fixing in removing proteins which are not structure-bound. The freezing-substitution method with subsequent paraffin embedding according to POST (1965) has been recommended. This method makes it possible to produce semi-thin sections and, in this way, to locate immune complexes more accurately (POLLAK *et al.*, 1973). After the rinsing operation, the dried frozen sections are coated with one to two drops of fluorescent reagent and incubated in a moist chamber, after which antiserum is rinsed off, the section rinsed again, and covered in glycerin: PBS 1:9. Microscopic analysis proceeds forthwith.

3. Fluorescence Microscopy and Photodocumentation

Immunofluorescence, whether with single cells or with tissues, is based on the fact that a substance with antigenic determinants is rendered visible by fluorescent-labeled antibodies that are specifically bound thereto. The fluorescence of the antibody (517 nm for FITC) is excited by ultraviolet radiation focused in the specimen plane. The maximum and optimum absorption values for fluorescein are between 490 and 500 nm. This wavelength is obtained with special selectivity by modern interference filters. Filters UG 1 and BG 12 have hitherto been used alternately, thereby permitting high-quality results to be achieved. Vertical incident illumination or transmittent illumination may be used in microscopy. In the conventional transmittent-light method, the immersed cardioid dark field condensor is used in immuno-histology to produce the lowest background brightness. Relatively greater fluorescence is achieved with vertical incident illumination with the objective lens serving simultaneously as the condensor (PLOEM, 1967). Minute amounts of immunofluorescence on the glomeruli can be detected much better with the aid of this technique and in particular may be photodocumented better.

Generally, the exposure times during routine examination and documentation are reduced considerably by vertical incident illumination microscopy. Reference must be made, however, to the fact that the background brightness (without dark field technique and with increased illumination) is higher and some may consider this a drawback to direct observation. The increased radiation energy also definitely results in intensive and rapid fading of the specific fluorescence. Prolonged observation and subsequent photography of the same object are therefore not possible for practical reasons. In spite of a gain in sensitivity in the vertical incident illumination microscope, the classical dark field observation of the renal biopsy remains a useful method.

Photodocumentation of all immunohistologic findings is the only way to permanently store observations for later comparison with histology or other biopsies. The specimen itself is only useful briefly. The findings are photographed on color film. Ektachrome High Speed daylight film is particularly suitable. If the film is developed accordingly, the automatic exposure may be set for a higher DIN (ASA) number than would correspond to the film. In particular, exposure times are shortened greatly for dark field microscopy.

III. The Immunohistologic Manifestations of Clinically and/or Histologically Defined Forms of Glomerulonephritis

Classification of the glomerulonephritides according to purely morphologic aspects is often unsatisfactory for the clinician. However, few clinical parameters exist which could improve classification. In a few cases, the clinical picture and, in particular, the progress of the disease is so dominant that the term "rapidly progressing glomerulonephritis", for example, is usually as fitting as the term "necrotizing glomerulonephritis". And even if different morphologic variations of rapidly progressing glomerulonephritis (intra- and extracapillary proliferative forms) can be shown, these may only be different degrees of severity of the same pathogenic process. On the other hand, there is no doubt that different etiologic factors may lead to the same clinical or pathomorphologic picture. It is therefore unwarranted to associate *a priori* clinical, immunohistologic, and pathomorphologic aspects in a fixed schematic relationship. Immunohistology is a method which employs neither morphologic nor clinical parameters. On the other hand, it is more closely related to pathogenesis than morphology or clinical observations (G. H. THOENES, 1973). The author therefore decided in this review to describe the immunohistologic phenomena of glomerulonephritis according either to the morphologic aspect *or* the clinical aspect that predominates in practice.

1. Rapidly Progressing (Subacute Glomerulonephritis, Necrotizing, Extracapillary, Crescentic) Glomerulonephritis

It appears to the author no accident that the most direct mechanism of tissue destruction caused immunologically—the nephrotoxic effect of antibodies on the basement membrane—produces the most severe clinical picture, that of rapidly progressing glomerulonephritis. The characteristic immunohistologic finding in rapidly progressing glomerulonephritis, is the sharply linear and brilliant basement membrane fluorescence (Fig. 2). In many cases, this finding is tantamount to the diagnosis of Goodpasture's syndrome (DUNCAN et al., 1965). The diagnosis may be confirmed immunohistologically by positive alveolar septa in lung biopsies (Plate I*D*). Cases of rapidly progressing glomerulonephritis, in which immunohistologic renal findings were not readily discovered, may be so advanced that positive basement membranes are no longer detectable. Even in large kidney sections after open biopsy, glomeruli are found rarely in which fragments of positive basement membranes prove the diagnosis (Plate I*A*). In exceptional cases, the tubular basement membranes are also dyed (Plate I *B*). The focal or diffuse deposition of fibrinogen (Plate I *C*) is described as typical (MOREL-MAROGER, 1973). Usually, but not always, complement C3 is detectable as a linear or less characteristic pattern. An explanation for the negative C3 findings is still wanting (MCPHAUL and DIXON, 1971; VERROUST *et al.*, 1974). It appears to the author, however, to be too sweeping to assume a nonimmunologic pathogenesis in such cases. Immunofluorescence in diabetic glomerulosclerosis, in which a linear pattern may also be observed occasionally (MCCLUSKEY, 1971), clearly differs quantitatively from classic Goodpasture cases as a rule (WILSON and DIXON, 1973). Although linear immunofluorescence has a high coincidence with the rapidly progressing course of the disease (LEWIS *et al.*, 1971) this does not apply exclusively. It must be assumed that—as is the case in animals (UNANUE and DIXON, 1967)—the degree of severity of the disease in humans is also determined by the amount of antibodies. Furthermore, antibasement-membrane nephritis without lung involvement (LERNER *et al.*, 1967; WILSON and DIXON, 1973) also exists. The antibodies involved reveal quantitative and qualitative differences as compared to Goodpasture cases (MCPHAUL and DIXON, 1970). On the other hand, a case has been described recently (LEWIS *et al.*, 1973; BRENTJENS *et al.*, 1974) in which pulmonary hemorrhagia and glomerulonephritis were not connected with an antibasement-membrane mechanism, but with an immune-complex deposition. Doubtless, the progress of the rapidly progressing form in all morphologic variations occurs under different preliminary etiologic signs (e.g. history of streptococcal infection). It is therefore not surprising that immunohistologic phenomena similar to poststreptococcal nephritis are observed in the rapidly progressing course of the disease. A granular or discontinuous linear pattern (Plate I *E*, *F*) is therefore considered to be evidence of another pathogenesis. It appears to be relevant in this context to quote the most recent experimental results of BRENTJENS *et al.* (1974). The antigen–antibody–complex mechanism resulting in glomerulonephritis, which is the same in principle, may also cause pneumonitis under certain circumstances.

Express reference was made by SCHREINER *et al.* (1973) to the clear prognostic differences in the progress of the rapidly progressing form. Moreover, primary vascular processes (Plate I *H*) result in glomerular changes with clear immunohistologic findings (Plate I *G*). The glomerulus appears to behave less as a functional unit, but rather simply as part of the vascular system.

The variability of the immunohistologic phenomenon in rapidly progressing glomerulonephritis is illustrated in Plate I. It is our impression, however, that the linear type of immunofluorescence is most prominent. The literature appears to confirm this fact (Table 1) (cf. also HEPTINSTALL, 1973 a).

2. Acute Glomerulonephritis (Postinfectious, Exudative, Endocapillary Proliferative, Mesangioproliferative, "Resolving")

Acute glomerulonephritis also constitutes for the clinican a disease entity (BALDWIN, 1973) and often has a close relationship to streptococcal infection.

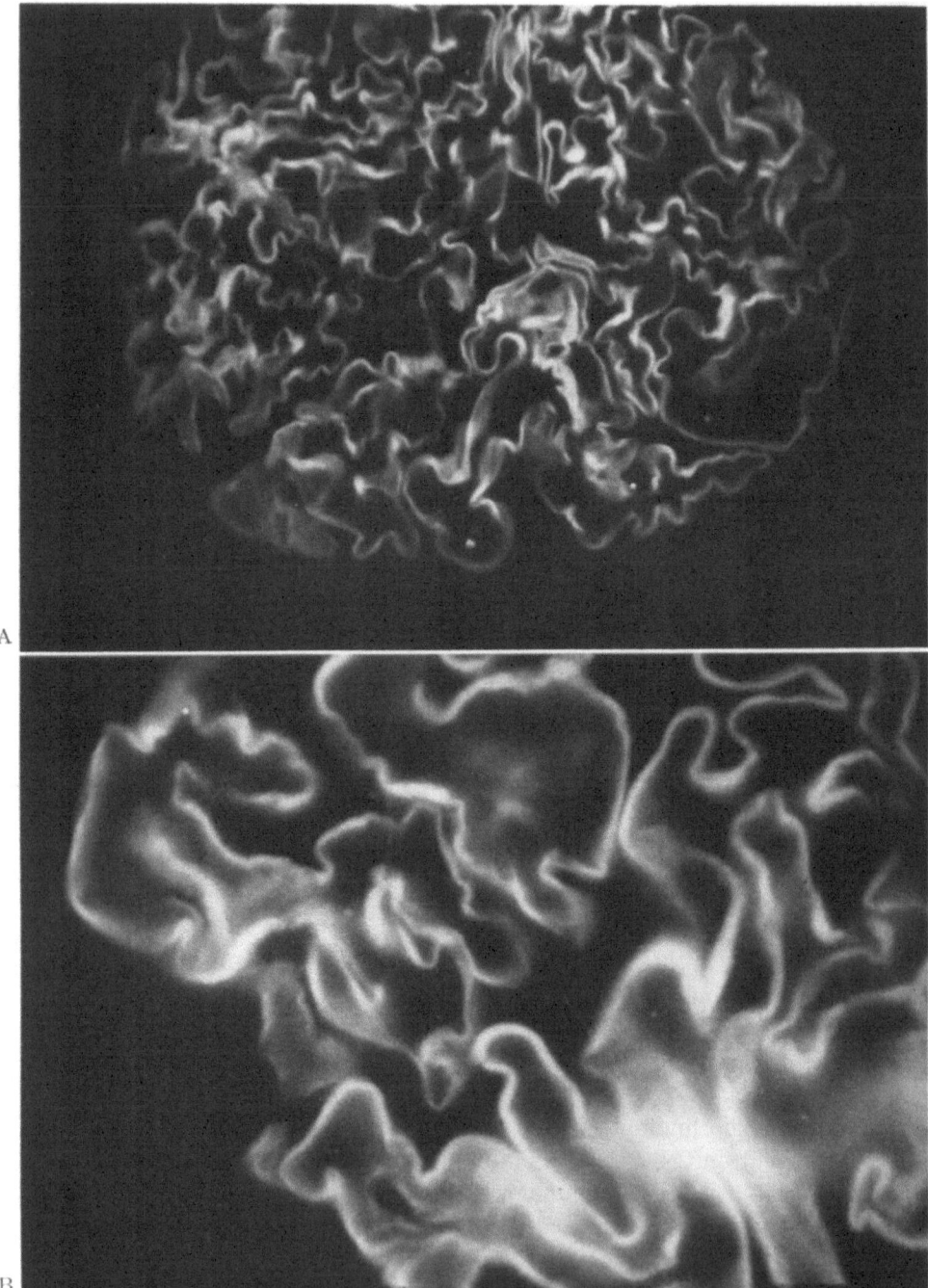

Fig. 2. *A* Glomerulus, showing a sharply linear and comprehensive staining of its basement membranes. Kidney biopsy from a patient who had only slight signs of pulmonary
and kidney involvement, suggesting a Goodpasture syndrome with unusually mild
incidence. IgG, ×583. *B* A larger magnification of a portion of a glomerulus, showing
the linear staining of basement membranes without any indications for immune deposits.
This is from a case with classical Goodpasture syndrome. IgG, ×1430

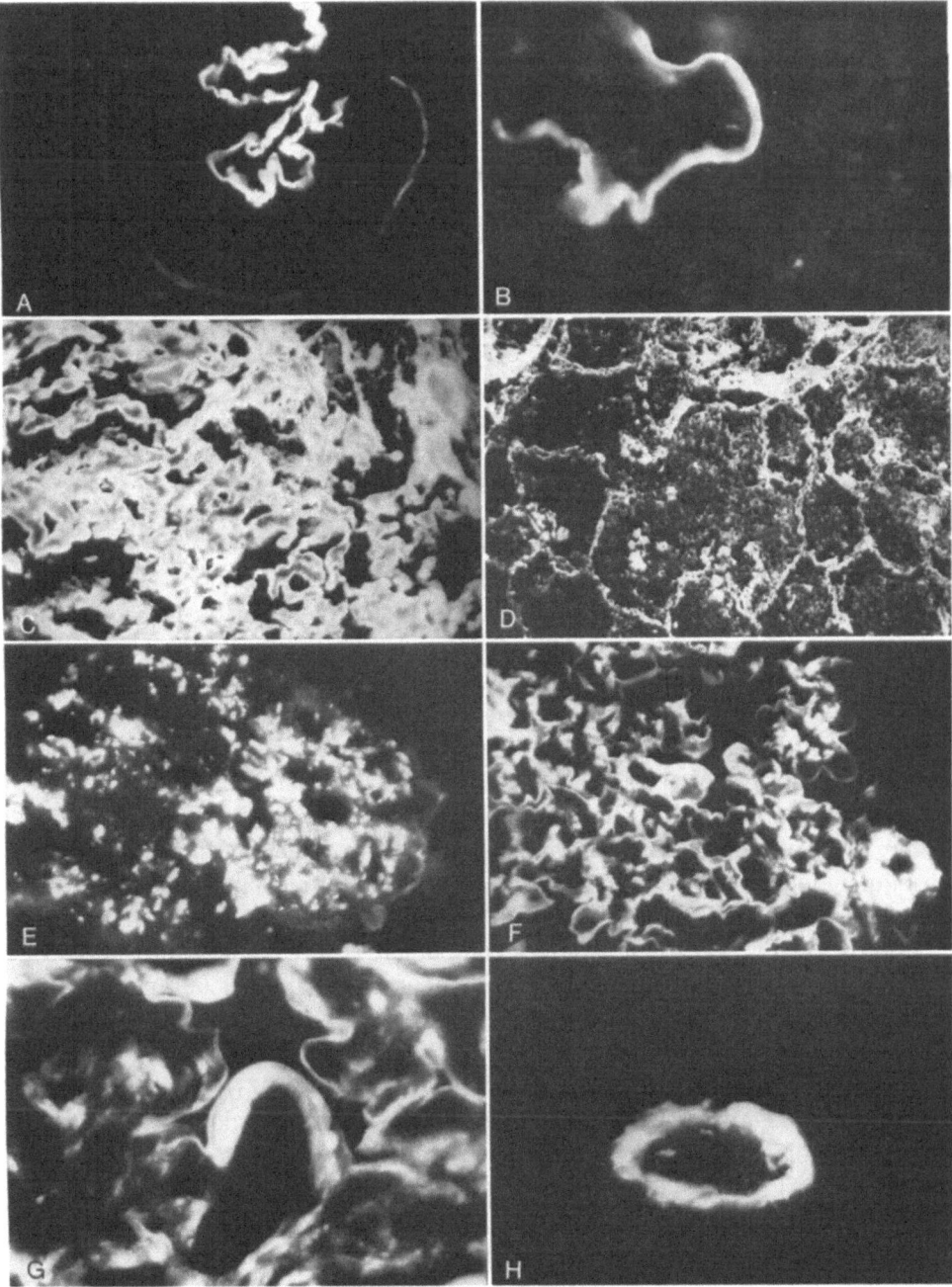

Plate I. The variable patterns of rapidly progressive glomerulonephritis. *A* The positive glomerular loops are moved aside by the negative capsular proliferation; note the faintly positive capsule. IgG, ×300. *B* A short fragment of a tubular basement membrane positive with C_3, ×300. *C* Glomerulus (Goodpasture) diffusely positive with Fibrinogen, ×300. *D* Lung biopsy (Goodpasture) with positive alveolar walls. IgG, ×74. *E, F* A granular pattern, in *F* mixed with discontinous-linear stainings, C_4, C_3, ×300. *G* Positive glomerular staining (C_3), associated with a rapidly progressive course of malignant nephrosclerosis; the vascular lesion is seen in *H* (IgM); ×736, ×300

Table 1. The frequency of linear fluorescence in cases of rapidly progressing
glomerulonephritis

	No. of cases	Linear	Other	Negative	Not incidated
CAMERON and OGG (1973)	22[a]	2	10	?	10
STRIKER et al. (1973)	10	2	—	8	—
LEWIS et al. (1971)	7[a]	6	1		—
MOREL-MAROGER et al. (1973)	33[a]	3	17	?	13
WILSON and DIXON (1973)	40[b]	31	—	2	7
THOENES, G. H. (unpublished)	16[a]	11	5	—	—
	128	55	33	10	30

[a] Identified by the authors as rapidly progressing glomerulonephritis.
[b] The groups of Goodpasture and non-Goodpasture patients required dialysis 0.1–18
(mean 3.5) months and 1–14 (mean 4.5) months respectively after onset of the disease.

This does not rule out the fact that primary chronic, extramembranous forms
may be concealed behind the clinical diagnosis in individual cases (HABIB,
1973; HINGLAIS et al., 1974). In most cases, however, practice shows that,
when viewed immunohistologically, acute glomerulonephritis has a characteristic appearance of a reticular, finely granulated type (Fig. 3 A). This
picture is so typical that the diagnosis of acute poststreptococcal nephritis
may be predicted with the aid of immunohistology, irrespective of pathologic
and clinical evidence. Frequently, the findings are relatively poor on a quantitative scale (Fig. 3 A), particularly with the IgG reagent.

Two variations of the immunohistologic pattern can be found in detail:
there is on the one hand the particularly clear representation of coarse and
irregular depots, the "humps" (Fig. 3 B). On the other hand, an interrupted
linear pattern (Fig. 3 C) is observed. It appears that, in the pattern with
"humps" in Fig. 3 B, the exudative component is predominant in the pathohistologic preparation. According to HERDSON et al. (1966), "humps" may be
detected by electron microscopy in the first 6 weeks after onset of the disease.
The pattern in Fig. 3 C is predominant in more proliferative glomerulonephritis. In contrast to the opinion of RICHET et al. (1973), who reported in
detail on the granular immunohistologic pattern in acute glomerulonephritis,
the immunohistologic appearance appears to us, as well as to others (VERNIER
et al., 1967; FISH et al., 1970), to be more differentiated. It is very probable
that the variations illustrated in Plates II and III express different stages
of disease and a different intensity during onset of the disease. Plate II shows
the granular variations, all cases being clinically acute diseases of the poststreptococcal nephritis type which were accompanied by a reduction in the
serum complement level (C3) (with the exception of G: normal C3, but patho-

Fig. 3. A The typical immunohistological pattern of acute, poststreptococcal glomerulonephritis. IgM, $\times 588$. B Large, irregular "humps" in extramembranous location, IgG,
$\times 1083$. C Interrupted linear pattern with few if any granular deposits. C_3, $\times 1083$

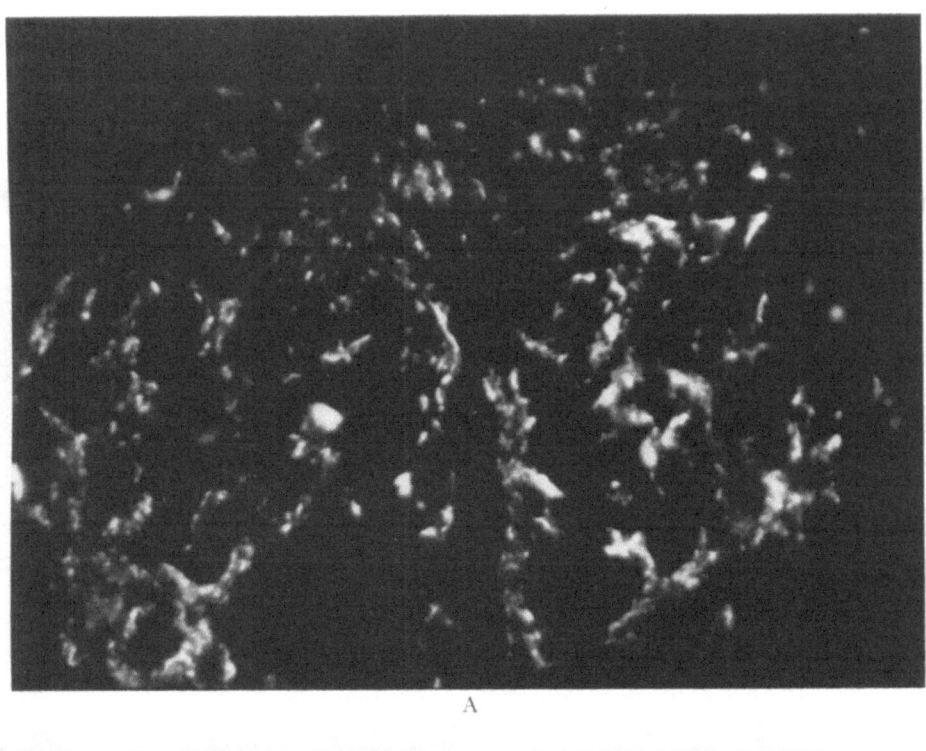

A

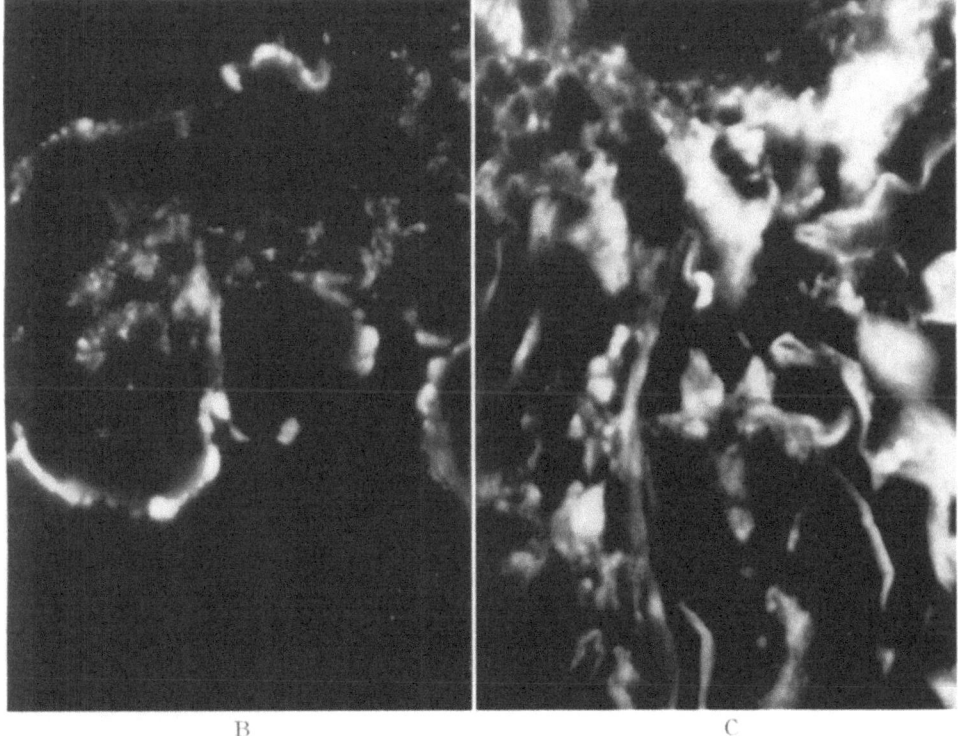

B   C

Fig.3 A—C

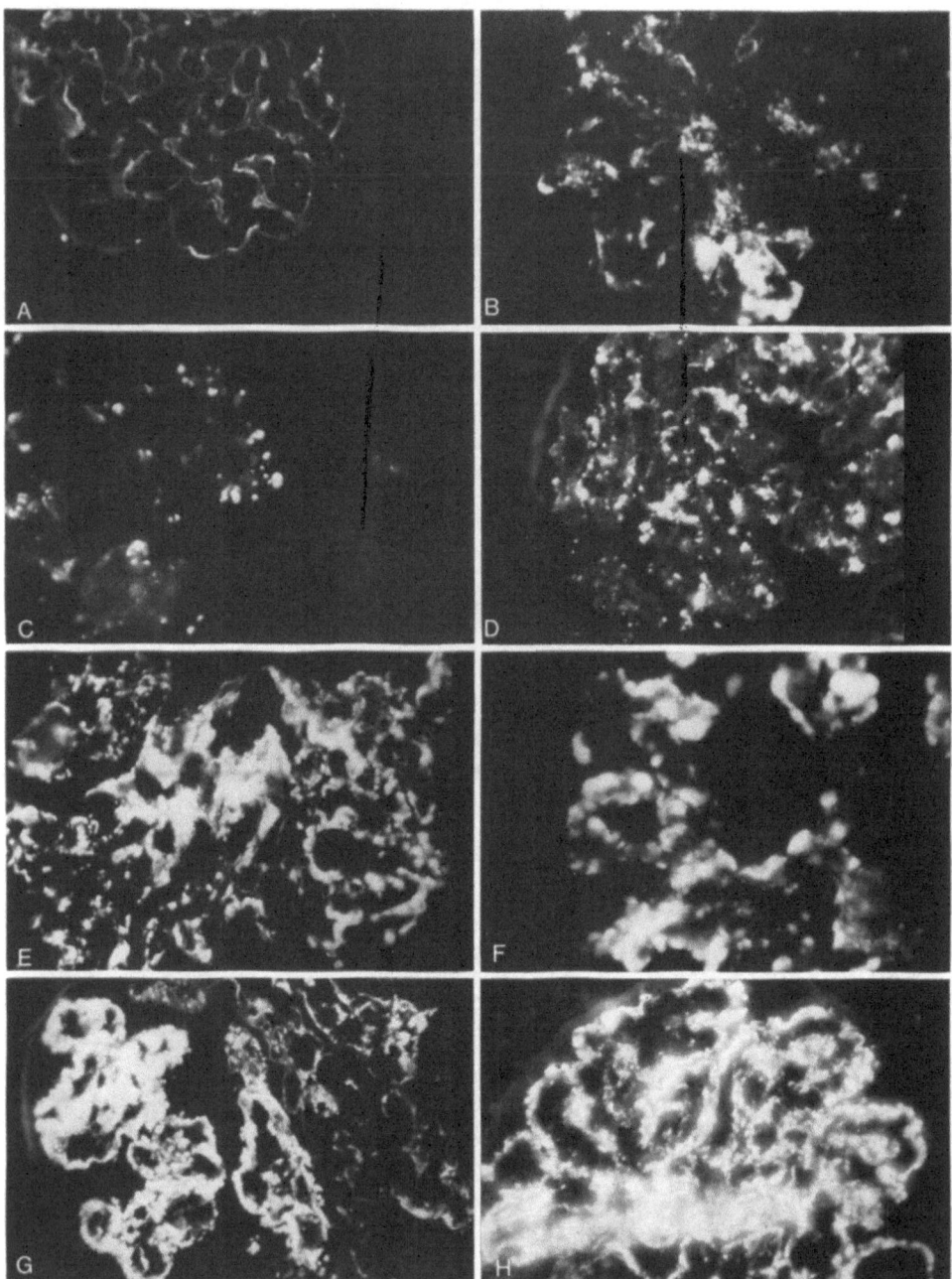

Plate II. The granular patterns in acute, poststreptococcal nephritis. They differ quantitatively from minimal (*A*) to very comprehensivly and tightly packed granulations (*H*),
Also note the segmental accentuation in *B* and *G*. *A* IgG, ×300. *B* C$_3$, ×300. *C* IgA
×300. *D* IgG, ×300. *E* IgG, ×300. *F* IgG, ×736. *G* IgG, ×300. *H* IgG, ×300

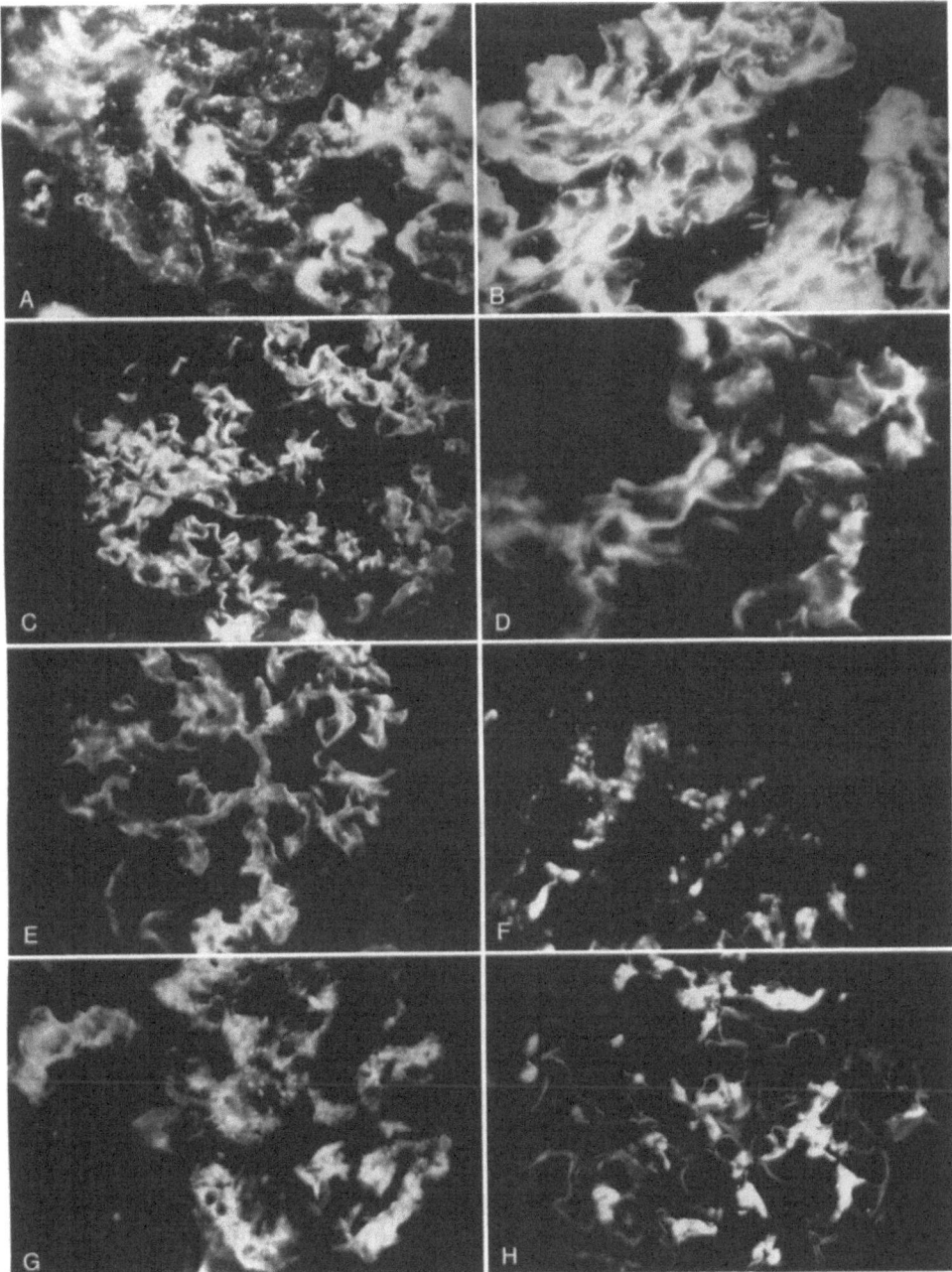

Plate III. The interrupted linear and mesangial patterns of acute, poststreptococcal nephritis, which are probably related to the later or resolving phases of the disease. The features range from an obvious involvement of all the capillary loops (A, B) and an almost continously linear appearance (B), to heavy mesangial stainings (G) or very small remnants in the mesangium (H). A IgG, $\times 300$. B C_3, $\times 300$. C C_3, $\times 300$. D IgG, $\times 736$. E C_3, $\times 300$. F IgG, $\times 736$. G C_3, $\times 300$. H C_3, $\times 300$

histologically a serious acute exudative proliferative glomerulonephritis;
cf. Tina et al., 1968), subsequent increase of the same, and indications of a
streptococcal infection (ASL, anamnesia). The illustrated patterns have no
exact correlation to the stage of disease. The impression is, however, that
distinctive granular forms coincide more closely with the early leukocytic
exudative phase of glomerulonephritis. On the other hand, Germuth and
Rodriguez (1973) emphasize that large confluent "humps" may also be seen
in the resolving phase. The timing of these findings together with the clinical
progress are still being contested.

Richet et al. (1973) attempted to follow sequential biopsies from the
same patient. In spite of considerable morphologic differences in the course
of the disease, they could not discover immunohistologic differences. We have
no explanation to offer, but believe with various other authors (Feldman
et al., 1965; Michael et al., 1966; Treser et al., 1968; Fish et al., 1970) that
the "interrupted linear" and, to an even greater extent, the mesangial
immunohistologic patterns (Plate III) are typical for a later phase of disease
which may already have begun to heal. However, it is not safe to draw prognostic conclusions from the immunohistologic picture (Burkholder and
Bradford, 1969). On the one hand, Richet et al. (1973) regard the outcome
of exudative glomerulonephritis (a predominantly granular type, Plate II) as
extremely doubtful. On the other hand, Treser et al. (1969) found a considerable number of positive immunohistologic findings in 19 out of 23 patients
2 years after commencement of the disease. The immunohistologic findings
later decreased in most cases, but nevertheless continued in some. In the light
of the importance of immunohistology, Treser should be quoted at this point:
"The immunologic and morphologic findings are often parallel, but, where
there is a discrepancy, the potential for continued activity, and consequently
the prognosis of the lesion, can probably be better determined by the information obtained by immunohistology than by light or electron microscopy"
(Treser et al., 1969).

Severe cases of exudative acute glomerulonephritis may show immunohistologic findings which are relatively unimpressive (Plate II B), but whose
prognosis is favorable. Excessive "humps" (Plate II G, H) in a proliferative
exudative histology may indicate a progressive course of the disease but do
not necessarily imply this. The correlation between immunohistologic and
electron-microscopic findings does not always exist (Burkholder and Bradford, 1969). It is beyond the scope of this article to become involved at length
with the problem of a link between acute and chronic (membrano proliferative)
glomerulonephritis, as suggested by the findlings of Glasgow and White
(1973). The predictive value of the immunohistologic pattern will depend on
much more experience collected independently from histology at individual
and sequential biopsies. From the (immuno)pathogenic point of view, however,
so much can be said that it seems illogical to attribute one type of glomerular
reaction pattern to one etiopathogenetic principle. On the other hand, we
still know far too little about the extent to which the various antigens cause

different immunohistologic phenomena. The pathogenic mechanism may vary in response to the nature of the antigen (e.g. "alternative way" of complement activation, WESTBERG et al., 1971; MCLEAN and MICHAEL, 1973; WEST et al., 1973). The role of cryoglobulins in acute poststreptococcal glomerulonephritis (GRUPE, 1968; MCINTOSH et al., 1969; MCINTOSH et al., 1971; VERROUST et al., 1971; ADAM et al., 1973) as another example remains to be clarified.

3. IgA Mesangioproliferative Glomerulonephritis
(IgA-IgG Mesangial Nephropathy, Focal Proliferative Glomerulonephritis with IgA, Recurrent (Gross) Hematuria)

The multiplication of mesangial cells is a general reaction of the glomerulus that may conceal very different etiologic principles. The term mesangio-proliferative glomerulonephritis is therefore a collective term for various clinical syndromes. IgA mesangial nephropathy, however, has become a domain of immunohistology and was first defined by BERGER (1969). Proof of IgA in typical, arborescent mesangial distribution (Fig. 4A, B) differentiates this form, for example, from the resolving poststreptococcal glomerulonephritis, another mesangio-proliferative syndrom. In most cases, IgA is the predominant immunoglobulin both qualitatively and quantitatively, but IgG and C3 are simultaneously detectable in almost all cases. The presence of fibrinogen in identical localization is not exceptional either.

Following the work of BERGER (1969), other papers have appeared (MCENERY et al., 1973; ROY et al., 1973b; LOWANCE et al., 1973; HYMAN et al., 1973; VAN DE PUTTE et al., 1974) which confirm that this IgA nephropathy (or IgA nephritis) is also a clinical disease. The immunohistologic diagnosis is due to the typical mesangial arrangement of the IgA (Plate IV A). On the basis of the immunohistologic findings, it does not appear to be justified to speak of focal glomerulonephritis, since all glomeruli are IgA positive (Plate IV B). Although the progress of the disease is immunohistologically slow, a low- (Plate IV C, D) and high-grade (Plate IV E, F) findings may be observed. It is not certain in all cases whether the IgA-C3 deposits are immune depots. The structure is often almost homogeneous (Fig. 4B). On the other hand, blot-like granulations (Fig. 4A) or toothed, double membrane-like fragments may be recognized. Fine granular markings in the depots are clearly visible in some areas (Plate IV G, H). The functions of the mesangium are poorly understood (MAUER et al., 1972; DAVISON et al., 1973) and therefore no definite statements can be made concerning the pathogenesis of IgA-mesangial disease. EVANS et al. (1973) believed that the complement sequence in focal mesangial nephritis is activated by the properdin system (alternate path).

The reader is reminded that GÖTZE and MÜLLER-EBERHARD (1971) reported that aggregated IgA can activate the complement sequence by the alternate path. Hence, IgA nephritis may be at least a secondary immunologic process. Irrespective of which pathogenesis is on record, proof of IgA contributes to a differentiation of the histologic picture of mesangioproliferative glomerulo-

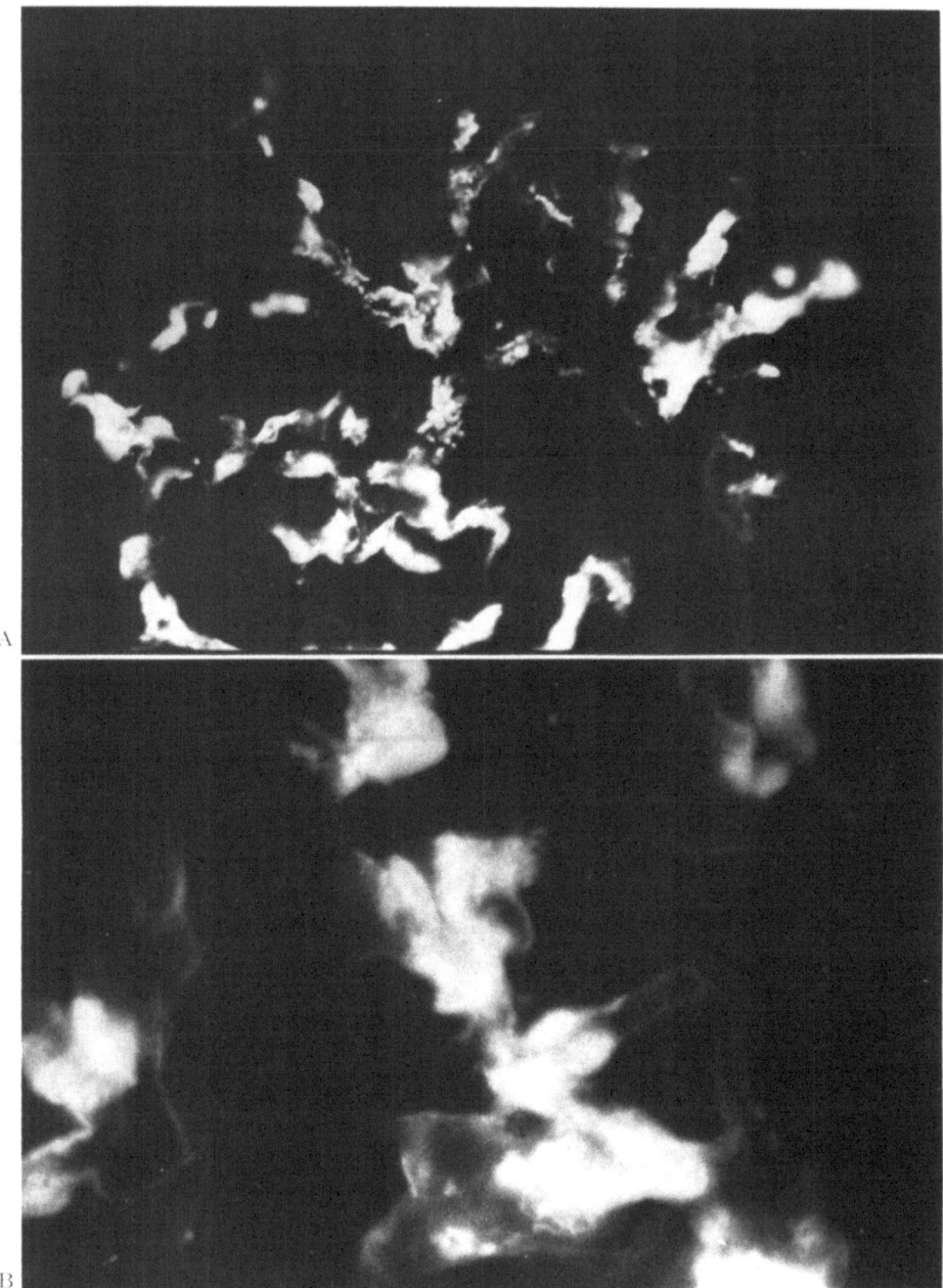

Fig. 4. *A* The distinctive, arborescent distribution of IgA in mesangial-proliferative glomerulonephritis. ×582. *B* The mesangial deposits are either granular or seem to be homogeneous, as is the case here. IgG, ×1430

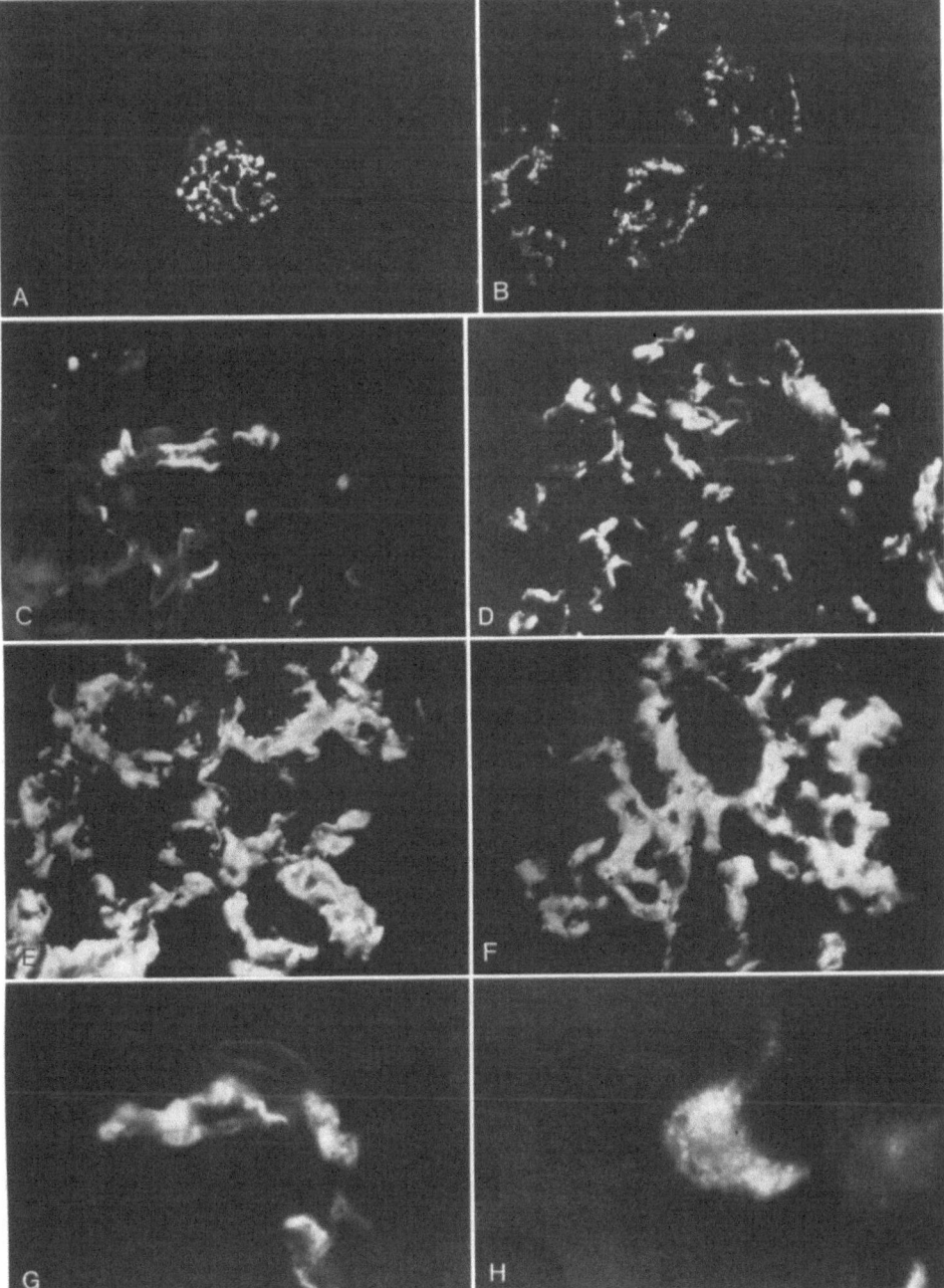

Plate IV. The various immunohistological correlates of mesangial-proliferative glomerulonephritis. The arborescent pattern (A) is seen diffusely in all glomeruli (not focal!) (B).
Small double-con⁺oured membranes (C, D) or solid mesangial tracks (E, F) occur. The
fine structure (G, H) does not always allow safe conclusions whether immune materials
are phagocytized or a direct anti-mesangial effect is involved. A Fibrinogen, ×74.
B IgA, ×74. C IgA, ×300. D IgG, ×300, E C₃, ×300. F C₃, ×300. G IgG, ×736.
H IgA, ×736

Table 2. The frequency of IgA-deposition and of IgA-nephropathy in relation to the total number of biopsies evaluated and the cases of mesangioproliferative glomerulonephritis

Renal Biopsies -total	IgA positive	Histology pure me-sangial-prolifera-tive	Immunofluorescence						
			Mesangial pattern		No specific pattern		Other specific pattern		Negative
			IgA-pos.	IgA-neg.	IgA-pos.	IgA-neg.	IgA-pos.	IgA-neg.	
696		180							
	132 (19%)		68 (37.8%)	7 (3.9%)	8 (4.4%)	36 (20.0%)	4 (2.2%)	30 (16.9%)	27 (15%

44.4% (80) of pure mesangioproliferative cases are IgA-positive

60.6% (80) of IgA-positive biopsies are pure mesangioproliferative

9.9% (68) of all kidney biopsies are IgA nephropathies.

nephritis. The close correlation of pure mesangial proliferation with IgA deposits is documented in Table 2. Almost 50% of all purely mesangio-proliferative cases are IgA-positive and 38% of those can be defined as IgA nephropathy. On the other hand, almost two-thirds of IgA-positive biopsies can be expected to be mesangioproliferative histologically. Finally, 10% of all kidney biopsies examined in our laboratory (without transplanted kidneys) could be defined as IgA nephropathies by combined immunohistology and histology.

4. Membranoproliferative Glomerulonephritis
(Mesangiocapillary, Lobular, Dense-Deposit Disease, Mixed Membranous, Hypocomplementemic Persistent Glomerulonephritis)

Membranoproliferative glomerulonephritis, as defined by its characteristic mesangial proliferation, the endo- and/or intramembranous alterations (ARAKAWA and KIMMELSTIEL, 1969; CAMERON et al., 1970) and the commonly depressed levels of serum complement factors (WEST et al., 1965), has become a disease entity (CAMERON et al., 1973a; CAMERON et al., 1973b; SCHÜRCH et al., 1972) for which immunohistology also presents certain diagnostic patterns (MICHAEL et al., 1971).

As shown in Fig. 5 A and B the garland-like accumulation of proteins in the peripheral areas of glomerular loops presents a destructive appearance. The involvement of the mesangium in the form of granular fluorescence is just as clear as the frequent partial linear appearance of the basement membrane. Our examination material has not yet revealed whether the linear basement-membrane representation is an immunologic equivalent for the variety of dense-deposit disease as suggested for example, by the electron-microscopic pictures of MacDonald (1973). It also seems to be obvious that the electron microscopist sees different types of membrane alterations, suggestive of replacement of the basement membrane by "linear deposits" (Cameron et al., 1973). On the other hand, Burkholder et al. (1970, 1973) differentiated this feature into three varieties of membranoproliferative glomerulonephritis, including also a form with typical extramembranous deposits. This view of an idiopathic membranous variety of membranoproliferative disease has not been generally accepted.

Plate V A–H is intended to show that the immunohistologic pattern of membranoproliferative glomerulonephritis is quite variable and could be the expression of different subgroups or of different stages of the disease as well. On the basis of the correct histologic diagnosis backed up by the low complement values, the exclusively membrane-oriented deposition of granular complexes can be observed (Plate V A). It is rarely possible with regular immunohistologic techniques to present exact information about the location of such deposits. Pollak et al. (1973) used semi-thin and freeze-substituted sections and localized most of the deposits in so-called mesangium-circumferential areas; only 1 patient in 9 showed a subepithelial deposition. A "mesangium-centrilobular" location is most common and is also seen in Plate V B, although the granular structure is less evident in some of those cases.

The involvement of the basement membrane is sometimes demonstrated especially well by antifibrinogen as shown in Plate V C. The destructive feature of "tram track-like" basement membranes can occasionally be detected (Plate V D), even by immunohistologic means. The so-called lobular variety of membranoproliferative glomerulonephritis simply shows a lobular pattern of the fluorescent structures as well (Plate V E). It seems evident from the higher magnification in Plate V F that mesangial granular deposits are the main components of the pattern. Sometimes there is in one case and even in one glomerulus an astonishing difference of immunofluorescent staining with different reagents as shown in Plate V G (anti-IgM) and H (anti-C3).

It is clear therefore that the typical pattern of membranoproliferative glomerulonephritis, again shown in Plate V G, does not become apparent with every reagent. It should be mentioned that the last two pictures represent a case in which the first biopsy made several months ago was classified as acute postinfectious glomerulonephritis by the clinician, histologist, and immunopathologist. This again touches upon the problem of transition from the (hypocomplementemic) acute postinfectious glomerulonephritis to the chronic (hypocomplementemic) membranoproliferative form. Glasgow and White (1973) recently reported such a case although others have presented evidence against an origin from acute poststreptococcal nephritis (Okuda et al., 1970) and it seems wise to keep an open mind on the issue (West et al., 1973 a).

Since Seegal et al. (1965) studied the role of streptococcal antigens in progressive glomerulonephritis the matter has remained doubtful although Zabriskie et al. (1973) have put forward an intriguing hypothesis relating the streptococcal infection to secondary autoimmune phenomena. Whatever

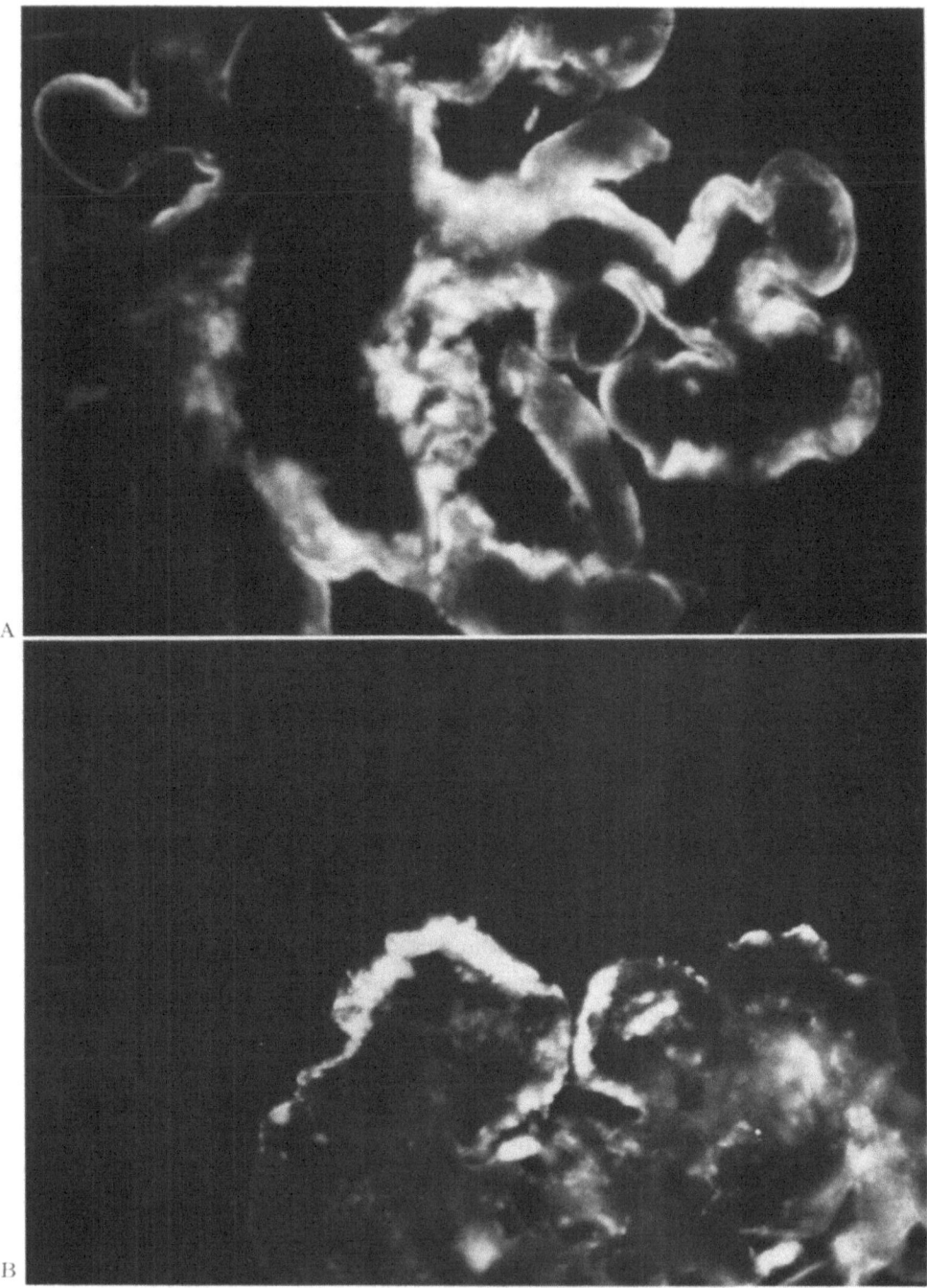

Fig. 5. *A* The distinctive pattern of membranoproliferative glomerulonephritis. The stained membranes with endo-membranous as well as mesangial deposition of fluorescent material is seen. C$_3$, ×582. *B* A garland-like staining of IgG in peripheral areas is characteristic for membranoproliferative glomerulonephritis. The central (mesangial) parts appear to be "empty". IgG, ×582

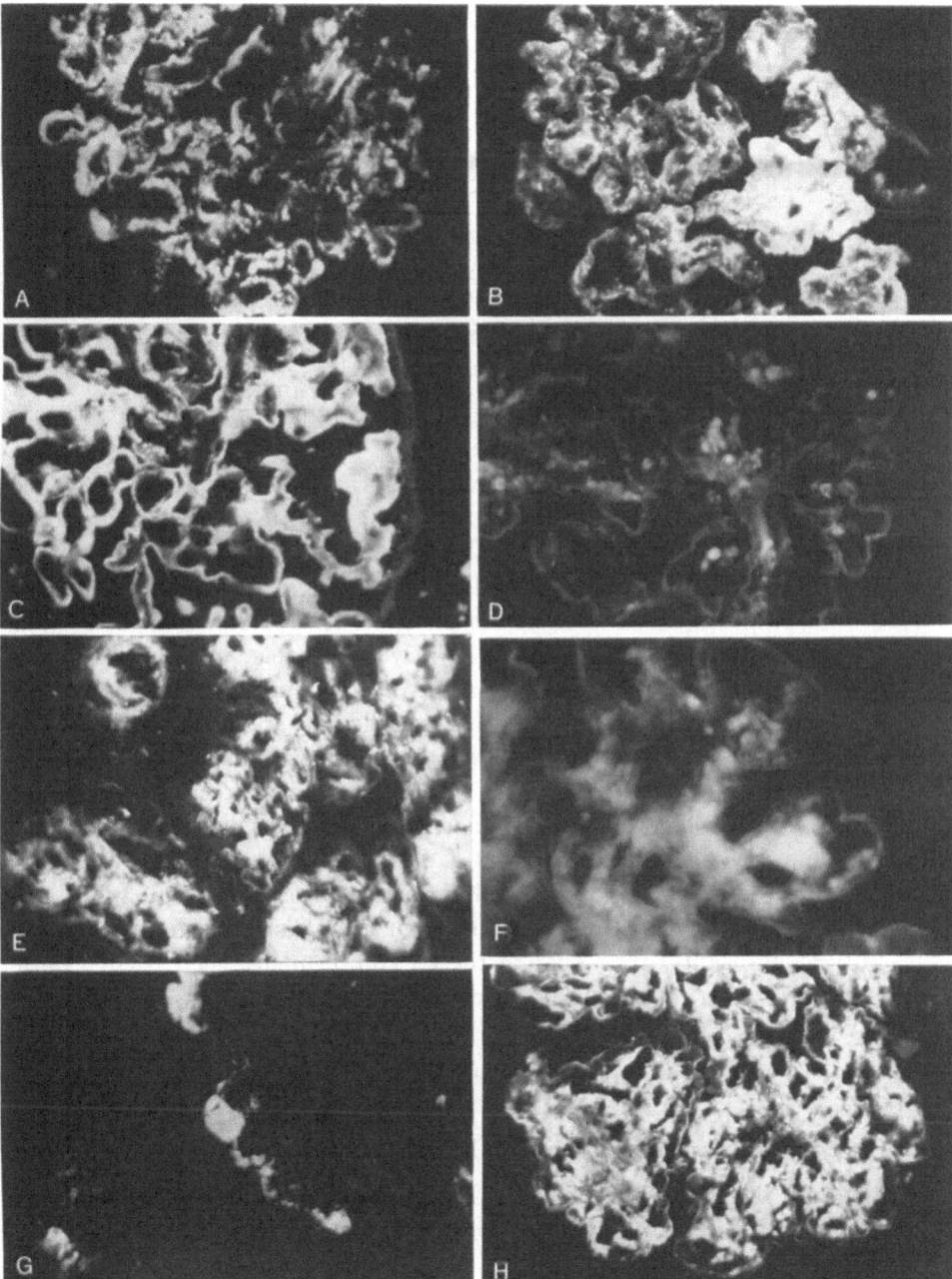

Plate V. The variable representation by immunofluorescence of membranoproliferative glomerulonephritis. The membrane-oriented granular deposits (A) are larger and more irregular than in (peri-) membranous nephritis. B "Centrilobular" location of immune deposits. Membrane staining with fibrinogen (C) and a "tram-track"-like feature of the membranes (D). Lobular configuration (E) with mesangial accumulation (F) of granular materials. The staining pattern sometimes depends on the reagent used (G and H). A IgG, ×300. B IgG, ×300. C IgG, ×300. D C$_3$, ×300. E IgG, ×300. F IgG, ×736. G IgM, ×300. H C$_3$. ×300

Table 3. The contribution of complement and immunoglobulins to the immunofluorescent
pattern of membranoproliferative glomerulonephritis

	No. of cases	Positive cases for	
		C_3	Immunoglobulins
MOREL-MAROGER, L. (1973)			
Membranoproliferative	32	29 (diffuse)	5 (diffuse), 24 focal-segmental
Lobular	5	4	(with IgM)
Dense-deposit disease	4	4	3 (IgM)
THOENES, G. H. (unpublished) (not further subdivided)	26	21	16 (IgG), 18 (IgM), 10 (IgA), 10 ($Fibrinogen$)
MICHAEL et al. (1971) (not further subdivided)	27	27	27 (IgG), 18 (IgM), 8 (IgA), 19 ($Fibrin$), 9 (C_1q), 7 (C_4), 11 ($Properdin$)

the etiology (see, for example, Waldenström's macroglobulinemia and mesangiocapillary glomerulonephritis, LIN et al., 1973) the membranoproliferative
or mesangiocapillary type of glomerular reaction is also a distinctive entity as
viewed by immunofluorescence. This does not rule out, for example, the fact
that the lupus pathogenesis often leads to a pattern of glomerular alterations
very closely resembling membranoproliferative glomerulonephritis.

It seems remarkable that only these three forms of glomerulonephritis—
membranoproliferative, acute, and lupus nephritis—are accompanied by a
more or less serious complement C3 and properdin depression (MCLEAN and
MICHAEL, 1973) which is suggestive of some pathogenetic relationship. Membranoproliferative glomerulonephritis has been associated with the alternate
way of complement activation. Indeed, C3 is involved in most cases whereas
C4 or Cl_q are much less frequent (Table 3). Moreover, immunoglobulins can
be seen in relatively high frequency although their distribution and location
may differ significantly from that of the C3 complement. Their pathogenetic
contribution awaits further clarification.

5. (Peri-) Membranous Glomerulonephritis
(Idiopathic Membranous Glomerulonephropathy,
Extramembranous Glomerulonephritis)

This form of glomerulonephritis is regarded as the prototype of immune-
complex nephritis in man. According to the classification of cases of glomerular
nephropathy (1368 cases) by HABIB (1973b), 4.3% of cases can be classified
as nonproliferative extramembranous or "membranous" glomerulonephritis.
Her biopsy specimens were presumably mainly from children. The frequency
distribution is similar to that found in our laboratory, which receives biopsy
specimens mainly, though not exclusively, from adults. In 701 cases of glomerular disease (first biopsies only) we found 5.9% perimembranous glomerulonephritis based on histology and 4.9% judged by the immunohistologic pattern (G. H. THOENES, unpublished). On the one hand—again according to

HABIB (1973 b)—diffuse proliferative glomerular lesions are observed about 5–6 times more often (25.6%) than nonproliferative membranous cases. In experimental models of glomerulonephritis, on the other hand, the extra-membranous localization of complexes is the rule. From these data two conclusions can be drawn: We do not have suitable experimental models for most of the quantitatively prevailing proliferative forms of glomerulonephritis. The minority of human, immune complex-related cases of perimembranous glomerulonephritis has some kind of experimental counterpart. It is, however, still uncertain to what extent the experimental model is comparable to idiopathic membranous glomerulonephritis in man (HEPTINSTALL, 1973 b). This relative exclusiveness of (peri-) membranous glomerulonephritis also seems to be expressed by the immunohistologic pattern which is the most typical of all (BARIÉTY et al., 1970). However, it also seems to involve the least variability.

As shown in Fig. 6A the granular deposition contrasts clearly with the other extreme type of pathogenesis, the linear type of immunofluorescence. It is not difficult to imagine that these granules can simulate a "broad-linear" type (MOREL-MAROGER et al., 1972) if they are close enough together or if a sandwich-type effect of complement over immunoglobulin obscures the single deposits. It is not always easy to decide whether or not the deposits are situated outside the membrane. Instead, another feature—a "carpet-like" arrangement of the fluorescent granules (Fig. 6B)—is typical for a peri-membranous nephritis. It is likely that this pattern is caused by tangential sectioning of the membranes. Since both types are not always found together, it could well be that one or the other reflects a more intramembranous allocation of complexes. The granular deposits commonly stain with anti-IgG and anti-C3 as well. IgM is seen occasionally; IgA is rare as is fibrinogen.

Very similar patterns can be seen in Figs. 7A and B which demonstrate the glomeruli of tubulus antigen-autoimmunized rats. This model experiment of so-called Heymann nephritis (HEYMANN et al., 1959; EDGINGTON et al., 1968; ALOUSI et al., 1969) supports the hypothesis of the immune-complex pathogenesis of (peri-) membranous glomerulonephritis. There are indications that at least in rats this form of glomerulonephritis remains essentially un-changed even when the nephritic kidney is transplanted into a healthy non-immunized syngeneic recipient (Fig. 7A, B) (STENGLEIN and THOENES, un-published). This may shed some light on the problem of permanent curability of (peri-) membranous glomerulonephritis (FRANKLIN et al., 1973; OLBING et al., 1973) and seems to indicate that the continual nephritic process is not necessarily dependent on further extrarenal stimulation. It is not known whether or not autoimmune processes are involved in human perimembranous glomerulonephritis, which is discussed in the last section. Based on the ex-perimental models, it will be interesting to learn if differences in immuno-histologic features can be detected for autoimmune nephritis on the one hand and heterologous antigen-induced perimembranous glomerulonephritis on the other.

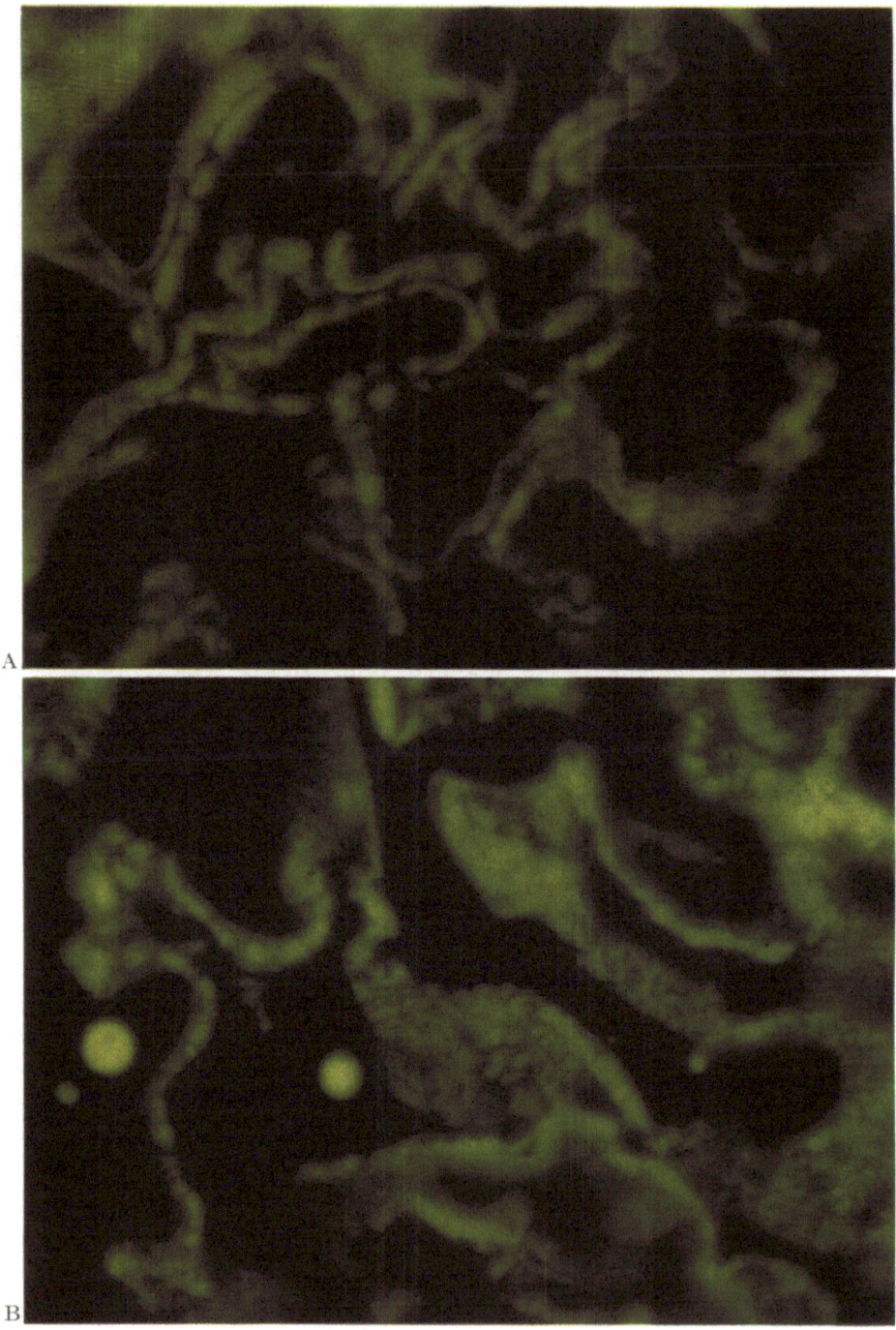

Fig. 6. *A* The granular pattern seen in (peri-) membranous glomerulonephritis. IgG, ×1320. *B* The "carpet-like" representation of immune complexes in tangential sections is especially characteristic. IgG, ×1320

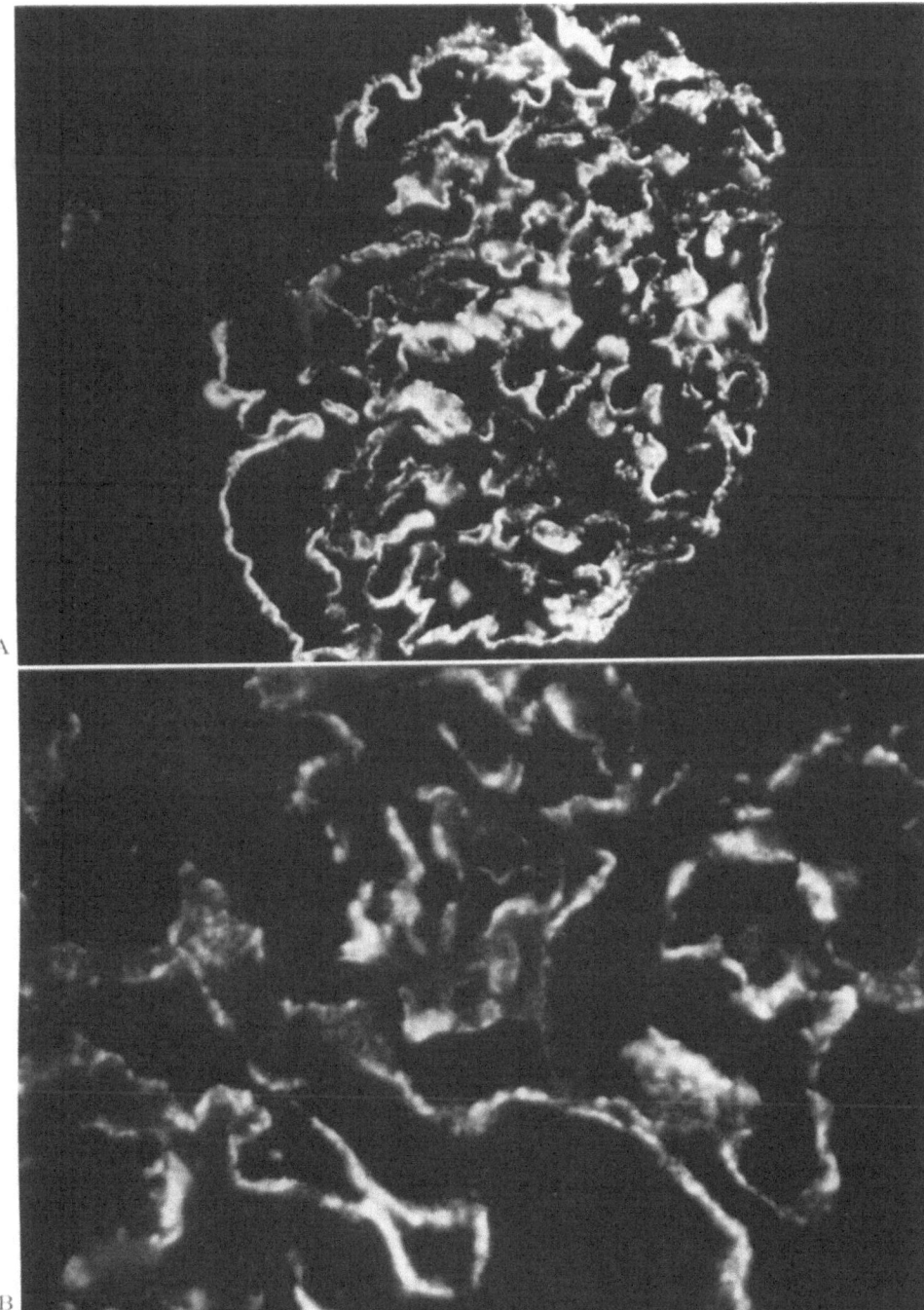

Fig. 7. *A* The immunofluorescence of experimental autoimmune glomerulonephritis with kidney tubular antigens in rats is shown for comparison. The pattern closely resembles that of human perimembranous glomerulonephritis. Here the continuance of the disease is demonstrated in a primary diseased kidney transplanted from the sensitized donor to a healthy recipient; 15 days post transplantation. Rat-IgG, ×582. *B* A larger magnification of the same glomerulus shows certain dissimilarities when compared with Figs. 6*A* and *B* from human cases. IgG, ×1430. (Both pictures from Dr. B. STENGLEIN, Munich)

6. Focal Segmental Sclerosing Glomerulonephritis (Glomerulopathy)
(Focal Sclerosis, Focal and Segmental Hyalinosis,
Global and Focal Fibrosis)

"More minute analysis of histological appearances will undoubtedly reveal significant differences between patients hitherto considered the same" (CAMERON, 1973). This statement has proved to be very true, especially in the case of the so-called lipoid nephrosis. The clinical syndrome of lipoid nephrosis has been found very often to have only minimal or no histologic correlates. The detection of focally distributed sclerotic lesions in mainly juxtamedullary glomeruli led to the definition of the new variant being causative for corticosteroid-resistant lipoid nephrosis (McGOVERN, 1964). Immunohistology has contributed to the "minute analysis" of the focal and segmental process in otherwise minimally changed glomeruli by being a sensitive diagnostic tool, described by McCLUSKEY (1971) as "a sort of special stain". By this, it is also meant that not everything shown up by immunofluorescence would indicate an *in vivo* immunologic reaction. Thus, in focal sclerosis, the distinct pattern of Fig. 8A, stained with anti-IgM or anticomplement factors is seen, but the picture does not show the regular immune pattern of granulation (Fig. 8B). However, the patchy appearance of the glomerular loops does not mean that less distinct deposits are not involved.

As shown by electron-microscopic examination, different kinds of deposits in different locations can be delineated in focal segmental sclerosing glomerulopathy including some minimally changed glomeruli (RUMPELT and W. THOENES, 1974). These authors also indicate that the glomeruli are diffusely altered when examined by electron microscopy. Accordingly, the immunhistologic pattern varies from minimal staining of loops (Plate VI *A*, *B*) and mesangial areas (Plate VI *H*) to complete segmental or global (comprehensive) changes (Plate VI *C–F*). Undoubtedly the major immunofluorescent findings are correlated to the sclerotic lesions of the glomeruli (HABIB and GUBLER, 1971). In contrast to these authors, however, we have observed either, slight but comprehensive (Plate VI *G*) or incipient (Plate VI *H*) immunofluorescent findings in otherwise minimally changed glomeruli (G. H. THOENES, 1974).

Irrespective of the later interpretation it seems justified to record minor immunofluorescent findings as well. In this regard one is reminded that, as early as 1955, ALLEN stated that "glomerular lesions may be disregarded by experienced observers often because they underrate the significance of intermediate degrees of change". According to HABIB and GUBLER (1973) and CHURG et al. (1970), in several cases a mesangial proliferation can be observed before the typical segmental sclerosis appears. Minor immunofluorescent findings, as seen in Plate VI *H*, should therefore be noted in this context of an unknown pathogenesis. Whereas DRUMMOND et al. (1966) described such cases of focal sclerosis staining with IgG and C3, it is generally accepted today (MOREL-MAROGER et al., 1972) that IgM is the major immunoglobulin involved. There is no definite evidence that this immunoglobulin, mostly associated

Table 4. Positive immunofluorescent cases of focal sclerosis and minimal-change disease

Focal sclerosis	Questionable minimal changes possibly focal sclerosis	Minimal changes
Strongly positive/total number of cases	Positive/total number of cases	Minimal positive/total number of cases
32/37	5/6	32/67

with complement factors, of course, indicates an immunologic pathogenesis. It may be cited, however, that GERMUTH and RODRIGUEZ (1973) experimentally induced segmental lesions with large IgM-immune complexes. The stronger lytic response of IgM antibodies could very well be responsible for an unusual nephrotoxic effect. MICHAEL et al. (1973) recently discussed the immunologic aspects of the nephrotic syndrome in general. Reports (HAMBURGER et al., 1973; HOYER et al., 1972) of recurrence of minimal-change nephrotic syndrome and focal sclerosis in kidney transplants are intriguing. It is likely that an extrarenal cause will be found for this disease entity and it might well be that even different pathogenic pathways will be detected, as suggested by the smooth linear fluorescence seen by the author (G. H. THOENES, 1974) in a few cases of focal segmental sclerosis and corroborated by the streak-like deposits reported by RUMPELT and W. THOENES (1974).

As HABIB and GUBLER (1973) discussed, the relationship between minimal-change nephrotic syndrome and focal sclerosis remains unsolved and it is the common view today to regard both forms as possibly separate diseases. This view, however, was recently strongly opposed by SIEGEL (1974). McGOVERN and LANER (1973) stated: "So far, it has not been possible to determine whether the two disorders are related or not." Doubtless most cases of corticosteroid-responsive nephrotic syndrome (minimal-change disease) are truly negative immunohistologically. On the other hand, most segmentally sclerosed glomeruli in focal sclerosis are massively positive by immunohistology (Table 4). What about the minimally changed glomeruli in focal sclerosis? Are *all* cases of minimal-change disease truly negative? It is our experience that in carefully studying the sections (preferably by vertical incident illumination fluorescence) minor fluorescent spots, dust-like or comma-like materials, or a weak linear staining in both sorts of minimally changed glomeruli are found (Table 4). These findings are usually faint and difficult to document by photography. WILSON and DIXON (1974) noted this "linear accentuation" of the basement membrane in quite a number of their biopsies but could not interpret it. The reader should be reminded that we do not fix our sections by acetone to avoid disturbing background phenomena and reduce unspecific protein remains. It should also be clearly understood that these observations do *not* necessarily imply an *immune* pathogenetic signi-

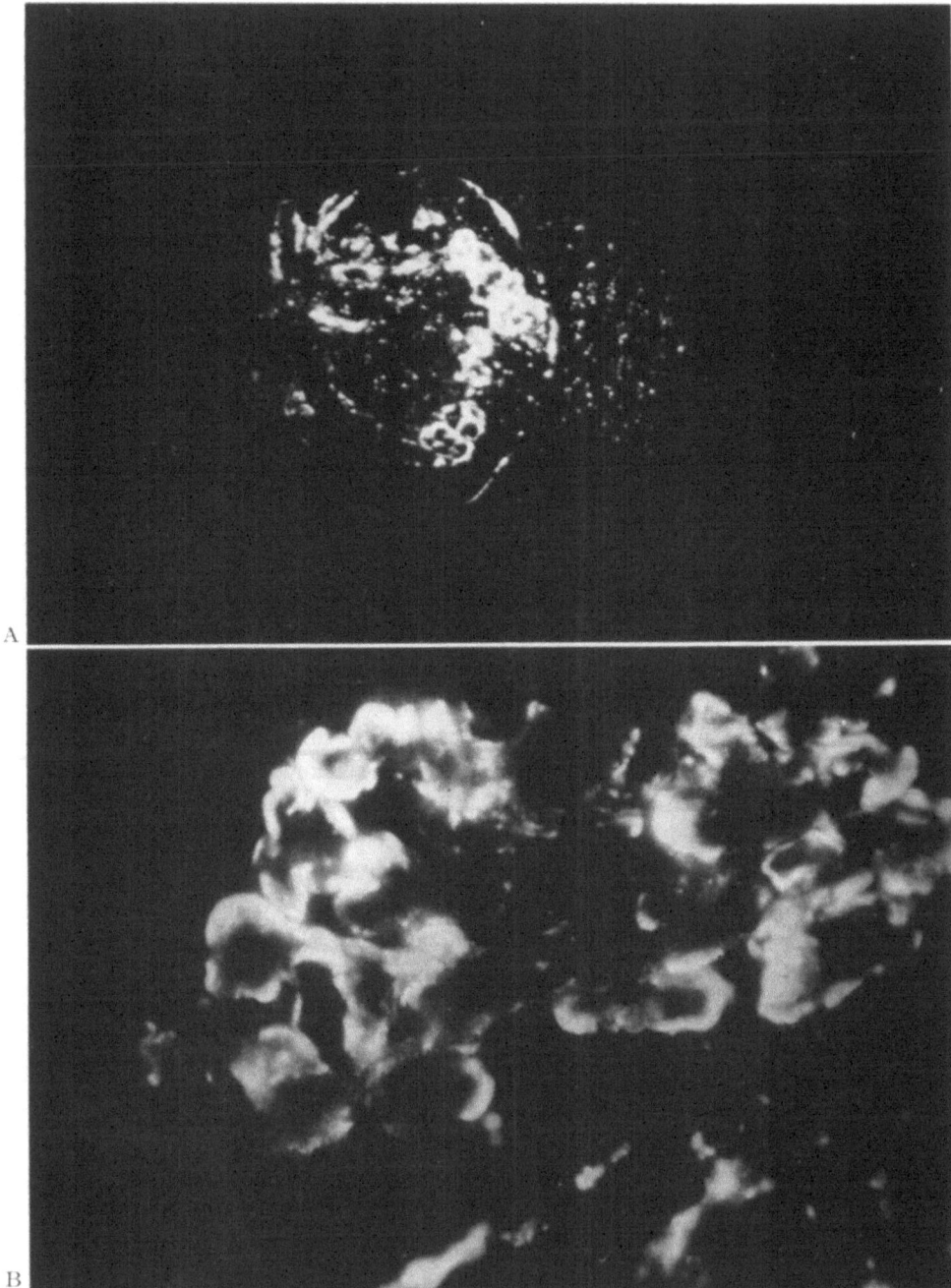

Fig. 8. *A* The distinctive pattern of focal-segmental sclerosis. C_3, ×143. *B* A large magnification of such segmental lesions does not show details which would resemble the usual immune patterns. As long as we do not have relevant experimental models we cannot guess whether or not an immune pathogenesis is involved. C_3, ×1430

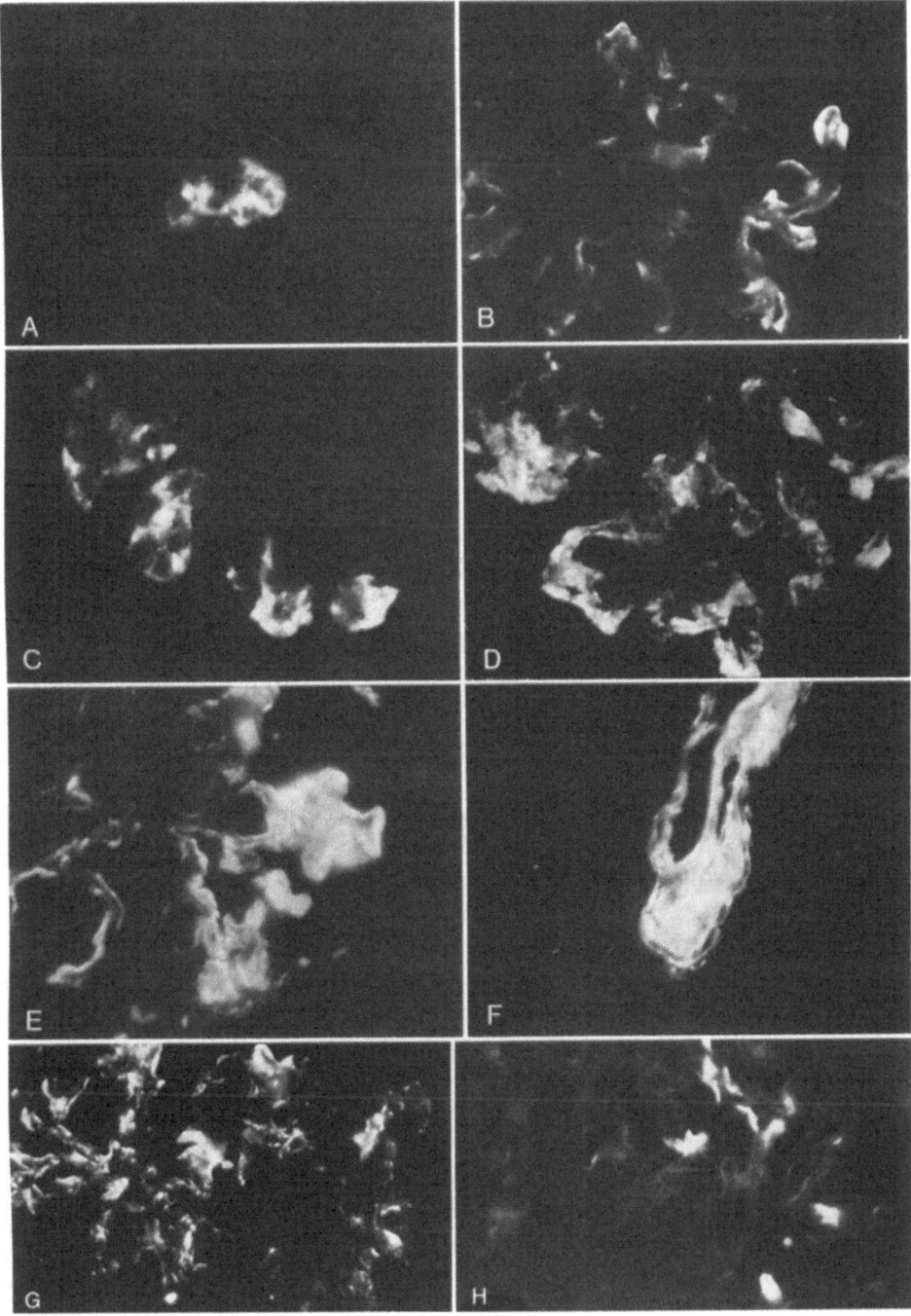

Plate VI. The variable patterns of focal-segmental sclerosis. *A* and *B* Incipient segmental lesions. *C–E* Full expression of the segmental lesions. *F* Positive vessel walls (complement) are not infrequently seen. Comprehensive (*G*) or minor (*H*) fluorescent stainings can also be observed in minimally changed glomeruli or parts of them. *A* IgM, ×300. *B* IgG, ×300. *C* IgM, ×300. *D* IgM, ×300. *E* C_3, ×300. *F* C_3, ×300. *G* IgG, ×300. *H* IgG, ×736

ficance. However, this could be an example to justify the increased application of immunofluorescence in biopsy examination. It can only serve as a "special stain" with high sensitivity in addition to its specific immunologic function. Finally, the "immunofluorescent minimal change" certainly does not indicate *at the present time* an inclination for progress to focal sclerosis. We observed some preference for IgM or C3 staining, but all other reagents could also be involved. We did not test for IgE. It must, however, be noted that the positive report of GERBER and PARONETTO (1971) could not be confirmed by ROY *et al.* (1973a) and LEWIS *et al.* (1973).

IV. Glomerular Lesions in Systemic Diseases

1. Systemic Lupus Erythematosus (SLE)

As early as 1957, VASQUEZ and DIXON investigated the "specific" lesions of such systemic diseases as rheumatic fever and SLE by immunofluorescence. Immunopathogenesis of SLE nephritis is well established (MELLORS *et al.*, 1957; PARONETTO and KOFFLER, 1965; KOFFLER and PARONETTO, 1965; KOFFLER *et al.*, 1967; SVEC *et al.*, 1967; KRISHNAN and KAPLAN, 1967; KOFFLER *et al.*, 1969; NATALI and TAN, 1972) and a wealth of references can be cited for the different forms of immunofluorescent appearance in SLE nephritis (BURKHOLDER, 1963; SVEC *et al.*, 1967; KOFFLER *et al.*, 1969; DUJOVNE *et al.*, 1972; AGNELLO *et al.*, 1973; MOREL-MAROGER *et al.*, 1973a). Histologically as well as by immunofluorescence, all kinds of glomerular alterations can be seen in SLE nephritis which cover almost the entire spectrum of patterns described in the foregoing sections. Since it has been possible to prove the immune-complex pathogenesis experimentally with DNA-anti-DNA antibodies (NATALI and TAN, 1972), the variability of the immunohistologic appearance in SLE seems to reconfirm the general hypothesis of the immune-complex pathogenesis of glomerular diseases (GERMUTH and RODRIGUEZ, 1973). These authors suggest that different sizes of complexes will localize in different places of the glomerulus and thereby initiate several patterns and histologic changes. Plate VII presents collectively the spectrum of immunohistologic patterns which can be observed in lupus nephritis. It ranges from faint mesangial stainings (VII *A* and *B*) and an acute proliferative type (VII *C*) to different forms of membranous involvement (VII *D–F*), lobular types (VII *G*) with obvious accumulations of complex structures in mesangial cells (VII *H*), perimembranous glomerulonephritis (VII *I, K*), and focal segmental alterations (VII *L, M*). The reader is referred to the histologic diagnosis given for each picture. At this time we can only speculate about the reasons for such diversity under the same etiologic principle. SLE should actually be considered as a suitable model in which different kinds of nuclear antigens, classes of antibodies, sizes of complexes, and effects of immunosuppressive therapy combine in varying degress and thus form the many patterns we might similarly see independent of lupus.

2. Contrasting Examples of Renal Involvement in Systemic Disease: Schönlein-Henoch Nephritis (Anaphylactoid Purpura)

This glomerulonephritis—another example of renal involvement in systemic disease—may have an immunologic basis, although nothing is known about the mechanism. URIZAR et al. (1968) thought that the pathogenetic process was mainly concentrated on the mesangium. This is clearly demonstrated on Plate VIII A, B. Most of our cases show this type of immunofluorescent pattern without defined circumscript immune complexes. It is a mesangial type which is frequently IgA-positive. Additionally, one finds fibrinogen deposited in segmental (C) or crescentic forms (D) (URIZAR and HERDMAN, 1970). Sometimes there is an interrupted linear pattern; HABIB (1973 c) mentioned two cases of membranoproliferative GN in her series. We can also contribute one case of Schönlein-Henoch nephritis with this histologic diagnosis and a low serum complement. In general however Schönlein-Henoch nephritis does not appear to be an immune-complex mediated process.

Amyloidosis

Because not infrequently a kidney biopsy turns up the unexpected diagnosis of amyloidosis instead of glomerulonephritis, the author presents its diagnostic immunohistologic pattern. Plate IX A and C show that immunofluorescence with anti-IgG or anti-C3 is very homogeneous and large. A more reticular but still homogeneous pattern is seen on Plate IX B and a typical amyloid vessel wall is depicted in D. As early as 1956, VASQUEZ and DIXON introduced the immunohistologic analysis of amyloid. To date there has been no convincing argument available for or against the immunopathogenesis of amyloid (cf. FRANKLIN and ZUCKER-FRANKLIN, 1972). The technique of immunohistology, however, can help once again to endorse the histologic diagnosis—even in cases where no clear-cut amyloid staining occurs.

V. Concluding Remarks

This paper intends to show that the distinctive marks of immunohistology permit an independent diagnostic application. The most definite patterns are schematically depicted in Fig. 10. However, the variables demonstrated in the preceding sections indicate quite readily that this diagnostic independence is only relative. In order to arrive at reliable conclusions, the evaluation of the biopsy has to rely on the fundamentals of histologic description. The author believes that most clinicians and pathologists have learned to value the access to information available through additional immunohistologic examination of their biopsies (SCHREINER, 1973). There is reason enough to interpret most findings as immunologic in nature. It should, however, be understood that positive immunofluorescence does not necessarily prove an immunologic pathogenesis. HAMBURGER (1973) has discussed this and other related problems.

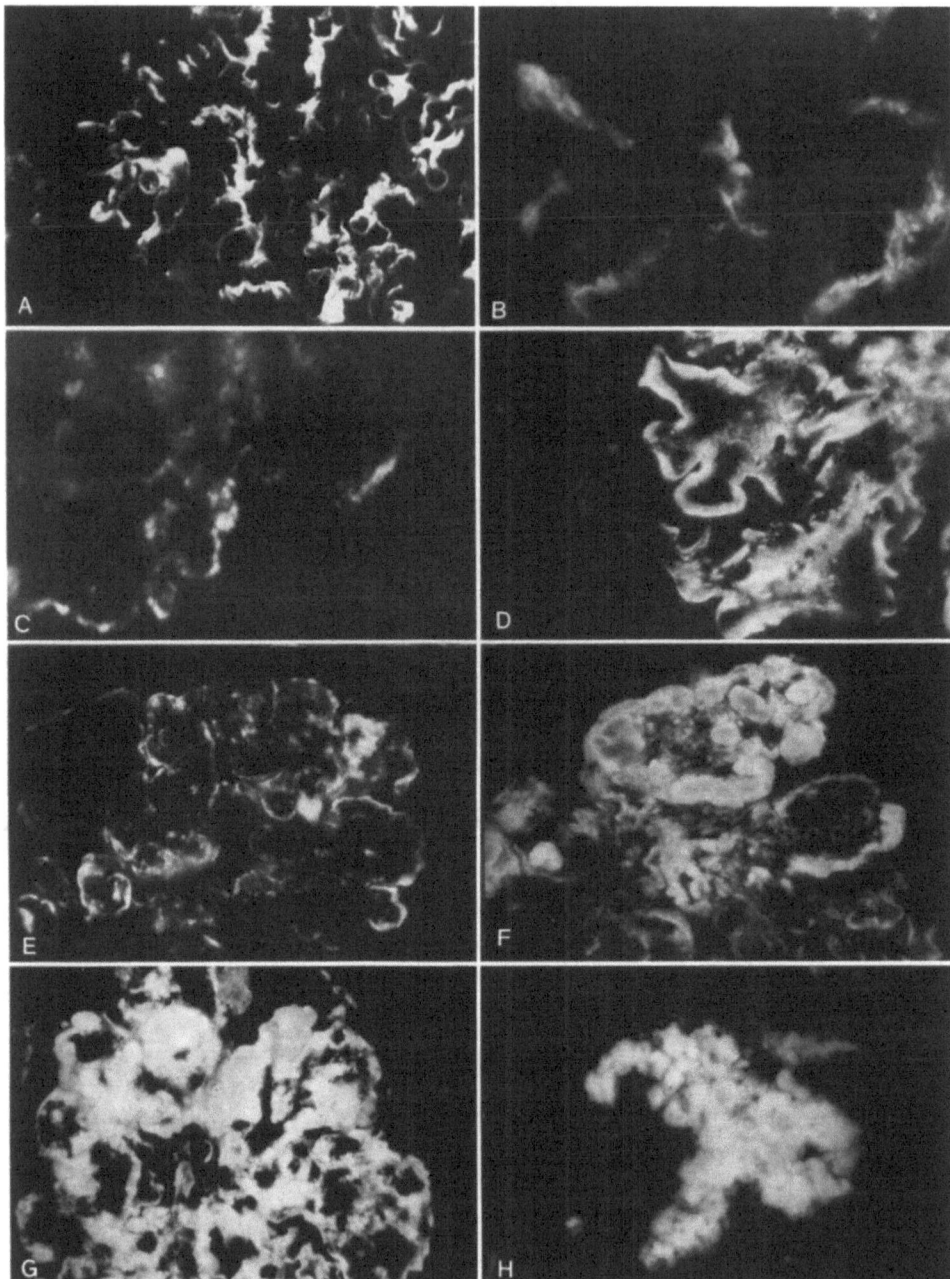

Plate VII A — H

Several questions may be raised from the view of immunohistology. In proving or disproving the notion of immunologic pathogenesis and/or etiology we should find means to routinely characterize the *antigens* involved. The basic task of immunofluorescence is to achieve this goal. However, it is

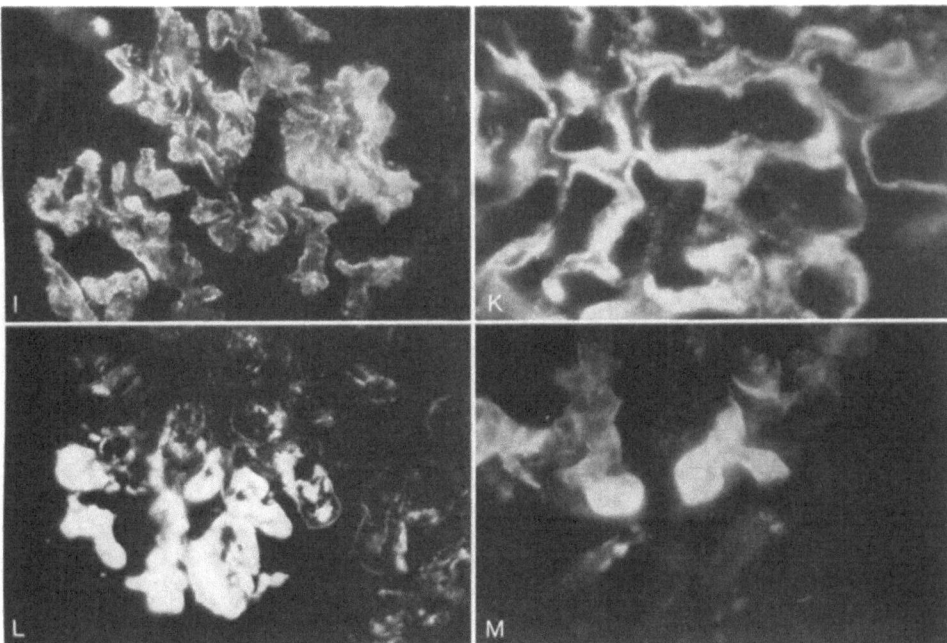

Plate VII. The highly variable immunofluorescent patterns seen in systemic disease with renal involvement: *Systemic lupus erythematosus*. Slight mesangial stainings (*A, B*), granular patterns as seen in acute glomerulonephritis (*C*), endomembranous depositions (*D*), features as typical for membrano-proliferative forms (*E*), with huge homogenous bodies (*F*), intensive mesangial participation (*G*) and clearly visible granulations in mesangial cells (*H*) are seen. Occasionally perimembranous patterns (*I, K*) occur and segmental findings (*L, M*) correlate to the known histological classification. *A* IgG, ×300. *B* IgG, ×736. *C* IgG, ×300. *D* IgM, ×300. *E* IgG, ×300. *F* IgG, ×300. *G* C$_3$, ×300. *H* IgG, ×736. *I* IgG, ×300. *K* IgG, ×736. *L* IgG, ×300. *M* IgG, ×300. *Histological diagnosis: A, B* Slight postacute, proliferative, glomerulonephritis (GN). *C* Specifically lobular, more recent glomerulonephritis. *D* Mesangial-proliferative GN. *E, F* Membrano-proliferative GN with crescent formations. *G, H* Focal-segmental proliferative GN. *I* Perimembranous GN. *K* Diffuse, focal-segmental, accented, proliferative GN with slight membranous components. *L* Intra-extra capillary, proliferative GN. *M* Moderate meangioproliferative GN

difficult because of the many possible agents. In individual cases, the antigens have been characterized by immunofluorescence. Such cases occur only individually but are nevertheless of great scientific importance. Most efforts have centered on streptococcal antigens. Using heterologous antibodies, SEEGAL et al. (1965) and ZABRISKIE et al. (1973) have been successful in demonstrating streptococcal antigen in cases of acute poststreptococcal glomerulonephritis. The appropriate use of homologous (patient's) fluoresceinated immunoglobulin (TRESER et al., 1969; TRESER et al., 1970) has also been convincing. We have also been successful with the same method (Fig. 9A). It can be seen, however, that the antigen and the other components of the presumed immune reaction (Fig. 9B) are not associated. This may be regarded as a typical example of the many unsolved problems in the pathogenesis of glomerulonephritis. There

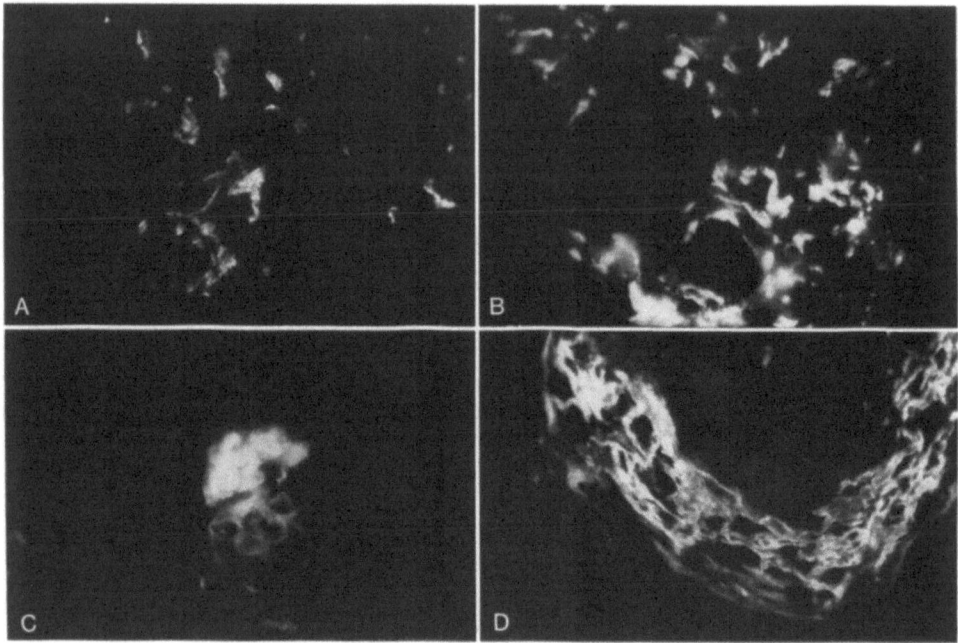

Plate VIII. The immunofluorescent findings in the kidney in Schönlein–Henoch's disease. *A* and *B* IgA deposits in mesangial areas, × 300. *C* and *D* Fibrinogen is positive in a glomerular loop and in capsular areas. × 300

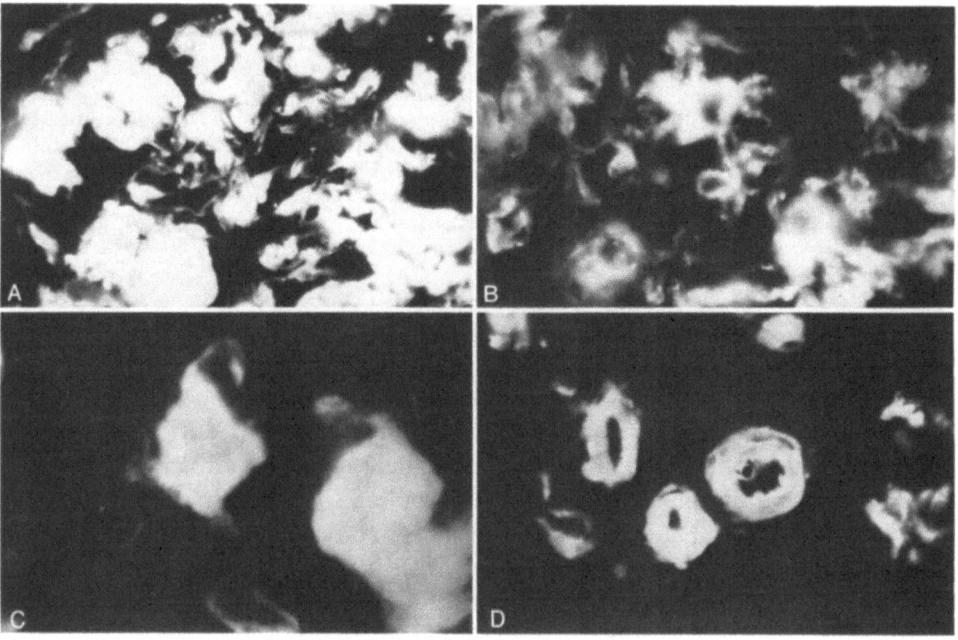

Plate IX. The immunofluorescent findings in kidney amyloidosis. Large and very homogeneous clumps of IgG/C_3-positive protein are deposited (*A, C*); sometimes the pattern is reticular, but still homogeneous (*B*) and vessel walls are found positive in the same manner. *A* C_3, × 300. *B* IgG, × 300. *C* C_3, × 736. *D* IgG, × 300

has been speculation that treponemal antigens could also be involved in immune-complex nephritis (BRAUNSTEIN et al., 1970).

Another well-investigated antigen is DNA in lupus nephritis. Its proven deposition in glomeruli has been connected with the viral etiology of LE and was discussed by COCHRANE and KOFFLER (1973). Specific indications have been reported in man for a deposition of Coxsackie virus B (BURCH et al., 1969) and measles antigen (TANNENBAUM et al., 1971). However, the hepatitis antigen has been more frequently described up to now (COMBES et al., 1971; GOCKE et al., 1970; EKNOYAN, 1972). Plasmodium has been of interest as a further living agent since ALLISON et al. (1969) investigated the close association between malaria and the nephrotic syndrome. Using the kidney elution procedure they indicated that malaria antigen forms the complex (see also BROWN, 1969). In addition to the many examples of heterologous antigens, one has to take into account the autoimmune pathogenesis of human glomerulonephritis. In the case of Goodpasture's syndrome, the antigen is not questionable (MARQUARDT et al., 1973) as is the mechanism of sensitization against glomerular basement membrane. The involvement of tubular basement membranes in kidney diseases is surprizingly rare, although several reports on possible immunologic tubular lesions have appeared recently (KLASSEN et al., 1972; McCLUSKEY and KLASSEN, 1973; MOREL-MAROGER et al., 1974). Turning again to immune complex-induced glomerular disease, it would seem likely to find tubular epithelial antigen deposited in man as well as in rats, as was described by EDGINGTON et al. (1968). A short positive report (NARUSE et al., 1973) awaits confirmation by others. Further autologous substances potentially leading to autoimmune reactions and/or glomerular deposition are thyroglobulin, tumor antigens (LEWIS et al., 1971), and cryoglobulins (FEIZI and GITLIN, 1969; MOREL-MAROGER and MERY, 1974; MOREL-MAROGER and VERROUST, 1974).

The author has only touched upon the problem of transplantation immunohistology in connection with recurrent glomerulonephritis. Indeed, in his opinion, the main interest of immunohistology is in this scientifically exciting area. The author's experience with about 70 transplant biopsies has been that the diagnostic value of immunohistology in relation to rejection processes is very limited. In addition to C3, IgM is involved not only in vascular lesions but also occasionally in glomeruli. This agrees with the results of MULLEN and HILDEMANN (1971) who showed the preferred cytotoxic effect of IgM compared with IgG. However, one should be aware of the so-called transplant-glomerulopathy (ZOLLINGER et al., 1973; PIELSTICKER et al., 1974) which must be differentiated from recurrent glomerulonephritis (McPHAUL et al., 1970; McPHAUL et al., 1973). Other reports in which a more positive view is expressed concerning immunohistology and transplant rejection may be found in ANDRES et al., 1970, and BUSCH et al., 1971.

The prevailing vascular processes in chronic transplant rejection, which could very well involve the glomeruli in a secondary manner, leads to the problem of secondary and "nonspecific" alterations of glomeruli and their

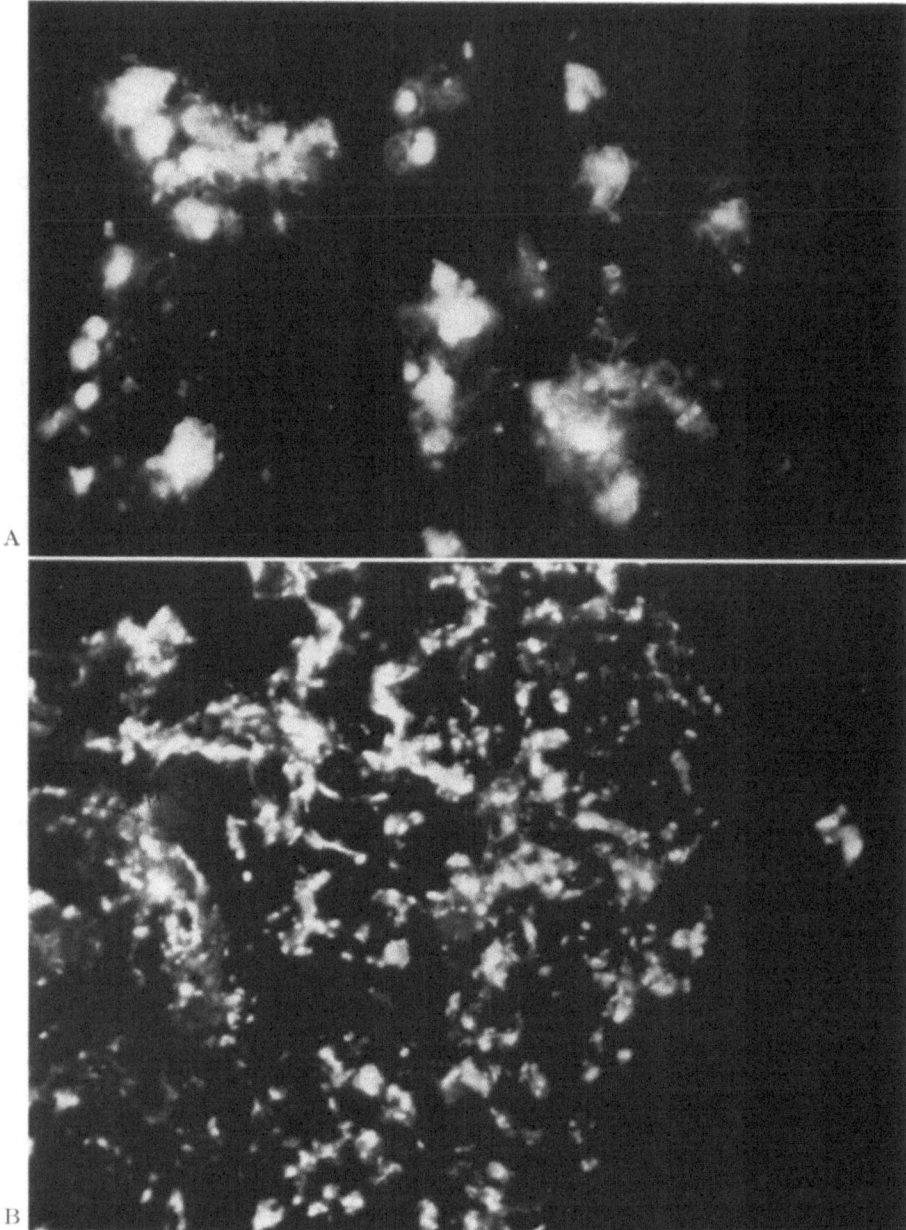

Fig. 9. Acute, poststreptococcal glomerulonephritis. *A* Glomerulus, stained with patient's IgG fraction (elevated AST); direct immunofluorescence. The spots represent streptococcal materials deposited. × 582. *B* With anti-C₃, the characteristic pattern of the acute-proliferative type is shown in the same glomerulus. × 582

Fig. 10. The distinctive marks of the foregoing major forms of human glomerulonephritis are schematically drawn in order to summarize and to abstract from the variability. (From G. H. Thoenes, 1973)

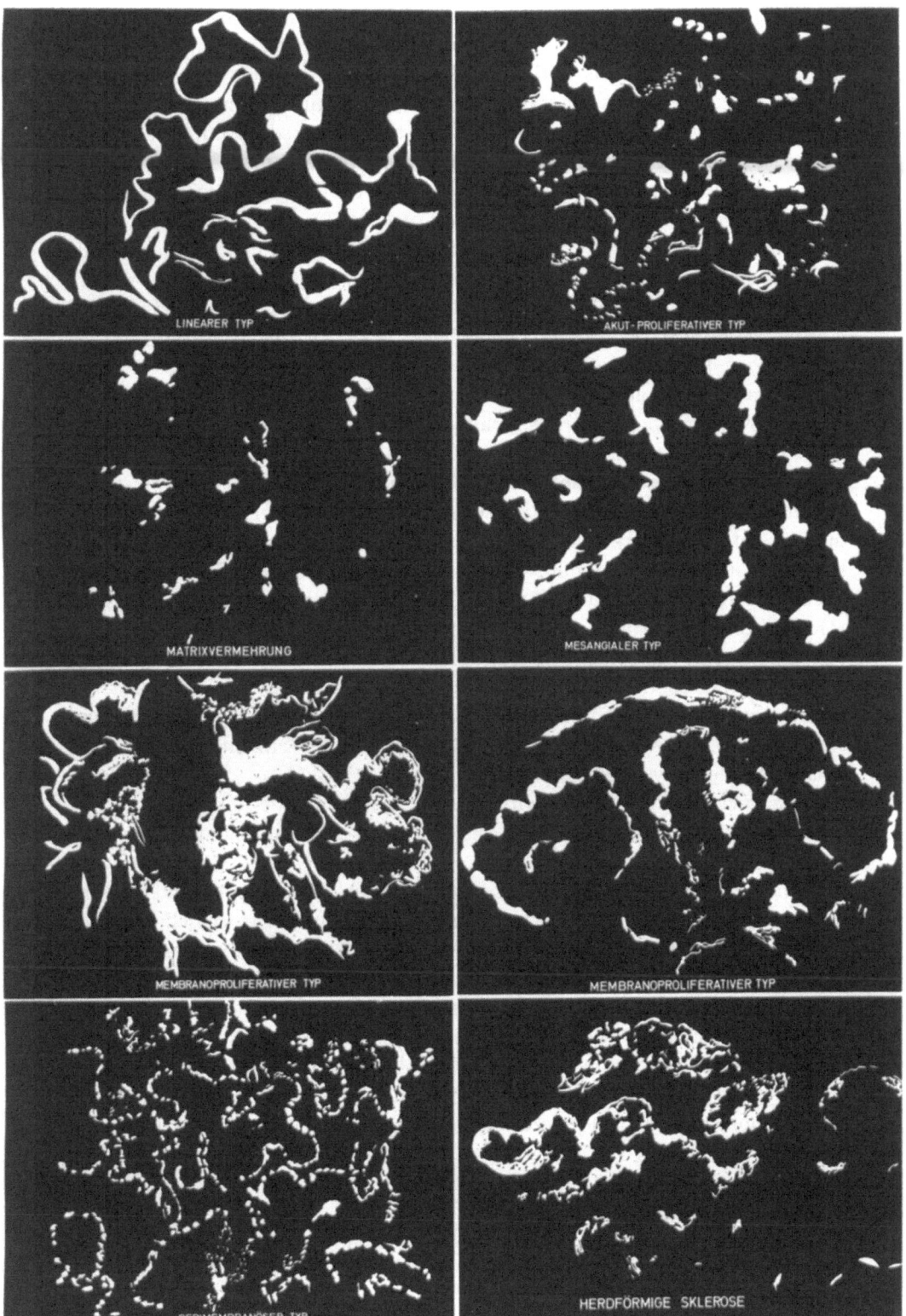

Fig. 10

immunohistologic correlates. Only minor glomerular immunofluorescent findings are normally observed in vascular diseases like periarteriitis nodosa or
malignant nephrosclerosis, although fibrinogen can be seen quite intensively
(Sraer et al., 1973). As long as we do not see distinct granular deposits we
suspect an unspecific protein imhibition of tissue altered by unrelated causes.
This seems to us to be the case with the very prominent vessels in primary
malignant sclerosis. Their walls are not only full of fibrinogen but often contain
IgM and complement as well (Burkholder, 1965). In periarteriitis nodosa
they are usually negative. This certainly does not exclude other cellular
immunologic processes.

Three further examples may be cited to illustrate why *we must maintain
a reserved attitude in judging immunologic specificity or nonspecificity.* The
faint linear fluorescence in diabetic glomerulosclerosis does not seem to
indicate an immunologic cause (Gallo, 1970), although Mauer et al. (1972)
could show somewhat different results in diabetic rats. The cause of diabetic
glomerulosclerosis, however is unknown. The so-called hereditary nephritis
(Alport's syndrome) does not seem to present any relevant immunohistologic
findings (Grünfeld et al., 1973). Undoubtedly, however characteristic glomerular alterations are found in this disease, reason enough to expect some
kind of unspecific immunofluorescence, which is not the case. The relationships
between renal-vein thrombosis and perimembranous glomerulonephritis and
the nephrotic syndrome, respectively, is unknown (Schwartz and Lewis,
1973). The great importance of extrarenal factors such as free blood and urine
flow, as is the case in this type of glomerulonephritis, has been demonstrated
in the experiments by Edgington et al. (1969). The accumulation of immune
complexes in transplanted kidneys of autoimmune recipient rats was significantly reduced by hydronephrosis.

This review will conclude with these examples in the hope that we have
contributed to the goal of keeping an open mind in glomerulonephritis
research.

When the *immunohistologist* sees a single granular deposit such as that
shown in Fig. 1, he is justified in giving this information to the clinician and
the pathologist. The *clinician* might accept this little spot as at least *one* small
confirmation of the *patient's clinical kidney findings*, but all those involved get
into trouble when the *pathologist* does not see anything by *light microscopy*.
However, it sometimes happens that the cooperative *pathologist* later reports
a single typical deposit in the only available glomerulus—by having applied
electron microscopy. The sensitivity of immunofluorescence and the significance
of immunohistological findings therefore should not be underestimated.

Acknowledgements

The author is indebted to the many clinicians whose collaboration was
the source of all our experience in kidney immunohistology. The personal
scientific contributions of those cited below seems to me admirable in view

of the predilection to balance scientific enthusiasm with care for the individual patient. I would personally like to thank Professors and Drs.:

EDEL, DOBBELSTEIN, and ALTMEYER, I. Medizinische Univ.-Klinik München
EIGLER, HELD, and BUCHBORN, II. Medizinische Univ.-Klinik München
DIEKER, Kreiskrankenhaus, Siegen
HÜBNER, Kinderklinik der Technischen Universität München
JOPPICH, Universitätskinderklinik, München
KLAUS, KLUMPP, Medizinische Univ.-Poliklinik Marburg
KRAMAR, Krankenhaus Linz/Austria
KUHLMANN, 6. Medizinische Abteilung des Städtischen Krankenhauses München-Schwabing
LANGE, Medizinische Univ.-Klinik Marburg
RENNER, REINHARDT and co-workers, Medizinische Klinik I, Köln-Merheim
SCHULZ, GESSLER and co-workers, 4. Medizinische Klinik Nürnberg
SIEBERTH, FREIBERG and co-workers, Medizinische Univ.-Klinik, Köln-Lindenthal

I would like to thank the pathologists Prof. A. BOHLE (Tübingen), Prof. W. THOENES (Marburg/Mainz), and Dr. K. PIELSTICKER (München) for their support and encouragement, Miss I. DOERING and Mrs. G. URBAN helped with enthusiasm and great technical ability. My colleague Dr. B. STENGLEIN assisted in evaluating the biopsies. Miss R. HAUSER and Miss A. KNÖDL kindly provided secretarial assistance.

References

ADAM, C., MOREL-MAROGER, L., RICHET, G.: Cryoglobulins in glomerulonephritis not related to systemic disease. Kidney Internat. **3**, 334–341 (1973)

AGNELLO, V., KOFFLER, D., KUNKEL, H. G.: Immune complex systems in the nephritis of systemic lupus erythematosus. Kidney Internat. **3**, 90–99 (1973)

ALLEN, A. C.: The clinicopathologic meaning of the nephrotic syndrome. Amer. J. Med. **18**, 277–314 (1955)

ALLISON, A. C., HOUBA, V., HENDRICKSE, R. G., DE PETRIS, S., EDGINGTON, G. M., ADENIHI, A.: Immune complexes in the nephrotic syndrome of African children. Lancet **1969I**, 1232

ALOUSI, M. A., POST, R. S., HEYMANN, W.: Experimental autoimmune nephrosis in rats. Amer. J. Path. **54**, 47–71 (1969)

ANDRES, G. A., ACCINI, L., HSU, K. C., PENN, I., PORTER, K. A., RENDALL, J. M., SEEGAL, B. C., STARZL, T. E.: Human renal transplants: III. Immunopathologic studies. Lab. Invest. **22**, 588–604 (1970)

ANTOINE, B., NEVEU, I., BERGER, J.: Applications de l'immunofluorescence en néphrology: I. Quelques problèmes de méthodologie. In: Actualités nephrologiques de l'Hôpital Necker II. p. 135. Paris: Flammarion 1967

ARAKAWA, M., KIMMELSTIEL, P.: Circumferential mesangial interposition. Lab. Invest. **21**, 276–284 (1969)

BALDWIN, D. S.: Discussion. In: Glomerulonephritis, p. 411. New York: Wiley 1973

BARIÉTY, J., DRUET, P.: Résultats de l'immunohistochimie de 589 biopsies rénales (transplantés exclus). Ann. Med. Intern. **122**, 63 (1971)

BARIÉTY, PH., DRUET, G., LAGRUE, P., SAMARCQ, P., MILLIEZ, P.: Les glomérulonéphrites "extramembraneuses". Etudè morphologique en microscopie optique electronique, et immunofluorescence. Path. Biol. **18**, 5–32 (1970)

BERGER, J.: IgA glomerular deposits in renal disease. Transplantation Proc. **1**, 939 (1969)

BERGER, J., NEVEU, T., MOREL-MAROGER, L., ANTOINE, B.: Applications de l'immuno-fluorescence en néphrologie. II. Localisation des immunoglobulines et du fibrinogene dans les lesions glomerulaires. In: Actualités Néphrologiques de l'Hôpital Necker, p. 161. Paris: Flammarion 1967

BRAUNSTEIN, G. D., LEWIS, E. J., GALVANEK, E. G., HAMILTON, A., BELL, W. R.: The nephrotic syndrome associated with secondary syphilis. An immune deposit disease. Amer. J. Med, 48, 643–648 (1970)

BRENTJENS, J. R., O'CONNEL, D. W., PAWLOWSKI, I. B., HSU, K. C., ANDRES, G. A.: Experimental immune complex disease of the lung. J. Exp. Med. 140, 105–125 (1974)

BROWN, I. N.: Immunological aspects of malaria infection. In: Advances in Immunology. New York: Academic Press 11, 267–348 (1969)

BURCH, G. E., CHU, K. C., COLOLOUGH, H. L., SOHAL, R. S.: Immunofluorescent localization of coxsackievirus B antigen in the kidney observed at routine autopsy. Amer. J. Med. 47, 36–42 (1969)

BURKHOLDER, P. M.: Complement fixation in diseased tissues. II. Fixation of guinea pig complement in renal lesions of systemic lupus erythematosus. Amer. J. Path. 42, 201–215 (1963)

BURKHOLDER, P. M.: Malignant nephrosclerosis: An immunohistopathologic study on localized γ-globulin and fixation of guinea pig complement in human kidneys. Arch. Path. 80, 583–589 (1965)

BURKHOLDER, P. M., BRADFORD, W. D.: Proliferative glomerulonephritis in children. A correlation of varied clinical and pathologic patterns utilizing light, immuno-fluorescence and electron microscopy. Amer. J. Path. 56, 423–446 (1969)

BURKHOLDER, P. M., HYMAN, L. R., KRUEGER, R. P.: Characterization of mixed membranous and proliferative glomerulonephritis. In: Glomerulonephritis, 557–589. New York: Wiley 1973

BURKHOLDER, P. M., MARCHAND, A., KRUEGER, R. P.: Mixed membraneous and proliferative glomerulonephritis. A correlative light, immunofluorescence and electron microscopic study. Lab. Invest. 23, 459–479 (1970)

BUSCH, G. J., REYNOLDS, E. S., GALVANEK, E. G., BRAUN, W. E., DAMMIN, G. J.: Human renal allografts. Medicine 50, 29–63 (1971)

CAMERON, J. S.: A clinician's view of the classification of glomerulonephritis. In: Glomerulonephritis, p. 63–79. New York: Wiley 1973

CAMERON, J. S., GLASGOW, E. F., OGG, C. S., WHITE, R. H. R.: Membranoproliferative glomerulonephritis and persistent hypocomplementaemia. Brit. Med. J. 4, 7–14 (1970)

CAMERON, J. S., OGG, C. S.: Rapidly progressive glomerulonephritis with extensive crescents. In: Glomerulonephritis, p. 736. New York: J. Wiley 1973

CAMERON, J. S., OGG, C. S., TURNER, D. R., WELLER, R. O., WHITE, R. H. R., GLASGOW, E. F., PETERS, D. K., MARTIN, A.: Mesangiocapillary glomerulonephritis and persistent hypocomplementemia. In: Glomerulonephritis, p. 541–556. New York: Wiley 1973a

CAMERON, J. S., OGG, C. S., WHITE, R. H. R., GLASGOW, E. F.: The clinical features and prognosis of patients with normocomplementemic mesangiocapillary glomerulonephritis. Clinical Nephrology 1, 8–13 (1973b)

CHURG, J., DUFFY, J. L.: Classification of glomerulonephritis based on morphology. In: Glomerulonephritis, p. 43–61. New York: Wiley 1973

CHURG, J., HABIB, R., WHITE, R. H. R.: Pathology of the nephrotic syndrome in children. Lancet 1299–1302 (1970)

COCHRANE, C. G., KOFFLER, D.: Immune complex disease in experimental animals and man. In: Advances in Immunology. New York: Academic Press 16, 186–264 (1973)

COMBES, B., STASTNY, P., SHOREY, J., EIGENBRODT, E. H., BARBERA, A., HULL, A. R., CARTER, N. W.: Glomerulonephritis with deposition of Australia antigen-antibody-complexes in glomerular basement membrane. Lancet 1971 II, 234–237

COONS, A. H., CREECH, H. J., JONES, R. N.: Immunological properties of an antibody containing a fluorescent group. Proc. Soc. Exp. Biol. (N.Y.) 47, 200–210 (1941)

COONS, A. H., KAPLAN, M. H.: Localization of antigen in tissue cells. II. Improvements in a method for the detection of antigen by means of fluorescent antibody. J. Exp. Med. 91, 1–13 (1950)

DAVISON, A. M., THOMSON, D., MacDONALD, M. K., UTTLEY, W. S., ROBSON, J. S.: The role of the mesangial cell in proliferative glomerulonephritis. J. Clin. Path. 26, 198–208 (1973)

DIXON, F. J., FELDMANN, J. D., VASQUEZ, J. J.: Experimental glomerulonephritis. The pathogenesis of a laboratory model resembling the spectrum of human glomerulonephritis. J. Exp. Med. **113**, 899–919 (1961)

DRUMMOND, K. N., MICHAEL, A. F., GOOD, R. A., VERNIER, R. L.: The nephrotic syndrome in childhood; immunologic, clinical, pathologic correlations. J. Clin. Invest. **45**, 620–630 (1966)

DUJOVNE, J., POLLAK, V. E., PIRANI, C. L., DILLARD, M. G.: The distribution and character of glomerular deposits in systemic lupus erythematosus. Kidney Internat. **2**, 33–50 (1972)

DUNCAN, D. A., DRUMMOND, K. N., MICHAEL, A. F., VERNIER, R. L.: Pulmonary hemorrhage and glomerulonephritis. Report of six cases and study of the renal lesion by the fluorescent antibody technique and electron microscopy. Ann. Intern. Med. **62**, 920–938 (1965)

EDGINGTON, T. S., GLASSOCK, R. J., DIXON, F. J.: Autologous immune complex nephritis induced with renal tubulus antigen. I. Identification and isolation of the pathogenetic antigen. J. Exp. Med. **127**, 555–572 (1968)

EDGINGTON, T. S., LEE, S., DIXON, F. J.: Persistence of the autoimmune pathogenetic process in experimental autologous immune complex nephritis. J. Immunol. **103**, 528–536 (1969)

EKNOYAN, G., GYORKEY, C., DICHOSO, C., MARTINEZ-MALDONADO, M., SUKY, W. N., GYORKEY, P.: Renal morphological and immunological changes associated with acute viral hepatitis. Kidney Internat. **1**, 413–419 (1972)

EVANS, D. J., WILLIAMS, D. G., PETERO, D. K., SISSONS, J. G. P., BOULTON-JONES, J. M., OGG, C. S., CAMERON, J. S., HOFFBRAND, B. I.: Glomerular deposition of properdin in Henoch-Schönlein syndrome and idiopathic focal nephritis. Brit. Med. J. **3**, 326–328 (1973)

FEIZI, T., GITLIN, N.: Immune complex disease of the kidney associated with chronic hepatitis and cryoglobulinaemia. Lancet **1969II**, 873–876

FELDMANN, J. D., MARDENEY, M. R., SHULER, S. E.: Immunology and morphology of acute poststreptococcal glomerulonephritis. Lab. Invest. **15**, 283–301 (1966)

FISH, A. J., HERDMANN, R. C., MICHAEL, A. F., PICKERING, R. J., GOOD, R. A.: Epidemic acute glomerulonephritis associated with type 49 streptococcal pyoderma. II. Correlative study of light, immunofluorescent and electron microscopic findings. Amer. J. Med. **48**, 28–39 (1970)

FRANKLIN, W. A., JENNINGS, R. B., EARLE, D. P.: Membranous glomerulonephritis: Long term serial observations on clinical course and morphology. Kidney Internat. **4**, 36–56 (1973)

FRANKLIN, E. C., ZUCKER-FRANKLIN, D.: Current concepts of amyloid. In: Advances in Immunology. New York: Academic Press, **15**, 249–304 (1972)

FREEDMAN, P., MARKOWITZ, A. S.: γ-globulin and complement in the diseased kidney. J. Clin. Invest. **41**, 328–334 (1962)

FREEDMAN, P., PETERS, J. H., KARK, R. M.: Localization of γ-globulin in the diseased kidney. Arch. Int. Med. **105**, 524–535 (1960)

GALLE, P., HINGLAIS, N., CROSNIER, J.: Recurrence of an original glomerular lesion in three renal allografts. Transplant. Proc. **3**, 368–370 (1971)

GALLO, G. R.: Elution studies in kidneys with linear deposition of immunoglobulin in glomeruli. Amer. J. Path. **61**, 377–386 (1970)

GERBER, M. A., PARONETTO, F.: IgE in glomeruli of patient with nephrotic syndrome. Lancet **1971I**, 1097–1099

GERMUTH, F. G., RODRIGUEZ, E.: Immunopathology of the Renal Glomerulus. Boston: Little, Brown 1973

GLASGOW, E. F., WHITE, R. H. R.: Acute poststreptococcal glomerulonephritis with failure to resolve. In: Glomerulonephritis, p. 345–361. New York: Wiley 1973

GOCKE, D. J., HSU, K., MORGAN, C., BOMBARDIERI, S., LOCKSHIN, M., CHRISTIAN, C. L.: Association between polyarteriitis and Australia antigen. Lancet **1970II**, 1149–1153

GÖTZE, O., MÜLLER-EBERHARD, H. J.: The C_3-activator system: An alternate pathway of complement activation. J. Exp. Med. **134**, 90s–108s (1971)

GRÜNFELD, J. P., BOIS, E. P., HINGLAIS, N.: Progressive and non-progressive hereditary chronic nephritis. Kidney Internat. **4**, 216–228 (1973)

Grupe, W. E.: IgG-β_1C cryoglobulins in acute glomerulonephritis. Pediatrics **42**, 474–482 (1968)

Habib, R.: Discussion, p. 1133. In: Glomerulonephritis. New York: Wiley 1973a

Habib, R.: Classification of glomerulonephritis based on morphology. In: Glomerulonephritis, p. 17–41. New York: Wiley 1973b

Habib, R.: Discussion, p. 411. In: Glomerulonephritis. New York: Wiley 1973c

Habib, R., Gubler, M. C.: Lés lesions glomérulaires focales des Syndromes néphrotiques idiopathiques de l'enfant. Nephron **8**, 382–401 (1971)

Habib, R., Gubler, M. C.: Focal sclerosing glomerulonephritis. In: Glomerulonephritis, p. 263–278. New York: Wiley 1973

Hamburger, J.: Foreword. In: Glomerulonephritis, p. V–VII. New York: Wiley 1973

Hamburger, J., Berger, J., Hinglais, N., Descamps, B.: New insights into the pathogenesis of glomerulonephritis afforded by the study of renal allografts. Clinical Nephrology **1**, 3–7 (1973)

Heptinstall, R. H.: Discussion. In: Glomerulonephritis, p. 765. New York: Wiley 1973a

Heptinstall, R. H.: Pathology of membranous glomerulonephritis. In: Glomerulonephritis, p. 415–427. New York: Wiley 1973b

Herdson, P. B., Jennings, R. B., Earle, D. P.: Glomerular fine structure in post-streptococcal acute glomerulonephritis. Arch. Path. **81**, 117 (1966)

Heymann, W., Hackel, D. B., Harwood, S., Wilson, S., Hunter, J.: Production of nephrotic syndrome in rats by Freund's adjuvant and rat kidney suspensions. Proc. Soc. Exp. Biol. Med. **100**, 660–664 (1959)

Hinglais, N., Garcia-Torres, R., Kleinknecht, D.: Long-term prognosis in acute glomerulonephritis. Amer. J. Med. **56**, 52–60 (1974)

Holborow, E. J.: Standardization in immunofluorescence. Oxford and Edinburgh: Blackwell 1970

Hoyer, J. R., Raij, L., Vernier, R. L., Simmons, R. L., Najarian, J. S., Michael, A. F.: Recurrence of idiopathic nephrotic syndrome after renal transplantation. Lancet **1972II**, 343–348

Hyman, L. R., Wagnild, J. P., Beirne, G. J., Burkholder, P. M.: Immunoglobulin-A distribution in glomerular disease: Analysis of immunofluorescence localisation and pathogenic significance. Kidney Internat. **3**, 397–408 (1973)

Klassen, J., Andres, G. A., Brenman, J. C., McCluskey, R. T.: An immunologic renal tubular lesion in man. Clin. Immunol. Immunopathol. **1**, 69–83 (1972)

Koffler, D., Agnello, V., Karr, R. I., Kunkel, H. G.: Variable patterns of immunoglobulin and complement deposition in the kidneys of patients with systemic lupus erythematosus. Amer. J. Path. **56**, 305–312 (1969)

Koffler, D., Paronetto, F.: Immunofluorescent localization of immunoglobulins, complement and fibrinogen in human diseases. II. Acute, subacute and chronic glomerulonephritis. J. Clin. Invest. **44**, 1665–1671 (1965)

Koffler, D., Schur, P. H., Kunkel, H. G.: Immunological studies concerning the nephritis of systemic lupus erythematosus. J. Exp. Med. **126**, 607–624 (1967)

Krishnan, C., Kaplan, M. H.: Immunopathologic studies of systematic erythematosus. II. Antinuclear reaction of globulin eluted from homogenates and isolated glomeruli of kidneys from patients with lupus nephritis. J. Clin. Invest. **44**, 1657 (1967)

Lachmann, P. J., Müller-Eberhard, H. J., Kunkel, H. G., Paronetto, F.: The localization of in vivo bound complement in tissue sections. J. Exp. Med. **115**, 63–82 (1962)

Lerner, R. A., Glassock, R. J., Dixon, F. J.: The role of antiglomerular basement membrane antibody in the pathogenesis of human glomerulonephritis. J. Exp. Med. **126**, 989–1004 (1967)

Lewis, E. J., Cavallo, T., Karrington, J. T., Cotran, R. J.: An immunopathologic study of rapidly progressive glomerulonephritis in the adult. Hum. Path. **2**, 185–208 (1971)

Lewis, E. J., Kallen, R. J., Rowe, D. S.: Glomerular localization of IgE in lipoid nephrosis. Lancet **1973I**, 1395

Lewis, E. J., Schur, P. H., Busch, G. J., Galvanek, E., Merrill, J. P.: Immunopathologic features of a patient with glomerulonephritis and pulmonary hemorrhage. Amer. J. Med. **54**, 507–513 (1973)

LEWIS, M. G., LONGHRIDGE, L. W., PHILLIPS, T. M.: Immunological studies in nephrotic syndrome associated with extrarenal malignant disease. Lancet 1971II, 134–135

LIN, J. H., OROFINO, D., SHERLOCK, J., LETTERI, J., DUFFY, J. L.: Waldenström's macroglobulinemia, mesangiocapillary glomerulonephritis, angiitis and myositis. Nephron 10, 262–270 (1973)

LINDEMANN, W.: Sur le mode d'action de certains poissons vénaux: Ann. Inst. Pasteur 14, 49 (1900)

LOWANCE, D. C., MULLINS, J. D., McPHAUL, J. J.: Immunglobulin A (IgA) associated glomerulonephritis. Kidney Internat. 3, 167–176 (1973)

MACDONALD, M. K.: Dense deposit disease. In: Glomerulonephritis, p. 515-530. New York: Wiley 1973

MARQUARDT, H., WILSON, C. B., DIXON, F. J.: Isolation and immunological characterization of human glomerular basement membrane antigens. Kidney Internat. 3, 57–65 (1973)

MASUGI, M.: Über die experimentelle Glomerulonephritis durch das spezifische Antinierenserum. Ein Beitrag zur Pathogenese der diffusen Glomerulonephritis. Beitr. Path. Anat. u. allg. Path. 92, 429–466 (1933/34)

MAUER, S. M., MICHAEL, A. F., FISH, A. J., BROWN, D. M.: Spontaneous immunoglobulin and complement deposition in glomeruli of diabetic rats. Lab. Invest. 27, 488–494 (1972)

McCLUSKEY, R. T.: The value of immunofluorescence in the study of human renal disease. J. Exp. Med. 134, 242 (1971)

McCLUSKEY, R. T., KLASSEN, J.: Immunologically mediated glomerular and interstitial renal disease. N. Engl. J. Med. 288, 564–570 (1973)

McCLUSKEY, R. T., VASALLI, P., GALLO, G., BALDWIN, D. S.: An immunofluorescent study of pathogenic mechanisms in glomerular disease. N. Engl. J. Med. 274, 696–701 (1966)

McENERY, P. T., McADAMS, A. J., WEST, C. D.: Glomerular morphology, natural history and treatment of children with IgA-IgG mesangial nephropathy. In: Glomerulonephritis, p. 305-320. New York: Wiley 1973

McGOVERN, V. J.: Persistent nephrotic syndrome: A renal biopsy study. Australian Ann. Med. 13, 306 (1964)

McGOVERN, V. J., LAUER, C. S.: Focal slerosing glomerulonephritis. In: Glomerulonephritis, p. 223-230. New York: Wiley 1973

McINTOSH, R. M., KAUFMANN, D. B., KULVINSKAS, C., GROSSMAN, B. J.: Cryoglobulins I. Studies on the nature, incidence, and clinical significance of serum cryoproteins in glomerulonephritis. J. Lab. Clin. Med. 75, 566–577 (1970)

McINTOSH, R. M., KULVINSKAS, C., KAUFMAN, D. B.: Cryoglobulins II. The biological and clinical properties of cryoproteins in acute poststreptococcal glomerulonephritis. Int. Arch. Allergy and Appl. Immunol. 41, 700–715 (1971)

McLEAN, R. H., MICHAEL, A. F.: Properdin and C_3 proactivator: Alternate pathway components in human glomerulonephritis. J. Clin. Invest. 52, 634–644 (1973)

McPHAUL, J. J. JR., DIXON, F. J.: Characterization of human anti-glomerular basement membrane antibodies eluted from glomerulonephritic kidneys. J. Clin. Invest. 49, 308–317 (1970)

McPHAUL, J. J. JR., DIXON, F. J.: Characterization of immunoglobulin G anti-glomerular basement membrane antibodies eluted from kidneys of patients with glomerulonephritis: II. IgG subtypes and in vitro complement fixation. J. Immunol. 107, 678–684 (1971)

McPHAUL, J. J. JR., DIXON, F. J., BRETTSCHNEIDER, L., STARZL, T. E.: Immunofluorescent examination of biopsies from long term renal allografts. N. Engl. J. Med. 282, 412–417 (1970)

McPHAUL, J. J. JR., THOMPSON, A. L. JR., LORDON, R. E., KLEBANOFF, G., COSIMI, A. B., DELEMOS, R., SMITH, R. B.: Evidence suggesting persistance of nephritogenic immunopathologic mechanisms in patients receiving renal allografts. J. Clin. Invest. 52, 1059–1066 (1973)

MELLORS, R. C., ORTEGA, L. G.: Analytical pathology. III. New Observations on the pathogenesis of glomerulonephritis, lipid nephrosis, periarteriitis nodosa, and secondary amyloidosis in man. Amer. J. Path. 32, 455 (1956)

MELLORS, R. C., ORTEGA, L. G., HOLMAN, H. R.: Role of α-globulins in pathogenesis of renal lesions in systemic lupus erythematosus and chronic membranous glomerulonephritis with an observation on the lupus erythematosus cell reaction. J. Exp. Med. **106**, 191–201 (1957)

MERRILL, J. P.: Glomerulonephritis. New Engl. J. Med. **290**, 257–381 (1974)

MICHAEL, A. F., DRUMMOND, K. N., GOOD, R. A., VERNIER, R. L.: Acute poststreptococcal glomerulonephritis: Immune deposit disease. J. Clin. Invest. **45**, 237–248 (1966)

MICHAEL, A. F., McLEAN, R. H., ROY, L. P., WESTBERG, N. G., HOYER, J. R., FISH, A. J., VERNIER, R. L.: Immunologic aspects of the nephrotic syndrome. Kidney Internat. **3**, 105–115 (1973)

MICHAEL, A. F., WESTBERG, N. G., FISH, A. J., VERNIER, R. L.: Studies on chronic membranoproliferative glomerulonephritis with hypocomplementaemia. J. Exp. Med. **139**, 208s–227s (1971)

MOREL-MAROGER, L.: Discussion, p. 1079. In: Glomerulonephritis. New York: Wiley 1973

MOREL-MAROGER, L., ADAM, C., RICHET, G.: The value of immunofluorescence in the diagnosis of glomerulonephritis not related to systemic diseases. In: Glomerulonephritis, p. 81–110. New York: Wiley 1973b

MOREL-MAROGER, L., KOURILSKY, O., MIGNON, F., RICHET, G.: Antitubular basement membrane antibodies in rapidly progressive poststreptococcal glomerulonephritis: Report of a case. Clin. Immunol. Immunopath. **2**, 185–194 (1974)

MOREL-MAROGER, L., LEATHEM, A., RICHET, G.: Glomerular abnormalities in non-systemic diseases: relationship between light microscopy and immunofluorescence in 433 biopsies. Amer. J. Med. **53**, 170–184 (1972)

MOREL-MAROGER, L., MÉRY, J. P.: Renal mixed IgG-IgM essential cryoglobulinemia. In: Proc. 5th int. Congr. Nephrol., Mexico 1972, **1**, 173–178. Basel:Karger 1974

MOREL-MAROGER, L., MÉRY, J. P., RICHET, G.: Lupus nephritis: Immunofluorescent study of 54 cases. In: Glomerulonephritis, p. 1183–1186. New York: Wiley 1973a

MOREL-MAROGER, L., VERROUST, P.: Glomerular lesions in dysproteinemias. Kidney Internat. **5**, 249–252 (1974)

MULLEN, Y., HILDEMANN, W. H.: Kidney transplantation, genetics and enhancement in rats. Transplantation Proc. **3**, 669–672 (1971)

NAIRN, R. C.: Fluorescent Protein Tracing, 2nd ed. Edinburgh and London: Livingstone 1964

NARUSE, T., KITAMURA, K., MIYAKAWA, Y., SHIBATA, S.: Deposition of renal tubular epithelial antigen along the glomerular capillary walls of patients with membranous glomerulonephritis. J. Immunol. **110**, 1163–1166 (1973)

NATALI, P. G., TAN, E. M.: Experimental renal disease induced by DNA-anti-DNA immune complexes. J. Clin. Invest. **51**, 345–355 (1972)

OKUDA, R., WATANABE, Y., YAMAMOTO, Y., WEST, C. D.: The origin of membranoproliferative nephritis. Evidence against an origin from acute poststreptococcal nephritis. Amer. J. Dis. Child. **119**, 291–295 (1970)

OLBING, H., GREIFER, I., BENNETT, B. P., BERNSTEIN, J., SPITZER, A.: Idiopathic membranous nephropathy in children. Kidney Internat. **3**, 381–390 (1973)

PARONETTO, F., KOFFLER, D.: Immunofluorescent localization of immunoglobulins, complement and fibrinogen in human diseases. I. Systemic lupus erythematosus. J. Clin. Invest. **44**, 1657–1664 (1965)

PIELSTICKER, K., EDEL, H. H., THOENES, G. H.: Glomerular lesions in renal transplants: Recurrent glomerulonephritis or transplant glomerulopathy. 10th Internat. Congr. Intern. Acad. Pathology, Abstract p. 37 (1974)

PLOEM, J. S.: The use of a vertical illuminator with interchangeable dichroic mirrors for fluorescence microscopy with incident light. Mikrosk. Technik **68**, 129–142 (1967)

POLLAK, V. E., MENDOZA, N., PIRANI, C. L.: Immunohistologic observations in mesangioproliferative glomerulonephritis. In: Glomerulonephritis, p. 633–640. New York: Wiley 1973a

POLLAK, V. E., PIRANI, C. L., DUJOVNE, I., DILLARD, M. G.: The clinical course of lupus nephritis: Relationship to the renal histologic findings. In: Glomerulonephritis, p. 1167–1181. New York: Wiley 1973b

Post, R. S.: A technique for cutting thin sections from solvent substituted paraffin embedded tissues. Cryobiology 1, 261 (1965)

Van de Putte, L. B. A., de la Riviere, G. B., van Breda-Vriesman, J. C.: Recurrent or persistent hematuria. New Engl. J. Med. 290, 1165–1170 (1974)

Richet, G., Chevet, D., Morel-Maroger, L.: Serial biopsies in diffuse proliferative glomerulonephritis in adults. In: Glomerulonephritis, p. 363–381. New York: Wiley 1973

Roy, P. L., Fish, A. J., Vernier, R. L., Michael, A. F.: Recurrent macroscopic hematuria focal nephritis, and mesangial deposition of immunoglobulin and complement. J. Pediatr. 82, 767–772 (1973b)

Roy, L. P., Westberg, N. G., Michael, A. F.: Nephrotic syndrome—no evidence for a role for IgE. Clin. Exp. Immunol. 13, 553–559 (1973a)

Rumpelt, H. J., Thoenes, W.: Focal and segmental sclerosing glomerulopathy(-nephritis). Virchows Arch. A. Path. Anat. and Histol. 362, 265–282 (1974)

Schreiner, G. E.: Summing up. In: Glomerulonephritis, p. 1225–1228. New York: Wiley 1973

Schreiner, G. E., Rakowski, T. A., Argy, W. P. Marc-Aurele, J., Maher, J. F., Bauer, H.: Natural history of oliguric glomerulonephritis. In: Glomerulonephritis, p. 711–725. New York: Wiley 1973

Schürch, W., Leski, M., Hinglais, N.: Evolution of recurrent lobular glomerulonephritis in a human kidney allotransplant. Virchows Arch. Abt. A Path. Anat. 355, 66–84 (1972)

Schwarz, M. M., Lewis, E. J.: Immunopathology of the nephrotic syndrome associated with renal vein thrombosis. Amer. J. Med. 54, 528–534 (1973)

Seegal, B. C., Andres, G. A., Hsu, K. C., Zabriskie, J. B.: Studies on the pathogenesis of acute and progressive glomerulonephritis in man by immunofluorescein and immunoferritin techniques. Fed. Proc. 54, 100–108 (1965)

Siegel, N. J.: Editorial. Lipoid nephrosis and focal sclerosis. Distinct entities or spectrum of disease. Nephron 13, 105–108 (1974)

Sraer, J. D., Beaufils, P., Morel-Maroger, L., Richet, G.: Vascular nephropathies with acute renal failure. In: Glomerulonephritis, p. 1035–1046. New York: Wiley 1973

Striker, G. E., Cutler, R. E., Huang, T. W., Benditt, E. P.: Renal failure, glomerulonephritis and glomerular epithelial cell hyperplasia. In: Glomerulonephritis, p. 662. New York: J. Wiley 1973

Svec, K., Blair, J. D., Kaplan, M. H.: Immunopathologic studies of systemic lupus erythematosus (SLE). I. Tissue bound immunoglobulins in relation to serum immunoglobulin in systemic lupus and in chronic liver disease with LE cell factor. J. Clin. Invest. 46, 558–568 (1967)

Tannenbaum, M., Hsu, K. C., Buda, J., Grant, J. P., Lattes, C., Lattimer, J. K.: Electron microscopic virus-like material in systemic lupus erythematosus: With preliminary immunological observations on presence of measles antigen. J. Urology 105, 615–619 (1971)

Thoenes, G. H.: Die Immunhistologie der Glomerulonephritis. Mittler zwischen Pathogenese und Morphologie. Klin. Wschr. 51, 739–747 (1973)

Thoenes, G. H.: Immunhistologische Befunde bei Minimalveränderungen und fokal sklerosierender Glomerulopathie mit nephrotischem Syndrom. Klin. Wschr. 52, 371–378 (1974)

Thoenes, W.: Pathomorphologische Prinzipien und Formen der Glomerulonephritis. Mschr. Kinderheilk. 122, 728–740 (1974)

Tina, L. U., D'Albora, J. B., Antonovich, T. T., Bellanti, J. A., Calcagno, P. L.: Acute glomerulonephritis associated with normal serum β_1C-globulin. Amer. J. Dis. Child. 115, 29–36 (1968)

Treser, G., Ehrenreich, T., Ores, R., Sagel, I., Wassermann, E., Lange, K.: Natural history of "apparently healed" acute streptococcal glomerulonephritis in children. Pediatrics 43, 1005–1017 (1969a)

Treser, G., Semar, M., McVicar, M., Franklin, M., Ty, A., Sagel, I., Lange, K.: Antigenic streptococcal components in acute glomerulonephritis. Science 163, 676–677 (1969b)

Treser, G., Semar, M., Ty, A., Franklin, M. A., Lange, K.: Partial characterization of antigenic streptococcal plasma membrane components in acute glomerulonephritis. J. Clin. Invest. **49**, 762–768 (1970)

Unanue, E. R., Dixon, F. J.: Experimental glomerulonephritis: Immunological events and pathogenetic mechanisms. Adv. Immunol. **6**, 1–90 (1967)

Urizar, R. E., Herdman, R. C.: Anaphylactoid purpura III. Early morphologic glomerular changes. Amer. J. Clin. Path. **53**, 258–266 (1970)

Urizar, R. E., Michael, A., Sisson, S., Vernier, R. L.: Anaphylactoid purpura: II. Immunofluorescent and electron microscopic studies of the glomerular lesions. Lab. Invest. **19**, 437–450 (1968)

Vasquez, J. J., Dixon, F. J.: Immunohistological composition of amyloid by the fluorescent technique. J. Exp. Med. **104**, 727–736 (1956)

Vasquez, J. J., Dixon, F. J.: Immunohistochemical study of lesions in rheumatic fever, systemic lupus erythematosus and rheumatoid arthritis. Lab. Invest. **6**, 205–217 (1957)

Vernier, R. L., Tinglof, B., Urizar, R., Litman, N., Smith, F.: Immunofluorescent studies in renal disease. In: Proc. 3rd Int. Cong. Nephrol., Washington 1966, vol. 3, p. 83–94. Basel, New York: Karger 1967

Verroust, P., Méry, J. P., Morel-Maroger, L., Clauvel, J. P., Richet, G.: Les lésions glomérulaires des gammo-pathies monoclonales et des cryoglobulinémies idiopathiques IgE-IgM. In: Actualités Néphrologiques de l'Hôpital Necker p. 167. Paris: Flammarion 1971

Verroust, P. J., Wilson, C. B., Cooper, N. R., Edgington, T. S., Dixon, F. J.: Glomerulonephritis. J. Clin. Invest. **53**, 77–84 (1974)

West, C. D., McAdams, A., McConville, J. M., Davis, N. C., Holland, N. H.: Hypocomplementemic and normocomplementemic persistent (chronic) glomerulonephritis; clinical and pathological characteristics. J. Pediatrics **67**, 1089–1112 (1965)

West, C. D., Ruley, E. J., Spitzer, R. E., Davis, N. C.: The natural history of membranoproliferative glomerulonephritis. In: Glomerulonephritis, p. 531–540. New York: Wiley 1973a

West, C. D., Ruley, E. J., Forristal, J., Davis, N. C.: Mechanisms of hypocomplementemia in glomerulonephritis. Kidney Internat. **3**, 116–125 (1973b)

Westberg, N. G., Naff, G. B., Boyer, J. T., Michael, A. F.: Glomerular deposition of properdin in acute and chronic glomerulonephritis with hypocomplementemia. J. Clin. Invest. **50**, 642–649 (1971)

Wilson, C. B., Dixon, F. J.: Anti-glomerular basement membrane antibody-induced glomerulonephritis. Kidney Internat. **3**, 74–89 (1973)

Wilson, C. B., Dixon, F. J.: Diagnosis of immunopathologic renal disease. Kidney Internat. **5**, 389–401 (1974)

Zabriskie, J. B., Utermohlen, V., Read, S. E., Fischetti, V. A.: Streptococcus related glomerulonephritis. Kidney Internat. **3**, 100–104 (1973)

Zollinger, H. U., Moppert, J., Thiel, G., Rohr, H. P.: Morphology and pathogenesis of glomerulopathy in cadaver kidney allografts treated with antilymphocyte globulin. In: Current Topics of Pathology, Vol. 57, p. 1–48. Berlin-Heidelberg-New York: Springer 1973

Division of Renal Pathology, Department of Pathology,
Mount Sinai School of Medicine, New York, N.Y. 10029
and Barnert Memorial Hospital Center, Paterson, N.J. 07514

Electron Microscopy of Glomerulonephritis*

J. Churg and E. Grishman

With 24 Figures

Contents

I. Introduction 107

II. Primary Glomerulonephritis 108
    1. Minimal-Change Disease (Lipoid Nephrosis) 108
    2. Focal Glomerular Sclerosis 111
    3. Membranous Nephropathy (Membranous Glomerulonephritis) 113
    4. Acute Proliferative Glomerulonephritis 118
    5. Extracapillary Glomerulonephritis 121
    6. Mesangiocapillary (Membranoproliferative) Glomerulonephritis 124
    7. Dense Deposit Disease 126
    8. Focal Glomerulonephritis 126
    9. Chronic Glomerulonephritis 131
    10. Hereditary Nephritides 131

III. Glomerulonephritis of Systemic Diseases 133
    1. Lupus Nephritis 133
    2. Hemolytic Uremic Syndrome and Thrombotic Thrombocytopenic Purpura 138
    3. Radiation Nephritis 140
    4. Hepatic Glomerulosclerosis 142
    5. Pre-eclamptic Nephropathy 143

IV. Transplantation 145

References 147

I. Introduction

The events occurring in glomerulonephritis produce a complex and compli-cated pattern of glomerular changes. Though these changes can be readily appre-ciated by light microscopy, many are too subtle to be clearly discerned. Only with the advent of electron microscopy did it become possible to describe the glomerular events with considerable accuracy and establish a basis for clinico-pathologic correlations. Many changes first discerned by electron microscopy were later seen also by light microscopy. Perhaps the most important contri-bution of electron microscopy was that it provided a means for distinguishing between the capillary wall and the mesangium and for describing in detail the structure of each. This information is available in standard textbooks and will be repeated here very briefly.

* Supported by Research Grant AM-00918 from the National Institute of Arthritis and Metabolic Diseases, U.S. Public Health Service.

The glomerulus can be conceived as a structure composed of three structural components and two spaces. The structural components are: Bowman's capsule, the capillary walls and the mesangium. The spaces defined by them are: Bowman's or the urinary space and the capillary lumina or blood spaces. The capillary wall consists of a basement membrane lined on the urinary side by visceral epithelial cells or podocytes and their foot processes, and on the capillary side by endothelium. The basement membrane in turn consists of three layers: the middle, lamina densa and the external and internal laminae rarae. These distinctions prove to be of considerable importance in the description of pathologic processes. The mesangium consists of cells and intercellular substance. The latter is known as mesangial matrix and although it resembles the basement membrane, it differs from the latter in a number of important properties (e.g. resistance to certain toxins).

This review will be devoted almost exclusively to the pathology of human glomerulonephritis. Brief mention of animal models will be made, and occasionally illustrated. Detailed review of the experimental immunologically induced nephritis will be found elsewhere in this volume.

II. Primary Glomerulonephritis
1. Minimal-Change Disease (Lipoid Nephrosis)

Lipoid nephrosis or minimal-change disease occurs most often in children and less frequently in adults. It is manifested by massive proteinuria and the nephrotic syndrome and has a relatively good prognosis, responding in the majority of cases to steroid or immunosuppressive therapy. Morphologic changes are most prominent in the tubules, which accumulate lipid and protein in the cell cytoplasm, leading to enlargement of the kidneys and imparting a pale yellow cast to the parenchyma. The glomeruli, in contrast, appear normal or near normal on light microscopy.

It is the study of minimal-change disease by electron microscopy that marks a milestone in the history of renal pathology. For the first time ultrastructural changes not visible by light microscopy were discovered in the glomeruli, thus establishing the glomerulus rather than the tubule as the primary site of pathology (Farquhar et al., 1957). The lesion, then discovered, involves the visceral epithelial cells, which show loss or "fusion" of their foot processes (Fig. 1) and gave the disease, at one time, the name "foot process disease". Since then, this finding has been confirmed by many authors (Movat, 1959; Kurtz, 1961; Churg et al., 1962) and, in the absence of significant proliferative changes, is considered to be the characteristic lesion of minimal-change disease.

In actuality, loss of foot processes is not due to fusion. Normally, foot processes of neighboring epithelial cells interdigitate, so that adjacent foot processes usually derive from two different epithelial cells (Simon and Chatelanat, 1969). In proteinuria, swelling of epithelial cytoplasm leads to

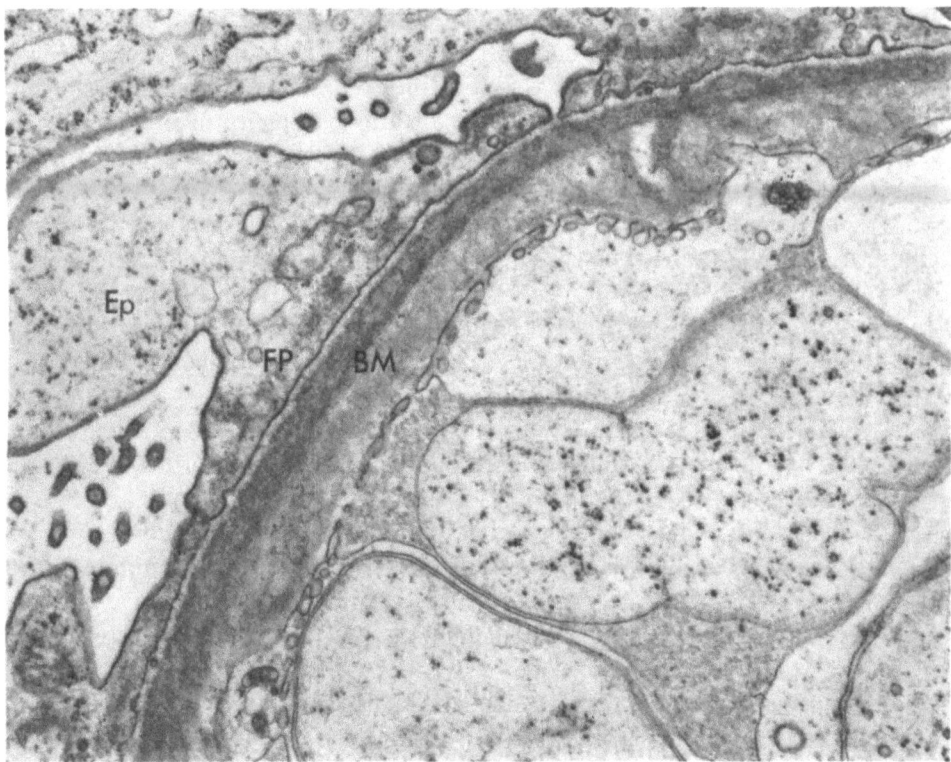

Fig. 1. Minimal-change disease (lipoid nephrosis). There is edema of epithelial cells, almost complete effacement of foot processes. The basement membrane shows considerable irregular widening of the lamina rara interna. ×22100

filling of the spaces between foot processes, while, at the same time, there is retraction of foot processes by the neighboring cell. This process has been visualized three-dimensionally by scanning electron microscopy (ARAKAWA, 1971). The cytoplasm of the swollen podocytes retains the dense material that is normally present in foot processes. This material is composed of microfibrils arranged in bundles and resembles myofilaments of smooth muscle cells. It has been suggested that these fibrils endow the cell with the ability to contract (KARNOVSKY and AINSWORTH, 1972). Similar fibrils are also present in the body of the podocyte, but in a much looser meshwork.

Loss of foot processes is usually accompanied by the appearance of numerous villi projecting from the free surface of the cells (CHURG, 1968). The loss may be limited to a few short stretches or may involve the entire capillary surface. In minimal-change disease, foot process loss is frequently reversible under the influence of steroid treatment. Foot process fusion is not

Abbreviations: BM = basement membrane; BMLM = basement membrane-like material; CL = capillary lumen; Cr = crescent; D = deposit; DD = dense deposit; En = endothelial cell; Ep = epithelial cell; F = fibrinoid material; FP = foot processes; L = leukocytes; MC = mesangial cell; MM = mesangial matrix; Y = yeast.

specific for lipoid nephrosis, but is also found in other conditions characterized by severe proteinuria and the nephrotic syndrome. It has not been established whether loss of foot processes is due to primary damage of epithelial cells or is secondary to increased permeability of the basement membrane. It is possible that under different circumstances either one of these mechanisms may come into action.

Other changes involving the podocytes in lipoid nephrosis consist of increase in number and size of cell organelles, e.g. Golgi membranes and endoplasmic reticulum, and the appearance of lipid and protein droplets (TRUMP and BENDITT, 1962; HAYSLETT et al., 1973). Conversely, there may be swelling of the cytoplasm with a diminished number of cell organelles indicating hypoactivity.

The endothelium usually shows only mild changes, such as edema and occasional bleb formation. The capillary lumen may contain fibrin and platelet aggregates (DUFFY et al., 1970).

Electron microscopic changes of the basement membrane consist of irregular widening of the lamina rara interna (Fig. 1), and minimal focal thickening and mottling (CHURG et al., 1965). However, in addition, there are probably changes in the basement membrane that are beyond the resolving power of the electron microscope. Alterations of morphologically normal glomerular basement membranes have been demonstrated in experimental aminonucleoside nephrosis in rats (KEFALIDES and FORSELL-KNOTT, 1970); they consist of decrease of hydroxyproline, hydroxylysine, and glycine, and increase of glucose.

It has been postulated that rearrangement of glomerular basement membrane molecules occurs, leading to enlargement of intermolecular pores, and thereby to increased permeability. This process, in turn, may be due to malfunction of epithelial cells that synthesize abnormal basement membrane (BERMAN and MISRA, 1972)

The mesangium in this disease usually shows little or no changes, though, occasionally, minimal increase of mesangial cells and matrix, either focal or diffuse, may be observed. For this reason, the names NIL-disease (nothing in light microscopy) or minimal-change disease have been variously applied. The latter term has now found general acceptance and the term "lipoid nephrosis," which was originally used by MUNK (1918) to designate a disease accompanied by lipiduria, is gradually being replaced.

All reports agree on the absence of electron dense deposits in minimal-change disease, and on the fact that this disease is not a precursor or in any way related to membranous nephropathy (HOPPER et al., 1970).

A condition resembling minimal change disease can be produced in rats by administration of aminonucleoside of puromycin. Glomerular changes bear considerable resemblance to those in man with lipoid nephrosis (FELDMAN and FISHER, 1959). However, prolonged administration of the chemical resulted in a progressive glomerular lesion reminiscent of focal sclerosis (see next section) (FELDMAN and FISHER, 1971).

2. Focal Glomerular Sclerosis

Focal glomerular sclerosis (FGS) was first observed about 50 years ago by FAHR (1925) who described it in some children with the nephrotic syndrome and suggested that it represented a step in progression to renal failure. RICH (1957) discovered that the lesion usually began in the juxtamedullary glomeruli. Recently, it has been noted that FGS is frequently associated with poor response to steroid treatment and an unfavorable clinical outcome (CHURG et al., 1970).

The light microscopic features have been described by a number of authors (HABIB et al., 1961; McGOVERN, 1964; HAYSLETT et al., 1969). The characteristic lesion is segmental, involving one or several lobules in a glomerulus, which take on a solid appearance. There is local increase in mesangial matrix, collapse of capillaries, adhesions to Bowman's capsule and, frequently, the appearance of hyaline material in involved areas. Slight diffuse increase in mesangial cellularity may sometimes be present. Frequently, there is hyperplasia and hypertrophy of the visceral epithelial cells, which may form small crescents over the sclerotic areas.

On electron microscopy, loss of foot processes is present in all glomeruli so that, in the stricter sense, the lesion represents a diffuse glomerular disease. In addition, the appearance of electron dense deposits has been described in the involved segments (HYMAN and BURKHOLDER, 1973) corresponding to fluorescence microscopic findings of immune globulins, especially IgM and complement (C3). Thickening of basement membranes and mesangial matrix were found by NAGI et al. (1971), and RUMPELT and THOENES (1972) described fine filamentous matrix-like material in the periphery of the capillary loop. Intracapillary fibrin and platelets are slightly more common in focal glomerular sclerosis than in minimal-change disease (DUFFY et al., 1970).

In our experience, most of the changes are rather nonspecific and consist of wrinkling and collapse of basement membranes and local increase of mesangial matrix and, occasionally, some mesangial cells (Fig. 2). Small dense deposits were found by us in 20 out of 48 cases. They are located between the basement membrane and endothelium, or under the basement membrane covering the mesangium. In addition, there are hyperplastic changes in the podocytes corresponding to those observed by light microscopy. They are characterized by swelling of cytoplasm with increase of rough endoplasmic reticulum. Occasionally, there is degeneration of podocytes causing breaks of the cell membranes in the early stages. Later, there may be detachment of podocytes from the basement membrane over shorter or longer stretches. The newly formed spaces may attain considerable width and become filled with thin layers of basement membrane and cell debris (Fig. 3). Such changes are found especially in young adult male patients who are also drug addicts (GRISHMAN and CHURG, 1975). These lesions resemble changes found in experimental radiation nephritis (MADRAZO et al., 1969) and those recently produced in rats made nephrotic by the injection of N,N'-diacetylbenzidine (CARROLL et al., 1974).

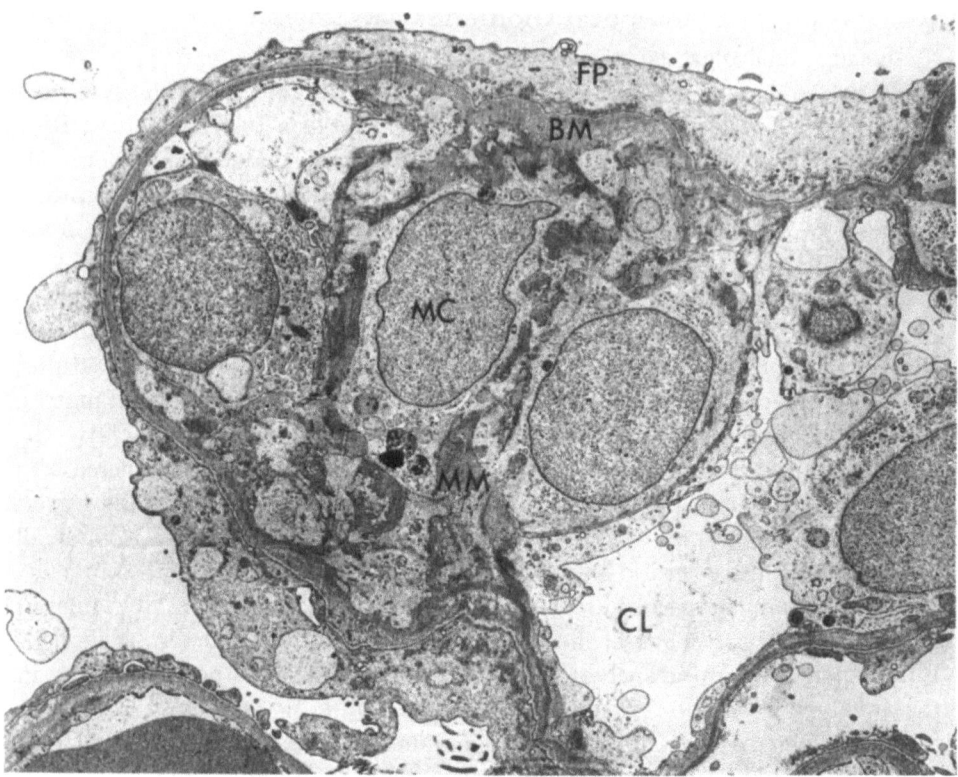

Fig. 2. Focal glomerular sclerosis. Mesangial expansion and partial capillary collapse
Note two mesangial cells. ×6000

Systematic semiquantitative methods of electron microscopic analysis
were applied by Jao et al. (1973) to separate patients with "minimal glomerular
changes only" from those with very subtle degrees of abnormality, such as
slight increase in mesangial matrix and slight wrinkling of glomerular basement membranes. By this means, the authors showed that patients with only
minimal glomerular changes apparently respond better to treatment with
steroids than those with minor mesangial or basement membrane changes.
However, this has not been conclusively proved.

The relationship between minimal-change disease and focal glomerular
sclerosis is still controversial. Most authors agree that the latter disease is
much less responsive to steroid treatment than pure lipoid nephrosis, but it
has not been established whether the two lesions represent two different
diseases or different stages of the same disease. Churg et al. (1970) postulated
two separate entities on the basis of light microscopic observations and clinical
data. A similar view is expressed by Jao et al. (1973), who found in their
series of patients that the duration of disease was no longer in patients with
FGS than in those with "minimal glomerular changes only." Recently,
Kashgarian et al. (1974) suggested, however, that "focal glomerular sclerosis

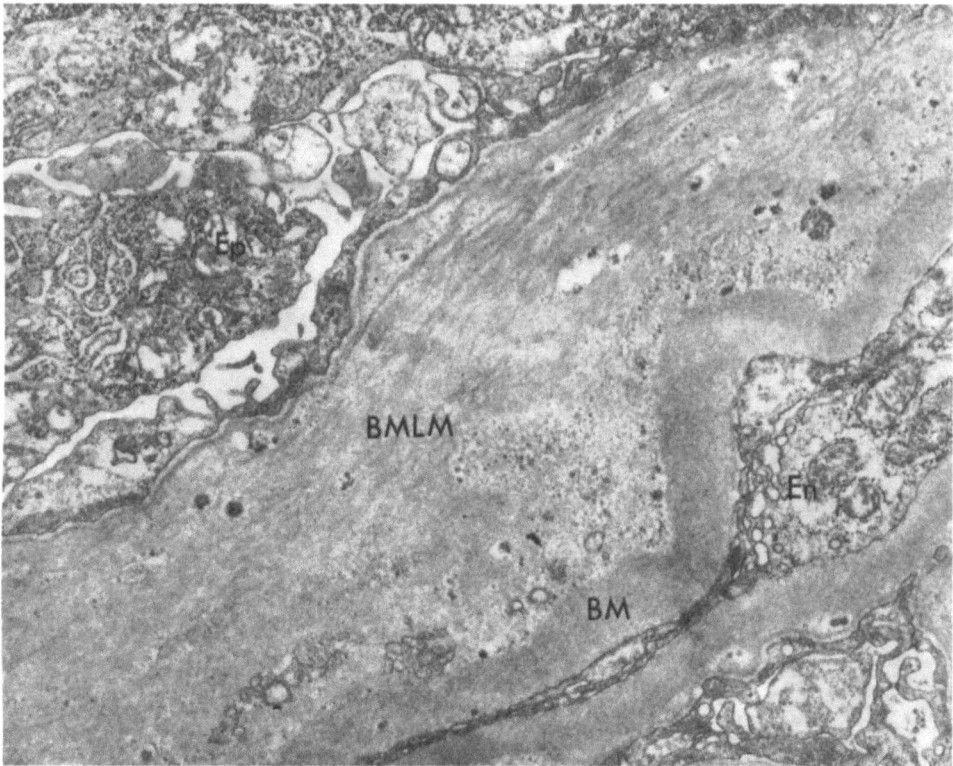

Fig. 3. Focal glomerular sclerosis. Detachment of epithelial cells from the basement membrane (see Text). ×13400

may be a stage in the evolution of the disease from minimal change to a more chronic form of glomerular damage." HABIB (1973) proposed that there are two populations of patients, namely those with FGS at the onset and steroid resistant disease, and those who develop FGS in previously normal kidneys and are more or less steroid-sensitive. Our own experience seems to support this concept (GRISHMAN and CHURG, 1975).

3. Membranous Nephropathy (Membranous Glomerulonephritis)

The term membranous glomerulonephritis was first applied by BELL in 1929 to cases that clinically presented themselves as idiopathic nephrotic syndrome and who, on histologic examination, showed thickening of capillary walls or capillary basement membranes in the glomeruli. BELL'S report was not easily substantiated partly because of inadequate (too thick) histologic sections generally in use at that time and partly because thickening of the capillary walls occurred only in some patients and was absent in others. With the use of thinner sections (2 to 3 μm or less) and the introduction of modern staining methods, such as PAS, silver methenamine, and improved trichrome, BELL'S findings were confirmed. It was possible to demonstrate that the

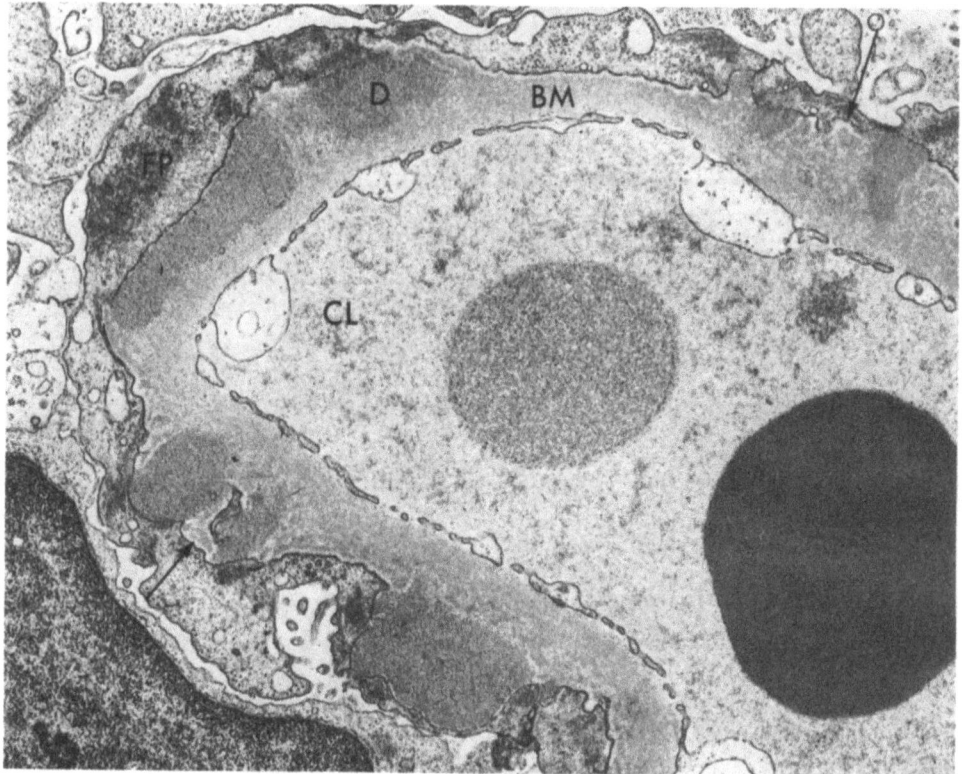

Fig. 4. Membranous nephropathy, early stage. Subepithelial deposits and "spikes" (the latter indicated by arrows). ×15600

thickening of the capillary wall was due to two elements: deposition of hyaline (protein) material between the epithelial cells and the basement membrane, and formation of "spikes" which stained in a manner similar to that of the basement membrane (Jones, 1957; Churg and Grishman, 1957). The details of these abnormalities could not be established accurately until the application of electron microscopy, supplemented by immunofluorescence microscopy. The typical appearance of "spikes and dome" was indeed found by electron microscopy to be due to deposits of proteins which included immunoglobulins— IgG, rarely IgM, and complement (C3).

The deposits are generally discrete and are separated from each other by projections of the basement membrane that constitute the spikes (Ehren-reich and Churg, 1968) (Fig. 4). The protein deposits are almost invariably homogeneous under low magnification electron microscopy and finely granular under high magnification. On very rare occasions they show an organized "fingerprint" pattern. The individual deposits are usually small and dome-shaped and are classified by immunofluorescence microscopy as granular.

The "spikes" arise from the underlying basement membrane and consist of structurally similar material, though, as a rule, they are less dense and less homogeneous than the original basement membrane. They vary in thickness and shape, sometimes being thicker at the tip, that is towards the epithelial cell, or more often at the base. The basement membrane itself appears little altered. The endothelial cells are often swollen and the epithelial cells show characteristic changes of massive proteinuria or nephrotic syndrome in the form of hyperplasia of the organelles or, alternately, edematous areas devoid of organelles, and the loss or "fusion" of foot processes.

In the early stages of the disease the protein deposits are the dominant feature. Very early, only small deposits may be present in some capillary loops. They are irregularly scattered in the glomeruli and cannot be seen by light microscopy though they can be recognized by immunofluorescence microscopy. At that time the spikes are absent or are very small and the appearance of the glomeruli suggests minimal-change disease. This appearance is probably the source of confusion in the older literature where cases have been reported showing transformation of minimal-change disease to membranous nephropathy. Actually no such cases have been authenticated. This early stage has been designated as Stage I (EHRENREICH and CHURG, 1968). Stage II is the previously described typical appearance of membranous nephropathy where deposits are numerous and are clearly separated by spikes. Stage III is characterized by progressive extension of the spikes, which eventually meet and entrap the deposits (Fig. 5). Deposits then seem to lie within a markedly thickened irregular basement membrane.

Formation of deposits is probably a continuous process. Some of them may be shed into the urinary space or are phagocytosed by the epithelial cells, and new deposits cross the basement membrane and are trapped under the epithelium. In this manner very complex patterns may be seen in Stage III. At the same time some of the entrapped deposits may undergo gradual dissolution with formation of "empty spaces." The latter eventually become filled with basement membrane material.

There is also a Stage IV where deposits disappear almost completely and the basement membrane becomes nearly homogenous and very thick, though sometimes still showing a tooth-comb appearance on the epithelial side. Stage IV represents healing by scarring. It is usually nonuniform, affecting some segments of capillary wall more prominently than others.

The glomerular mesangium shows comparatively little change. There may be minimal increase in cellularity and perhaps also slight increase in amount of mesangial matrix. Occasionally these two processes are more prominent, leading to confusion with the membranous nephropathy of systemic lupus erythematosus. Sometimes mesangial changes signify a process which is akin to focal sclerosis (see previous section): In addition to enlargement of the mesangium there is collapse of the capillaries with solidification of the whole lobule. This is apparently a progressive process, which eventually leads to the picture of chronic glomerulonephritis. Even in the advanced stage, it is still possible to recognize the nature of the disease by the presence of spikes in at least some of the capillaries. Crescents do occasionally occur in association

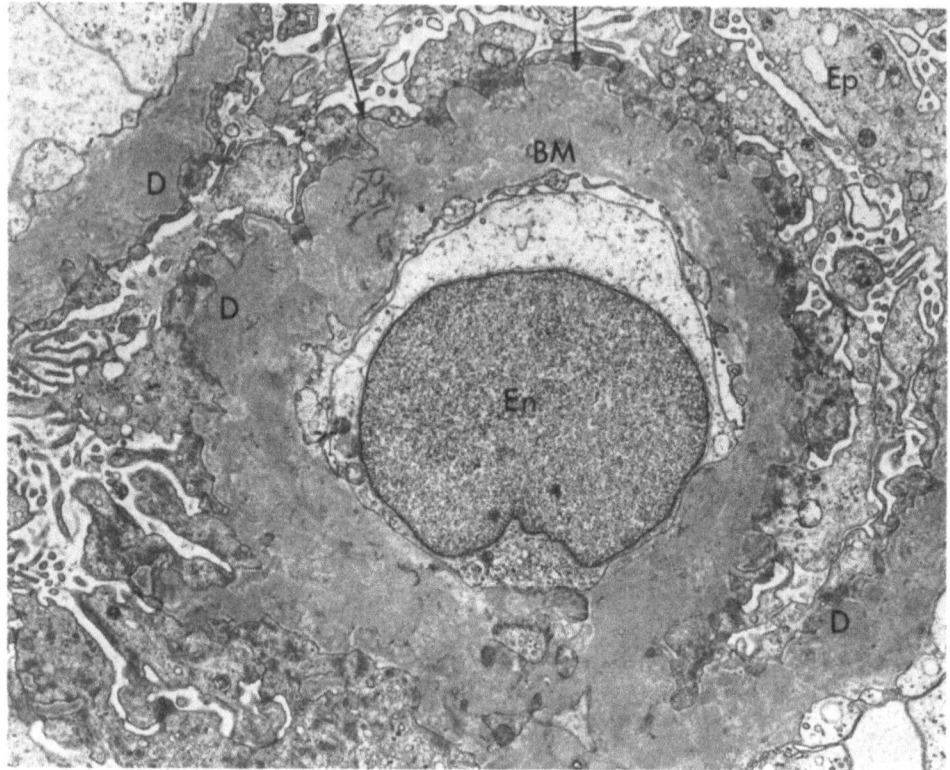

Fig. 5. Membranous nephropathy, advanced stage. The basement membrane shows a complex pattern of projections (arrows) and deposits. ×7500

with membranous nephropathy. They may signify a change in the nature of the disease from an immune complex process to antiglomerular basement membrane disease (Klassen et al., 1974), and they definitely accelerate the development of renal failure.

Clinically, membranous nephropathy is manifested primarily by the nephrotic syndrome, that is, massive proteinuria, edema, and hypoalbuminemia. If the disease is encountered at an early stage, only proteinuria may be present, but edema develops almost invariably in due course. Microscopic hematuria is not uncommon though gross hematuria is rare. Hypertension is often present but it may predate the membranous nephropathy. The disease affects males and females at about the same rate and is much more common in adults than in children.

There is a fairly good clinical correlation between the histologic stage and the course of the disease. Most patients in Stage I either recover or improve, though some show progression which may be quite rapid. When the patients are in Stage II, they show fewer recoveries but considerable incidence of improvement. There are cases on record of complete or nearly complete resolution of the glomerular lesions (Laver and Kincaid-Smith, 1973). In Stage III the majority of patients do not improve and often progress to renal failure. Stage IV, as mentioned, is a healing stage. It is an uncommon outcome of the disease. Such patients may be totally free of symptoms, though it is likely that they have decreased renal reserve.

The nature of membranous nephropathy is unknown. Because of the presence of immunoglobulins and complement, it is thought to represent an immune-complex disease. This is probably true of some cases of secondary membranous nephropathy (see below) and perhaps also true of the idiopathic form, though further data are needed for the latter. There is evidence that in at least some cases, the antigen is derived from the renal tubules (NARUSE et al., 1973). Some instances apparently follow acute proliferative glomerulonephritis (RICHET et al., 1974). Whatever the origin of the protein deposits, it is obvious that they consist of molecules of the proper size, shape, and charge, which are able to cross the basement membrane but are unable to easily cross the epithelial cell membrane. Because of this property, they remain for a long time within the capillary wall and apparently set up a reactive process that leads to formation of additional basement membrane material, most likely by the overlying epithelial cells. One must assume that if the basic disease process abates, healing can take place either by removal of the deposits or by incorporation into the basement membrane. If the disease continues, there may be irreversible progression to renal failure.

In addition to the idiopathic membranous nephropathy there are several forms associated with or secondary to other diseases. Membranous nephropathy is not too rare in pregnancy where it runs a course similar to that of the idiopathic group. It appears to be incidental rather than related to the pregnancy. Certain drugs and chemicals are capable of producing nephrotic syndrome with histologic changes of membranous nephropathy, among them heavy metals (gold or mercury), penicillamine, and organic solvents. Allergic reactions to beesting or to poison ivy can also be followed by membranous nephropathy. Certain infectious processes such as secondary or congenital syphilis may lead to nephrotic syndrome with membranous nephropathy. These forms tend to respond to specific therapy. Membranous nephropathy also occurs in combination with glucose dysmetabolism either in the form of frank diabetes or chemical diabetes (high fasting blood sugar or abnormal glucose tolerance test). As mentioned earlier there is a membranous form of lupus nephritis, which will be discussed in that section. Renal vein thrombosis has been suggested as a cause of membranous nephropathy. The available evidence, however, favors the view that thrombosis is secondary to membranous nephropathy, or more specifically, to the nephrotic syndrome (DUFFY et al., 1973). Experimental constriction of renal veins in animals leads to proteinuria and nephrotic syndrome but without membranous changes in the glomeruli (FISHER et al., 1968). On the other hand, membranous nephropathy is not uncommon in animals, such as dogs and cats (MURRAY et al., 1971; SCOTT et al., in press).

Experimentally, membranous nephropathy has been produced by administration of heavy metals (iron, mercury) (DACHS and CHURG, 1965;

Bariety et al., 1971) or kidney suspension (Heymann nephritis) (Heymann et al., 1959). Membranous glomerulonephritis also follows repeated injections of foreign protein (Dixon et al., 1961) or a single injection of a nephritogenic glycoprotein (Shibata et al., 1972). In the last two instances the resulting glomerular disease resembles membranous lupus nephritis rather than idiopathic membranous nephropathy.

4. Acute Proliferative Glomerulonephritis

Acute diffuse proliferative glomerulonephritis most often follows streptococcal infection, but may also be associated with other bacteria (e.g. staphylococcus) and probably with virus, or it may be caused by noninfectious agents, such a foreign protein. Clinically it is manifested by the "nephritic syndrome," that is, hematuria, proteinuria, hypertension, and salt and water retention.

The characteristic histologic features are enlargement of the glomerular tuft with increase in the number of cells and compression of the capillaries. The cells are of two types: rather large mononuclear cells and polymorphonuclear leukocytes. In addition, there may also be proliferation of the cells lining Bowman's capsule with formation of crescents. The polymorphonuclear leukocytes are mostly neutrophils (Figs. 6 and 7) though some eosinophils may be encountered. The number of leukocytes is related to a degree to the severity of the disease process and the stage of development. Leukocytes are more numerous in the early stages and tend to disappear later. They may be present in the capillary lumen, in the mesangium, and in the urinary space. Those in the lumina tend to adhere to the capillary wall, either to the endothelium or to the denuded basement membrane (Fig. 7) and sometimes can be seen wandering through the wall. They are particularly prominent in the areas of subepithelial deposits (see below). The mononuclear cells tend to occupy the mesangium, expanding the lobular stalks. However, some may also be found in the capillary lumina. Some of the cells are undoubtedly blood monocytes. However, the majority of cells appear to be of local origin, representing predominantly the proliferated mesangial cells (Fig. 6).

Older concepts dating from the days of light microscopy view these cells as endothelial. Though differences between endothelial and mesangial cells in the normal glomerulus are readily perceived, in disease the proliferating cells lose some of their characteristics and the recognition of the cell type is often impossible by the morphologic appearance alone. What is crucial is the relation of the cells to the capillary lumina and to the mesangial matrix. The endothelial cells undergo considerable swelling with constriction of the lumen. They face the lumen on at least one aspect and are attached to each other by junction complexes. The mesangial cells on the other hand are separated from the lumen and from the endothelial cells, as well as from each other, by strands of mesangial matrix. This separation is usually incomplete so that over small areas the mesangial cell can be in contact with the endothelial cell and even form protrusions ("blebs") in the capillary lumen through or between

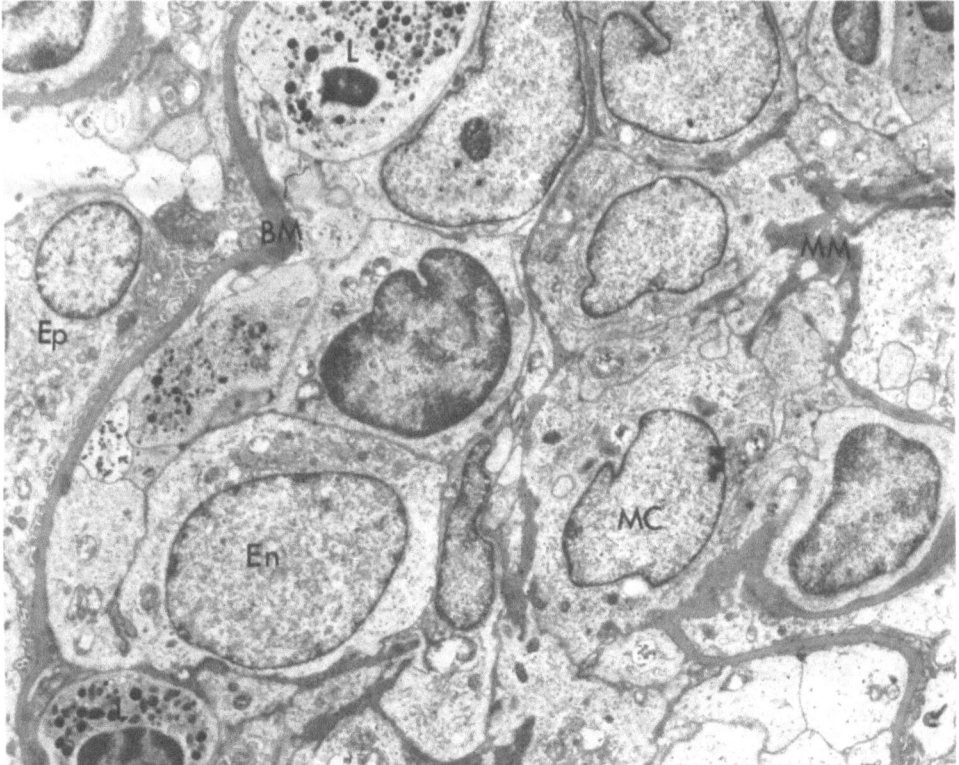

Fig. 6. Acute proliferative glomerulonephritis. There is marked increase in the number of mononuclear cells, most of which are mesangial but some, endothelial. The mesangial cells are separated by thin strands of mesangial matrix. Note polymorphonuclear leukocytes under the basement membrane. × 3 560

the endothelial cells. However in any plane of section, the mesangial cells are clearly demarcated by the mesangial matrix which surrounds them, while the endothelial cells contact the matrix only over their basal portions.

A degree of endothelial proliferation may be encountered in some capillary loops (Fig. 6), but their contribution to the total cellularity is generally small. More conspicuous endothelial proliferation may accompany capillary embolism and thrombosis, particularly during the stages of organization and regeneration.

The second important feature that was recognized by electron microscopy and later confirmed by immunofluorescence and even by light microscopy is the presence of protein deposits (CHURG et al., 1962; KIMMELSTIEL et al., 1962). These deposits are most often seen between the basement membrane and the visceral epithelial cells (podocytes). The deposits in this location (Fig. 7) are generally small, "hump-like," dome or flame-shaped, usually discrete, but occasionally confluent. On electron microscopy they may be homogeneous under low magnification and finely granular with high magnification, but sometimes they are nonhomogeneous showing lighter and darker areas (CHURG and GRISHMAN, 1972). The latter type of deposit is more often seen in the more

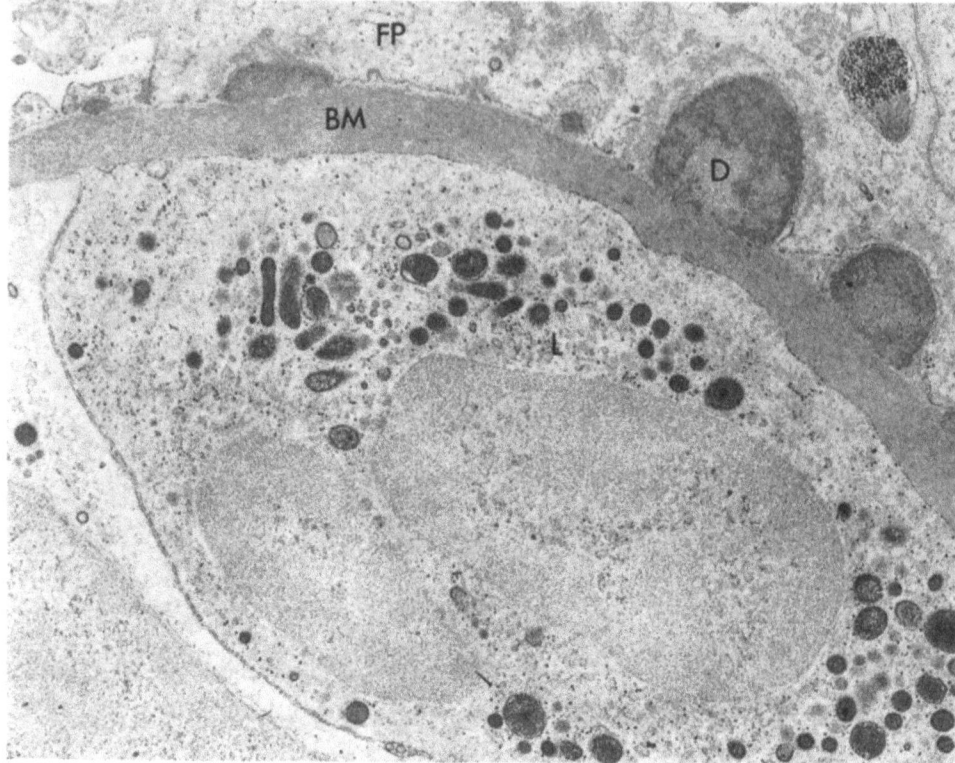

Fig. 7. Acute proliferative glomerulonephritis, higher magnification. Deposits (so-called "humps") are seen on the epithelial side of the basement membrane. They vary in size and are non-homogeneous. A polymorphonuclear leukocyte adheres to the basement membrane on the endothelial side. ×15 860

advanced stages of the disease. Andres et al. (1963) noted that in serum sickness nephritis in animals the denser areas in the deposits contain gamma globulins and the lighter areas do not. Whether a similar explanation applies to the deposits in man is unknown. The foot processes over the deposits are usually effaced, but the underlying basement membrane is unchanged or at most slightly indented.

In addition to the subepithelial deposits, small subendothelial deposits may be present. These also tend to be nonhomogeneous. Deposits in the mesangium are rarely seen by electron microscopy but sometimes may be demonstrated by immunofluorescence microscopy. Immunofluorescence also shows that the deposits contain immune globulins, especially IgG and complement. In some instances streptococcal antigens have been demonstrated by immune ferritin techniques (Andres et al., 1967), mainly in the mesangial deposits but not in the subepithelial deposits. Though poststreptococcal glomerulonephritis is believed to be an example of immune complex disease, the absolute proof of this is not yet available.

The number and density of the deposits vary considerably from case to case. In severe cases they are numerous and may be confluent; in mild cases they may be completely absent (HINGLAIS *et al.*, 1974). The deposits persist for only a short time even in the severe cases, at most for several weeks, and later disappear despite the persistence of the disease. On rare occasions they may be present for many months or even years though it is not certain whether they are actually the original deposits or are newly formed. When deposits are present for a long time they may be accompanied by focal thickening or projections of basement membrane ("spikes"). There are also cases on record where deposits are accompanied by numerous spikes so that the appearance of the capillary wall is similar to that of membranous nephropathy.

With resolution of the disease the proliferated cells decrease in number and eventually disappear, the newly formed mesangial matrix is resorbed, and restitution to normal follows. This process may take several weeks or months. As the capillaries reopen, the remaining cells can be clearly localized to the mesangium and the term "mesangial glomerulonephritis" is sometimes applied in this situation. This mesangial proliferation may not be uniform and without the knowledge of previous history, one may think of focal glomerulonephritis. In some patients the resolution is very slow, and mesangial cellularity may be present many months or many years after the acute episode. Immunoglobulins may also be found along the mesangial cells. Such patients often have mild clinical symptoms in the form of trace proteinuria or microscopic hematuria, but eventually tend to become symptom-free. It is not certain whether this healing occurs by complete resolution or by scarring and obliteration of the few more severely damaged glomeruli. In severe attacks, in addition to marked cellular proliferation and the subepithelial deposits, thrombi may occur in the capillary lumina and crescents may form in Bowman's space. The presence of one or both of these elements aggravates the prognosis and when the crescents are very numerous, severe and prolonged renal failure may ensue, sometimes ending in death. The structure of the crescent will be described in a subsequent section.

Experimentally a picture closely resembling acute proliferative glomerulonephritis occurs in serum sickness and can be produced by injection of foreign protein (e.g. bovine serum albumin) into animals (DIXON, 1965). Despite the morphologic similarity, the pathogenetic identity of serum sickness nephritis and poststreptococcal nephritis is still uncertain.

5. Extracapillary Glomerulonephritis

This form of glomerulonephritis is also known to the clinicians as "rapidly progressive glomerulonephritis." It is characterized clinically by the nephritic syndrome, sometimes insidious in onset, by anemia which may be severe, and by rapid progression (weeks or months) to renal failure. The histologic hallmark of the disease is the presence of crescents, which are large and numerous. Crescents may accompany changes in the capillary tuft or may be the sole

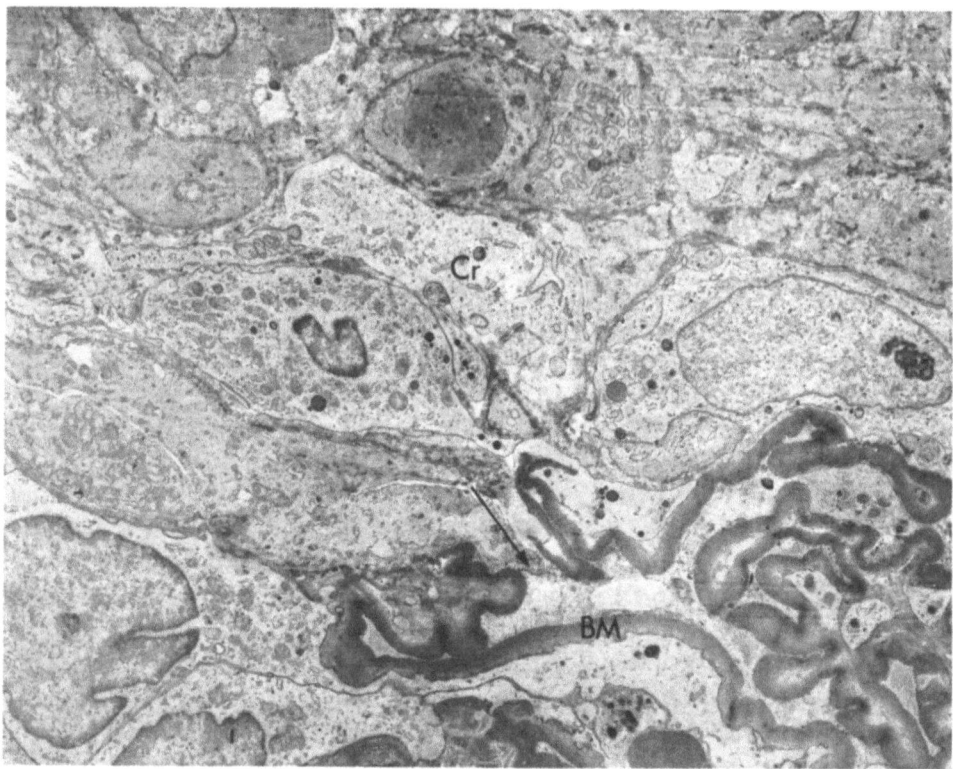

Fig. 8. Extracapillary glomerulonephritis. Cellular crescent occupies the upper part of the picture. Collapsed glomerular capillaries are seen in the lower right corner. The arrow indicates a break in the basement membrane. ×3400

or the major change in the glomerulus. The combination of extracapillary and intercapillary changes is seen in such diseases as poststreptococcal and other infectious glomerulonephritides, in lupus nephritis, occasionally in membranous nephropathy, in mesangiocapillary or lobular glomerulonephritis, and a variety of other glomerular diseases. Pure extracapillary glomerulonephritis may be either idiopathic or associated with systemic diseases such as periarteritis nodosa, Goodpasture's syndrome, or Wegener's granulomatosis.

The structure of the crescent is similar in all of these conditions with the possible exception of that in focal sclerosis (MORITA et al., 1973a). The crescent begins by proliferation of the cells of Bowman's capsule. These cells are normally flat but under the stimulus of the disease, they first become cuboidal and then form multiple layers which arrange themselves into a crescentic structure (Fig. 8). The cell cytoplasm tends to vary in appearance from very light, containing a very small number of organelles, to dark with abundant rough-surfaced endoplasmic reticulum. The cells are attached to each other by intercellular junctions but may be separated by narrow clefts containing precipitated protein material. In addition, erythrocytes and fibrin may be found between or near the proliferating cells.

There has been some question whether the visceral epithelial cells, the podocytes, participate in crescent formation. Recent studies suggest that the answer is in the affirmative (MORITA et al., 1973 a). Usually the proliferating podocytes contribute only a small fraction of the volume of the crescent though they assume the same appearance as the proliferating cells of Bowman's capsule. In some situations such as focal sclerosis, it is the podocytes which predominate in the crescents.

The purely cellular crescent is rapidly transformed into mixed (fibrocellular) form. The intercellular protein precipitates, and other debris is replaced by intercellular fibers. These at first have the appearance of branching basement membranes and stain positive with PAS method. Soon they are either transformed or are augmented by deposition of gradually thickening collagen fibers which do not stain with PAS. The typical fibrocellular crescent consists of a fine framework of fibers surrounding single and small groups of crescentic cells. With further progression the intercellular fibers increase in thickness and size, gradually compressing the cells and eventually transforming the crescent into a fibrous, acellular, or nearly acellular structure. This process may take a few weeks or a few months.

Crescents have a profound effect on the structure and function of the capillary tuft. This effect depends in part on the size of the crescent, the rapidity of its development, the concurrent changes in the capillary tuft and, as far as the function of the kidney as a whole, on the percentage of glomeruli involved by the crescentic formation. In those conditions where the disease is primarily extracapillary, the tuft responds mainly by collapse of the capillaries. However, if there is intercapillary proliferation in the tuft, the capillaries appear to resist the pressure of the crescent and may eventually recover. In pure extracapillary glomerulonephritis the presence of crescents in 50% of the glomeruli is a poor prognostic sign. In poststreptococcal glomerulonephritis recovery is possible even with 75% involvement.

The changes in the capillary tuft in the "pure" extracapillary glomerulonephritis are not limited to the collapse of capillaries but also take the form of protein deposits in and around the basement membrane. In some cases such as Goodpasture's syndrome, the deposits are distributed in a diffuse linear pattern affecting basement membranes of all capillaries. In other conditions the deposits show varying patterns of short linear stretches or irregular lumps (CHURG et al., 1973; STRIKER et al., 1973). In poststreptococcal glomerulonephritis and in other diseases in which crescents are incidental, the pattern of deposits is typical for the disease concerned.

A very interesting finding is the demonstration by electron microscopy of breaks or defects in the capillary basement membranes (MORITA et al., 1973 a; MIN et al., 1974) (Fig. 8). Such breaks occur in nearly all cases of pure extracapillary glomerulonephritis and in a lesser percentage of those associated with intercapillary proliferation. The breaks are of several morphologic varieties. Some of them may be secondary to crescent formation and some appear to precede crescent formation. It has been suggested that the early

breaks are part of the disease process and that they are responsible for leakage
of red blood cells and proteins including fibrinogen into Bowman's space.
The breaks may be caused by the action of antibasement membrane antibodies
and perhaps also by the action of leukocytes. Once red blood cells and fibrin
escape into Bowman's space they induce a proliferative reaction on the part
of the epithelial cells. This is the current explanation for the formation of
crescents, though probably any substance which is deposited in Bowman's
space through the leaking capillary walls or by disintegration of the capillary
because of necrosis and thrombosis, can produce a similar reaction.

The experimental equivalent of extracapillary glomerulonephritis is sometimes thought to be represented by Masugi (antikidney serum) nephritis
(Churg and Grishman, 1959), especially because of the linear deposits ot
immunoglobulins in the glomeruli (Dixon et al., 1971). Crescents indeed do
occur in this disease, but mesangial proliferation and capillary thrombosis
are also present (Churg et al., 1960). None of the experimental models is
identical to "pure" extracapillary glomerulonephritis in man.

6. Mesangiocapillary (Membranoproliferative) Glomerulonephritis

The term mesangiocapillary glomerulonephritis (Churg et al., 1970) denotes
a form of glomerular disease that is manifested by proteinuria often accompanied by the nephrotic syndrome, by frequent hematuria and hypertension, and by low complement levels in the blood. It is also commonly called
membranoproliferative glomerulonephritis (Habib et al., 1961), hypocomplementemic glomerulonephritis (West et al., 1965) and for certain histologic
forms, lobular glomerulonephritis. The disease occurs mainly in young people.
It is slowly progressive, ending in renal failure. However, occasional cases with
clinical and histologic recovery have been reported (Kincaid-Smith, 1973).

On light microscopy the glomeruli are large, show considerable cellularity
with enlargement of the mesangium and thickening of the capillary walls.
If the mesangium in the lobular centers is strikingly enlarged, a picture of
lobular glomerulonephritis is obtained. The term membranoproliferative
glomerulonephritis was introduced by light microscopists who thought that
they were dealing with a combination of proliferative changes and basement
membrane thickening. However, the true nature of the pathologic changes
is revealed by electron microscopy.

The characteristic feature of mesangiocapillary glomerulonephritis is the
extension of the mesangium into the capillary wall between the endothelium
and the basement membrane (Churg et al., 1965) (Fig. 9). This extension
may consist mainly of cells but is usually accompanied by mesangial matrix
and also by formation of protein deposits. The mesangial layer in the capillary
wall completely encircles the lumen or forms shorter or longer stretches along
the basement membrane. Its thickness varies considerably depending upon the
number of cells and especially the amount of matrix. The inner layer of matrix
adjoining the endothelial cells often forms a more or less continuous line which

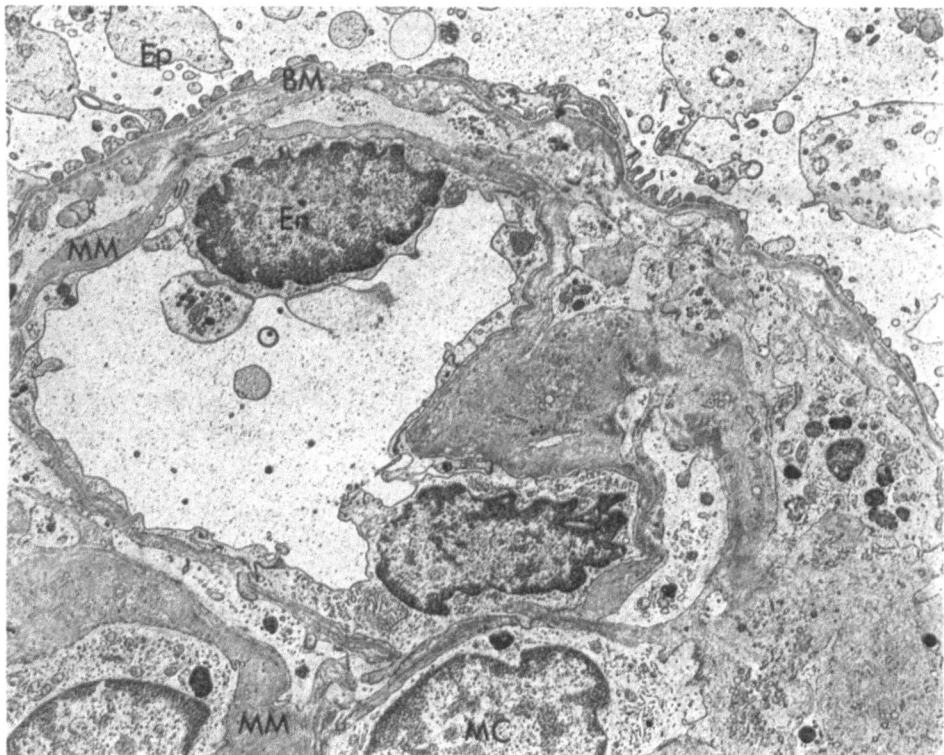

Fig. 9. Mesangiocapillary glomerulonephritis. A narrow space encircles the capillary, separating the basement membrane from a subendothelial layer of mesangial matrix. The space contains cytoplasm of mesangial cells. Proliferating mesangium occupies the right corner and lower part of the picture. ×4900

on light microscopy gives the impression of splitting or reduplication of the basement membrane. However, the latter appears quite normal by electron microscopy with perhaps slight irregularities in the outline and density. The epithelial foot processes are usually absent over shorter or longer stretches of the capillary wall. This is generally related to the degree of proteinuria and the nephrotic syndrome. The mesangium in the areas of the glomerular stalk shows proliferation of cells and deposition of matrix. Occasionally a few polymorphonuclear leukocytes may be present, but this cannot be related to the severity or duration of the disease.

The second important feature of mesangiocapillary glomerulonephritis is protein deposits. These may be found in several locations. The most striking and most common location is the subendothelial space, or more precisely the subendothelial mesangium. Such deposits are usually discontinuous, forming smaller and larger "lumps" and sometimes attaining considerable dimensions. On electron microscopy they appear homogeneous or very finely granular. By immunofluorescence they are shown to contain the C3 component of complement, and less constantly and in smaller amounts gamma globulins such as IgG and IgM and sometimes also IgA (HERMAN et al., 1970). Similar deposits may also be found in the stalk within or next to strands of the mesangial matrix. The deposits may also be present within the basement membrane, where they often assume a particularly dense appearance (see following section). Occasionally deposits filter across the basement membrane and appear in the subepithelial space.

The origin of mesangiocapillary glomerulonephritis is unknown. It sometimes begins in a manner similar to acute proliferative postinfectious glomerulo-nephritis though there is no clear-cut evidence of streptococcal etiology in most cases. It is known that in severe acute proliferative glomerulonephritis the mesangium may extend into the capillary wall, suggesting that persistence of this phenomenon may lead to mesangiocapillary glomerulonephritis. How-ever, it must be remembered that subendothelial extension of the mesangium is not specific for any disease and may be seen in a variety of situations such as lupus nephritis, hemolytic-uremic syndrome, or hepatic glomerulosclerosis.

7. Dense Deposit Disease

Dense deposits in the glomerular basement membrane were first described by BERGER and GALLE (1963). The name is suggested by their electron micro-scopic appearance. On light microscopy they stain brightly with eosin, im-parting a ribbon-like character to the capillary walls. On electron microscopy they are nearly black (Fig. 10) and often completely fill the basement mem-brane, which is no longer recognizable as such. Such basement membranes vary in thickness and outline but may show areas free of deposits. In other cases the dense deposits occupy only part of the width of the basement mem-brane or form short interrupted stretches.

Dense deposits are frequently associated with mesangiocapillary glomerulo-nephritis (HABIB et al., 1973). However there are cases where they appear to constitute the primary glomerular change, or where they accompany other forms of glomerulonephritis (JENIS et al., 1974). Dense deposits are not limited to the glomeruli but occur also in and around the tubular basement mem-branes. Their nature is presently unknown. BERGER and GALLE (1963) sug-gested that they may include glycoproteins. On immunofluorescence they sometimes contain complement (C3) but in other instances immunofluorescence microscopy gives completely negative results. The peritubular deposits contain C3 more often than the glomeruli. Dense deposits stain well with thioflavin T but this is a nonspecific reaction.

Patients with dense deposits eventually develop renal failure. It had been demonstrated that at least in some cases the deposits reappear in the transplant though at first they do not cause any obviously glomerular damage (GALLE et al., 1971). The eventual fate of such transplants is presently unknown.

8. Focal Glomerulonephritis

Focal glomerulonephritis is defined as an inflammatory process affecting only some glomeruli, while others remain normal. If some segments of glomeruli

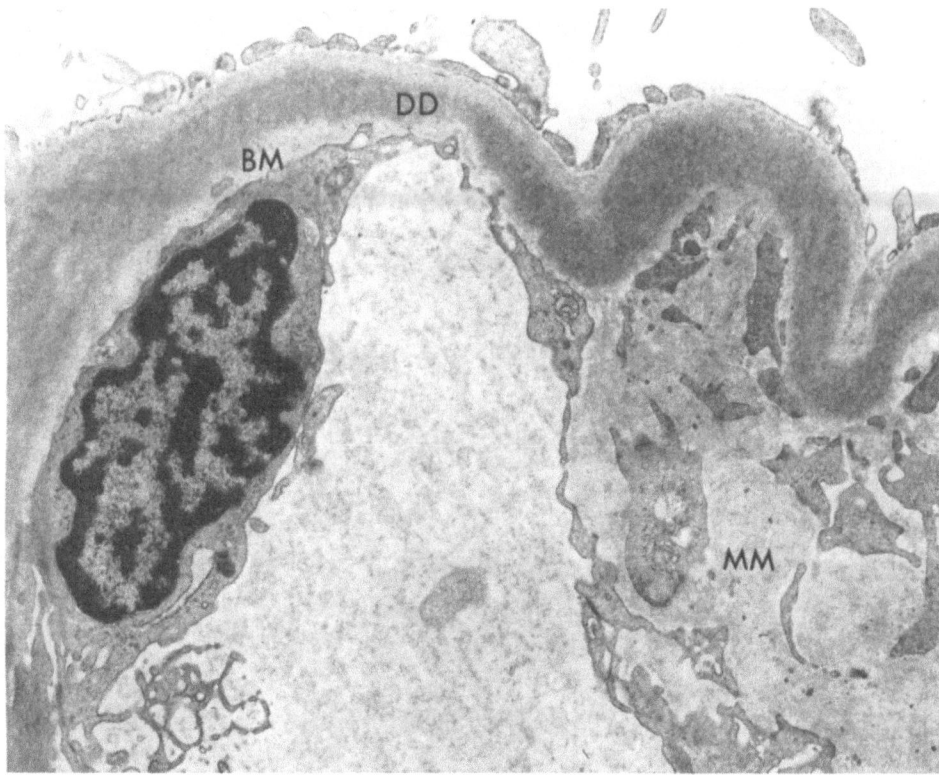

Fig. 10. Dense deposit disease. Dense deposit occupies the central part of a widened basement membrane. Proliferating mesangium is seen on the right side of the picture.
× 10660

are involved, with the remainder of the lobules being unchanged, the term "segmental" applies. Usually the lesions are both focal and segmental. The term "focal glomerulonephritis" is descriptive. The lesion may occur as a disease limited to the kidneys, or it may be part of a systemic affection. The etiology and pathogenesis vary with the disease.

Several histologic types of focal glomerulonephritis are recognized, although there may be some overlap.

Focal suppurative glomerulonephritis occurs in patients with septicemia caused by virulent microorganisms, such as *Staphylococcus aureus* (ZOLLINGER, 1966). It is characterized by polymorphonuclear leukocytic infiltration of part of a glomerulus, but soon leads to abscess formation and destruction of the whole glomerulus and surrounding tissue.

Focal proliferative glomerulonephritis is similar to diffuse proliferative, showing increase in mesangial cells and matrix. However, this proliferation is limited to only some glomeruli and to segments of these glomeruli. An example is glomerulonephritis in rheumatic fever. In this disease, focal segmental glomerulitis was observed in 2 of 22 patients; it consisted of slight segmental

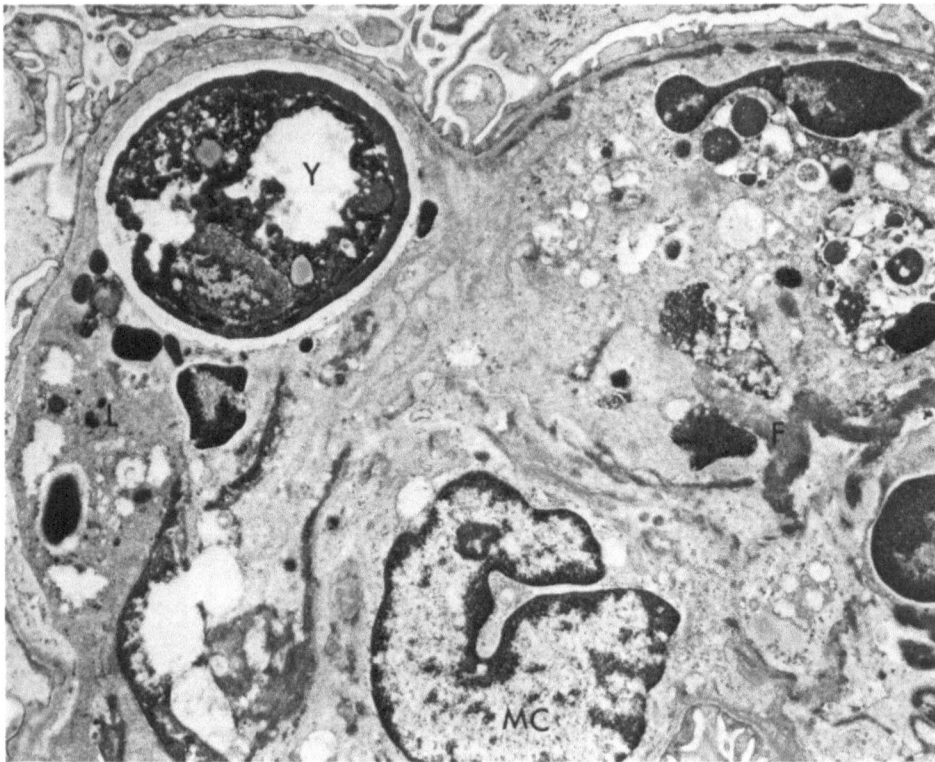

Fig. 11. Focal glomerulonephritis induced by yeast. A yeast body (upper left corner) is located in a polymorphonuclear leukocyte. Other leukocytes are also present in the picture. Fibrinoid material lies in the capillary under the endothelium along the basement membrane (upper right corner). Mesangial cell is seen at the bottom of the picture (reproduced from: Acute Focal Glomerulonephritis in the Rabbit Induced by Injection of Saccharomyces cerevisiae by Wiliam H. Johnston and Harrisson Latta, Lab. Invest. **26**, 741–754, 1972, with permission of the authors and the International Academy of Pathology). ×10000

proliferation of mesangial cells and a few small dense deposits in the mesangial matrix (Grishman et al., 1967).

An experimental model of focal glomerulonephritis in the rabbit has been produced by Johnston and Latta (1972), who injected a suspension of *Saccharomyces cerevisiae* into the renal artery. The resulting lesion resembled both the suppurative and the proliferative focal glomerulonephritis (Fig. 11) and sometimes led to focal or diffuse necrosis of the glomerulus.

The focal glomerulonephritis of *IgA-nephropathy*, first described by Berger and Hinglais (1968), is also mainly proliferative. Patients suffering from this disease have asymptomatic attacks of microscopic or gross hematuria, which are often associated with respiratory infections. On light microscopy, there may be diffuse widening of mesangial areas, but frequently there is focal or segmental proliferative glomerulonephritis involving mainly mesangial cells, while other glomeruli appear normal. Immunofluorescence microscopy shows

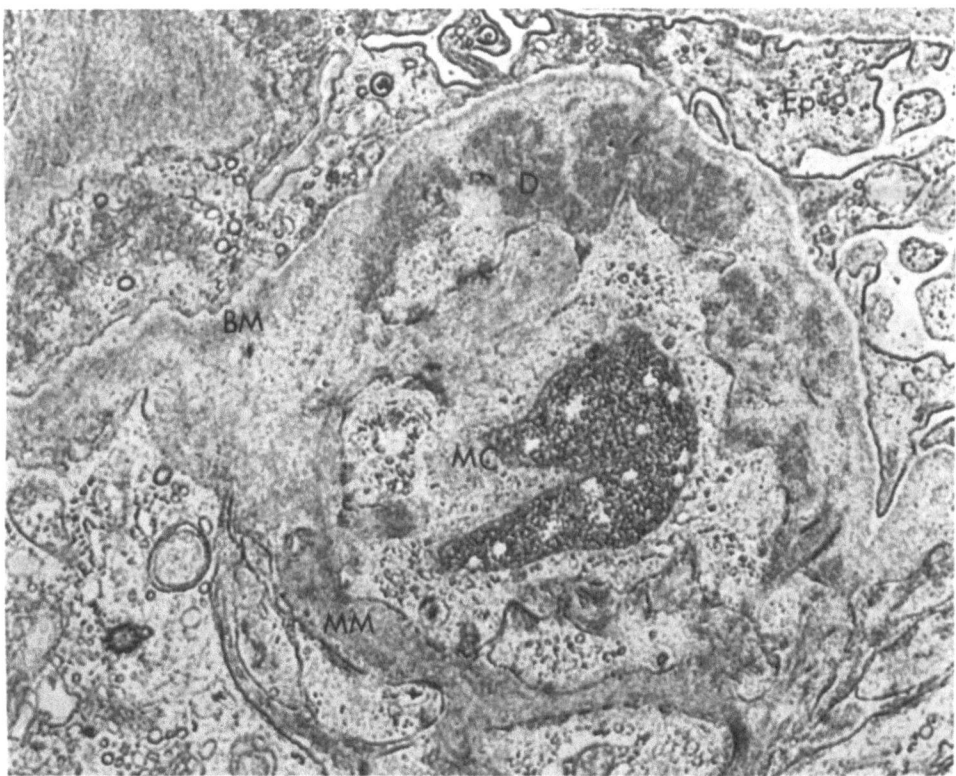

Fig. 12. Berger's disease (IgA-IgG). Fluffy deposits in the mesangium along the basement membrane. ×21 300

the presence of diffuse mesangial deposits of IgA, and sometimes IgG and C3. On electron microscopy, there is an increase of mesangial cells and matrix with "woolly" electron dense deposits in the mesangium (Fig. 12), and basement membrane of capillary loops (DAVIES *et al.*, 1973). In addition, there may be deposits in Bowman's capsule and in the arterioles entering the glomerular hilum (McCoy *et al.*, 1974). Epithelial and endothelial cells are usually unremarkable. McENERY *et al.* (1973) found deposits mainly on the mesangial side of that portion of the basement membrane that is nonfiltering. Mesangial cells are described as proliferative with an increased number of organelles and an increase in cytoplasmic mass. There is general agreement that the diagnosis of IgA-nephropathy can only be made by means of immunofluorescence microscopy.

Another form of focal, segmental proliferative glomerulonephritis was observed by VAN DE PUTTE *et al.* (1974) in a group of 22 patients with hematuria. The glomerular lesion was also associated with mesangial dense deposits which, however, on immunofluorescence microscopy contained mainly IgM, C3 and C1q.

Focal necrotizing glomerulonephritis may represent a more severe form of the preceding types. However, necrosis is most often due to capillary thrombosis and probably follows damage or destruction of the endothelium. Patients suffering from so-called *benign recurrent hematuria*, an intrinsic renal disease, frequently present focal and segmental glomerulonephritis which is characterized on light microscopy by localized areas of cellular proliferation, or small foci of necrosis and intravascular thrombosis (HEPTINSTALL, 1973). Electron microscopic studies of focal glomerulonephritis in five patients with recurrent hematuria were described by LANNIGAN and INSLEY (1965), who found focal increase of mesangial matrix, folding and thickening of basement membranes and, in one case, electron-dense mesangial deposits. In another study of 31 children (SINGER *et al.*, 1968) many dense deposits were observed, usually related to the basement membrane, either subepithelial, intramembranous, or subendothelial. Since none of these studies includes immunofluorescence examinations, it is possible that some cases actually belong in the group of IgA-nephropathy.

The classic example of a systemic disease associated with focal necrotizing glomerulonephritis is that occurring in patients with *subacute bacterial endocarditis*. This lesion was first described by LÖHLEIN (1910) as focal embolic glomerulonephritis. It was called thrombocapillaritis by ZOLLINGER (1966). Because of antibiotic treatment of the underlying endocarditis, the active lesion has become rare in recent years, and there are no conclusive reports of its electron microscopic appearance.

A histologically similar lesion may be seen in patients with *anaphylactoid purpura*. This disease, occurring mainly in children, affects the small blood vessels of the skin, gastrointestinal tract, and frequently the glomeruli. The glomerular lesions are segmental and characterized by foci of hypercellularity, sometimes associated with intracapillary thrombosis, necrosis, and small crescents. Electron microscopy reveals endothelial cell hyperplasia, increase of mesangial matrix, focal foot process fusion, and platelets and fibrin in capillary lumina. Electron dense deposits are partly mesangial, partly subendothelial, and have a fluffy, granular, and fibrillar appearance (URIZAR *et al.*, 1968). They often contain IgA in addition to IgG, C3, and fibrin.

The glomerular lesion occurring in patients with *Wegener's granulomatosis* is also segmental and necrotizing. The additional finding of granulomas and vasculitis on light microscopy may be helpful in differentiating it from other types of focal necrotizing glomerulonephritis, but these lesions may be absent in the kidney. HORN *et al.* (1974) examined 18 renal biopsies from patients with Wegener's granulomatosis by electron microscopy; they found microfocal sclerosis and subepithelial dense deposits which they interpreted as immune complexes; the antigen remains, however, unknown. The deposits correspond to coarse granules that can be visualized by staining with fluorescinated anti-IgG and complement (ROBACK *et al.*, 1969).

Polyarteritis, which is closely related to Wegener's granulomatosis, may involve the larger arteries, or sometimes the microvasculature of glomeruli. In the latter, the microscopic form of polyarteritis, the glomerular lesions are often segmental with fibrinoid necrosis and podocyte reaction, and resemble those seen in Wegener's granulomatosis.

Focal sclerosing glomerulonephritis may be the end result of focal proliferative or necrotizing glomerulonephritis, e.g. in patients with treated subacute bacterial endocarditis or healed Henoch-Schönlein syndrome. By definition, it represents an inactive process and is characterized by acellular glomerular segments showing collapse of capillaries, ingrowth of collagen fibers and adhesions to Bowman's capsule. It must be distinguished from a somewhat similar, but active disease, termed focal glomerular sclerosis.

Focal proliferative and sclerosing glomerulonephritis may on occasion be the outcome of an incompletely resolved diffuse proliferative glomerulonephritis.

The renal changes in systemic lupus erythematosus, Goodpasture's syndrome, and hereditary nephritis may, at times, be focal or segmental. These lesions are discussed in other sections.

9. Chronic Glomerulonephritis

Chronic glomerulonephritis is a term broadly applied to various advanced glomerular diseases characterized by predominance of sclerosis over cellular proliferation. Chronic glomerulonephritis may be the result of acute proliferative glomerulonephritis, mesangiocapillary glomerulonephritis, membranous nephropathy, or a variety of other diseases. Sometimes specific features may be recognized in at least some glomeruli; e.g., advanced membranous nephropathy may still show subepithelial spikes and deposits in a few capillary loops. On electron microscopy the mesangial matrix is abundant, forming thick strands and masses. It is sometimes nonhomogeneous, containing vacuoles, fragments of cytoplasm, lipid and protein deposits, and often fibrils of collagen. The process of sclerosis is irreversible and ends in total loss of glomerulus, frequently followed by absorption of Bowman's capsule and of the collapsed capillary walls.

10. Hereditary Nephritides

Of the several forms of hereditary nephritis, two show rather specific changes on electron microscopy. One of these is Alport's syndrome, which is characterized by progressive glomerular damage, especially evident in males. It begins in childhood with manifestations of hematuria and ends in renal failure at a relatively young age. Women generally do better and can survive to old age. Children usually show no significant changes on light microscopy or at most a minor thickening of capillary basement membranes. By electron microscopy this thickening is often found to be caused by extensive longitudinal splitting of the glomerular basement membrane with small dark particles located between the split layers (HINGLAIS et al., 1972; SPEAR and SLUSSER, 1972; CHURG and SHERMAN, 1973) (Fig. 13). The nature of the dark particles is uncertain; they may possibly represent trapped lipid droplets. In more severe cases disruption of the basement membrane and actual breaks

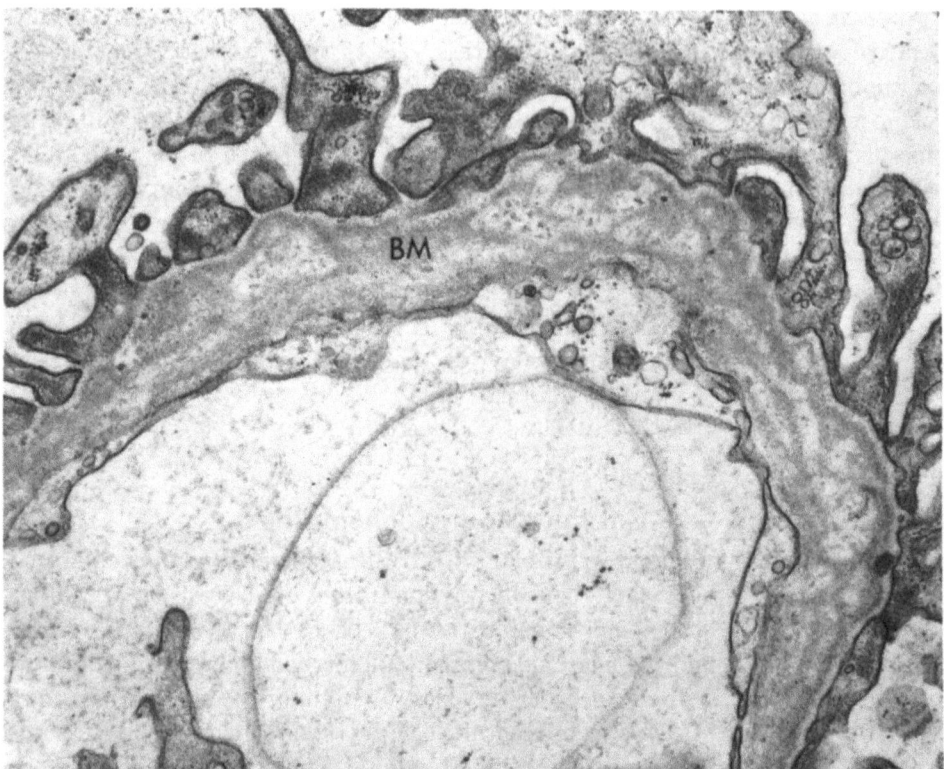

Fig. 13. Hereditary nephritis. There is longitudinal splitting of the basement membrane with clear spaces and small dark particles. ×18 700

may be seen. The lesion is probably nonspecific but when it is seen in a specific clinical setting and is associated with no, or only minimal changes by light microscopy, it may be considered diagnostic of Alport's syndrome. The basement membranes of Bowman's capsule and of the tubules may also show splitting and accumulation of lipid. Such lesions cannot be distinguished from those seen in nephrotic syndrome of various etiologies. However, they may be considered significant if the blood lipid levels are normal.

The second disease that shows characteristic electron microscopic changes is the nail-patella syndrome. In addition to changes in the bones and joints, these patients sometimes show progressive renal disease which in its advanced stages resembles chronic glomerulonephritis. In the early stages the only visible lesion may be thickening of glomerular basement membranes. On electron microscopy the thickening is due to deposition of thick bundles of collagen within the lamina densa (Fig. 14). Similar bundles may also be seen in the mesangial matrix (Ben-Bassat *et al.*, 1971; Morita *et al.*, 1973 b) (Fig. 14).

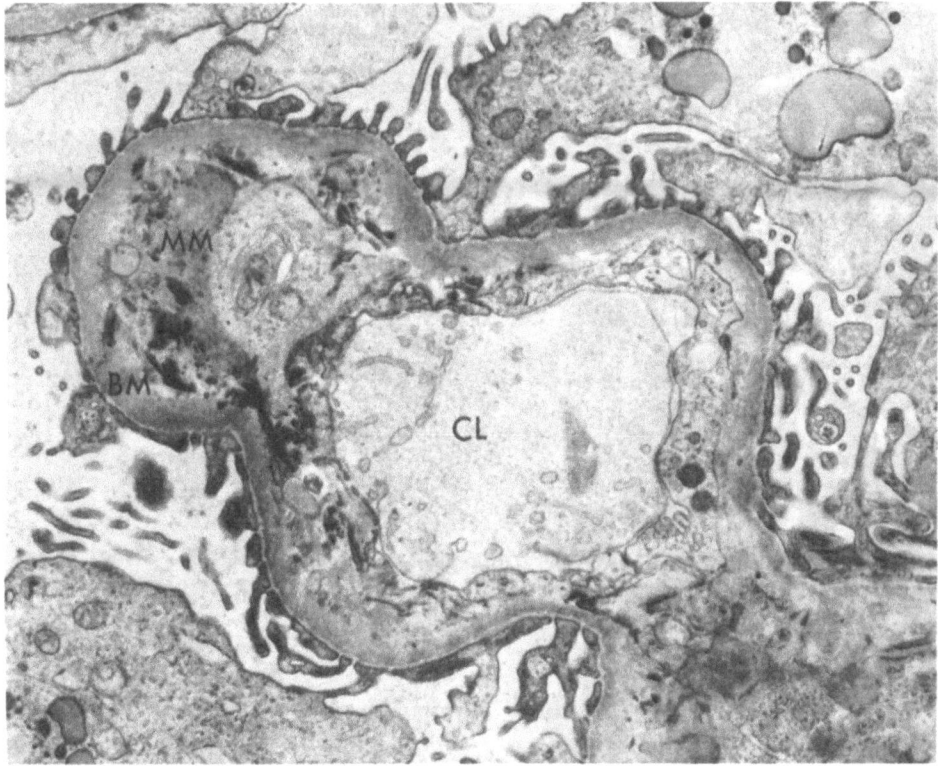

Fig. 14. Nail patella syndrome. Widening of basement membrane with dark bundles of collagen in the basement membrane and in the mesangial matrix. Phosphotungstic hematoxylin stain. ×7 000

III. Glomerulonephritis of Systemic Diseases

1. Lupus Nephritis

The study of lupus nephritis by electron microscopy has contributed greatly to the understanding of this disease. Lupus nephritis is one of the classic immune complex nephritides, antigen and antibody having both been recovered from the kidney (KOFFLER et al., 1967). It is presumed that these are combined into complexes and appear structurally as electron dense deposits (EDD) which correspond to immune globulins and complement demonstrated by fluorescence microscopy (MELLORS et al., 1957). Dense deposits were visualized for the first time by FARQUHAR et al. (1957) who correlated them with fibrinoid seen by light microscopy. Electron microscopy serves to localize these deposits in relation to cellular and extracellular components of the glomerulus. Thus, it was found that EDD may be present in the mesangium, and in the subendothelial and the subepithelial spaces. The amount and localization of the deposits are probably responsible for the type of lupus nephritis in an individual patient.

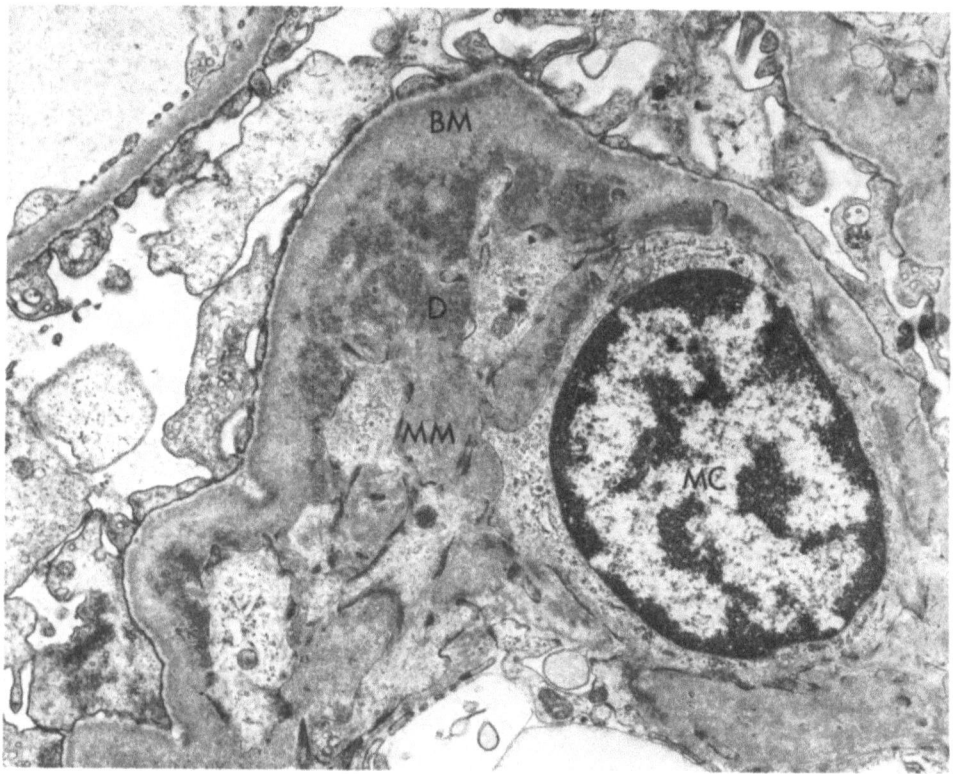

Fig. 15. Lupus nephritis. Mesangial deposits along the basement membrane and the mesangial matrix. ×12200

We distinguish five forms of lupus nephritis: minimal, focal, mesangial, diffuse, and membranous (McClusky, 1970; Koffler et al., 1969). In the first two groups there are usually few (or no) deposits. Mesangial lupus nephritis shows mainly mesangial deposits; the membranous form, subepithelial and mesangial deposits, and diffuse lupus nephritis, a mixture of subendothelial, subepithelial, and mesangial deposits. The presence of this mixture of deposits is highly suggestive, though not absolutely diagnostic, for lupus nephritis. It has been postulated that the localization of deposits depends on the molecular size of the immune complexes (Germuth and Rodriguez, 1973).

Mesangial deposits (Fig. 15) are the most common, are often present even in asymptomatic minimal disease, and are probably caused by the phagocytic activity of the mesangial cells which remove these complexes from the circulation. "Wire loops" are massive subendothelial deposits of proteins (Fig. 16) and were originally recognized on light microscopy as a characteristic feature of lupus nephritis (Klemperer et al., 1941). They are usually found in active diffuse lupus nephritis and connote a poor prognosis (Dujovne et al., 1972; Comerford and Cohen, 1967; Grishman et al., 1973). Comerford and Cohen (1967) were the first to correlate the localization of deposits with the clinical presentation of the disease. It has also been shown that the number of deposits

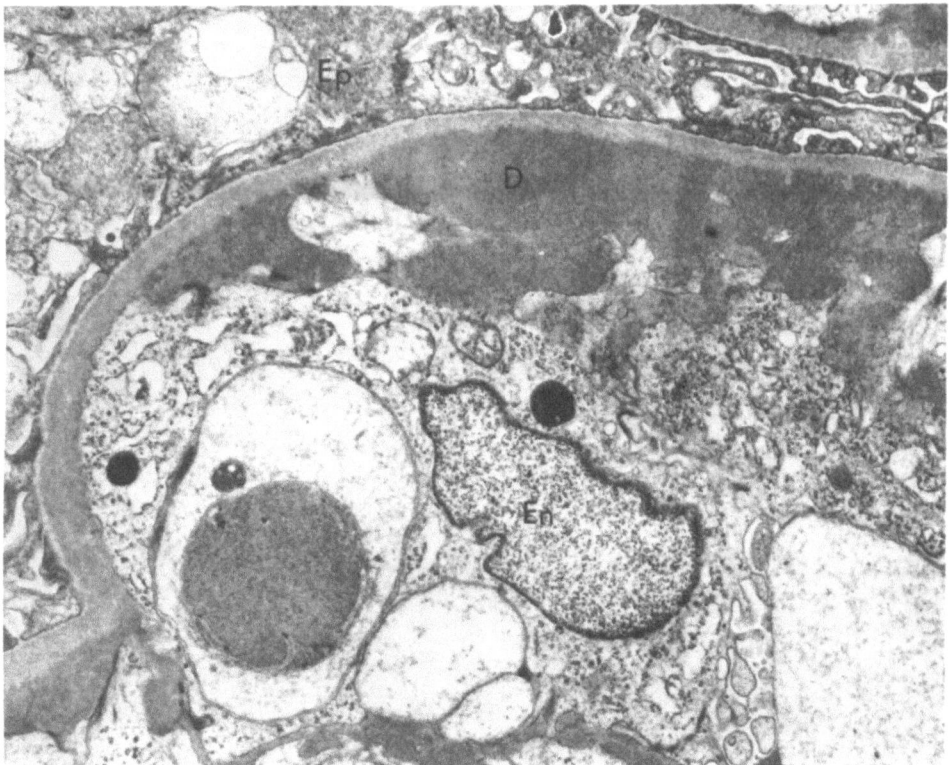

Fig. 16. Lupus nephritis. Large subendothelial deposit ("wire-loop"). ×13800

can be related to the outcome. In general, patients with few deposits have better prognosis than those with large, massive deposits, who often show progression of the disease.

Membranous lupus nephritis resembles membranous nephropathy clinically and histologically, but is usually accompanied by mesangial deposits, which are extremely rare in nonspecific membranous nephropathy. Patients with this type of lesion are usually nephrotic and may have a prolonged course lasting many years. While the pure membranous form of lupus nephritis is rare (5% in our experience), focal subepithelial deposits are common, occurring in about 25% of cases. Electron dense deposits, especially subendothelial, often decrease after immunosuppressive treatment, but this does not usually prevent the nonspecific mesangial proliferation and scarring (DUJOVNE et al., 1972; GRISHMAN et al., 1973). If patients die in renal failure after many years of steroid therapy, the kidneys are usually small and show the picture of nonspecific chronic glomerulonephritis with few deposits.

Electron dense deposits in varying amounts are also found around tubular basement membranes, capillaries, and in the wall of larger blood vessels.

Most of the deposits appear finely granular, but occasionally they show organized "fingerprint-like" structures (Fig. 17) (Grishman et al., 1967) which

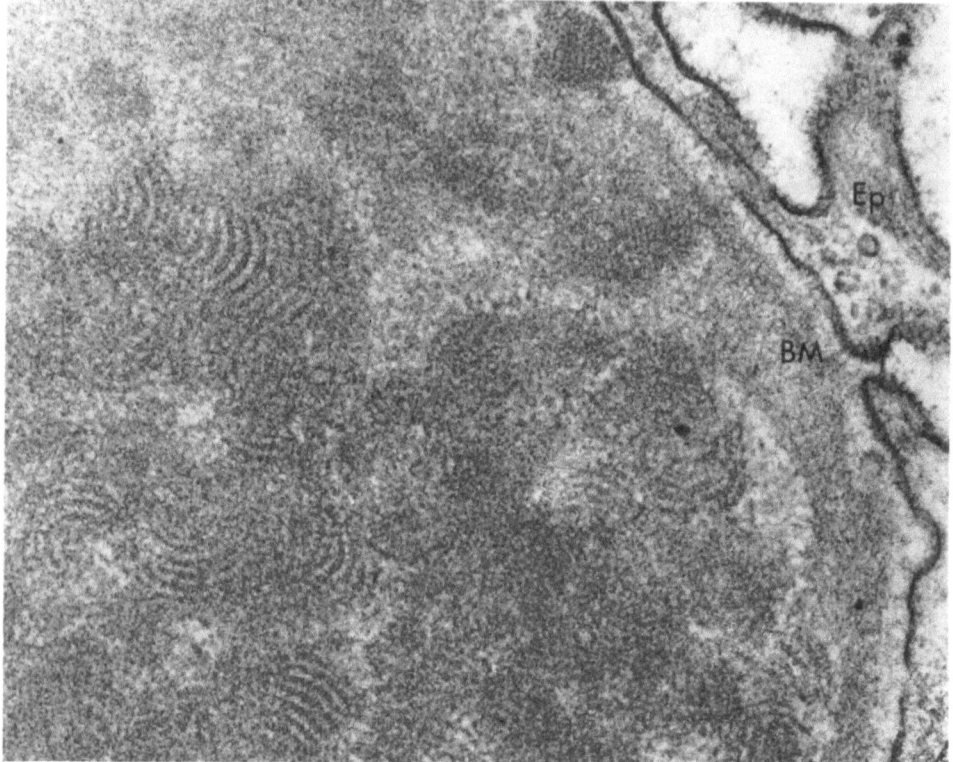

Fig. 17. Lupus nephritis. Subendothelial deposit of "fingerprint" pattern. ×65000

are possibly due to the presence of phospholipids (WOOD, 1972) and have been experimentally produced by repeated immunization of mice with egg albumin (OKUMURA, 1973). Though most of the fingerprint-like deposits are found in patients with systemic lupus erythematosus, they are not specific for this disease, having been observed also in patients with other types of glomerulonephritis.

Cellular changes found in lupus nephritis consist of increase and enlargement of mesangial cells, swelling of endothelial and epithelial cells and, in patients with marked proteinuria, loss of foot processes. All cells show abundant cytolysosomes and prominent mitochondria. Frequently, there is circumferential subendothelial extension of mesangial cells resembling mesangiocapillary glomerulonephritis. It is believed that most of these cellular changes are a secondary response to the deposition of immune complexes. The glomerular basement membrane is frequently thickened.

Another electron microscopic feature found in almost all cases of lupus nephritis is membrane-enclosed tubular arrays within the cytoplasm of endothelial and sometimes other cells (GYORKEY et al., 1972) (Fig. 18). If a sufficient number of glomeruli are examined, tubular arrays may be found in close to 100% of patients. They may also be found in endothelial cells of intertubular capillaries, as well as skin, muscle, and liver capillaries (DUBOIS and ARTER-

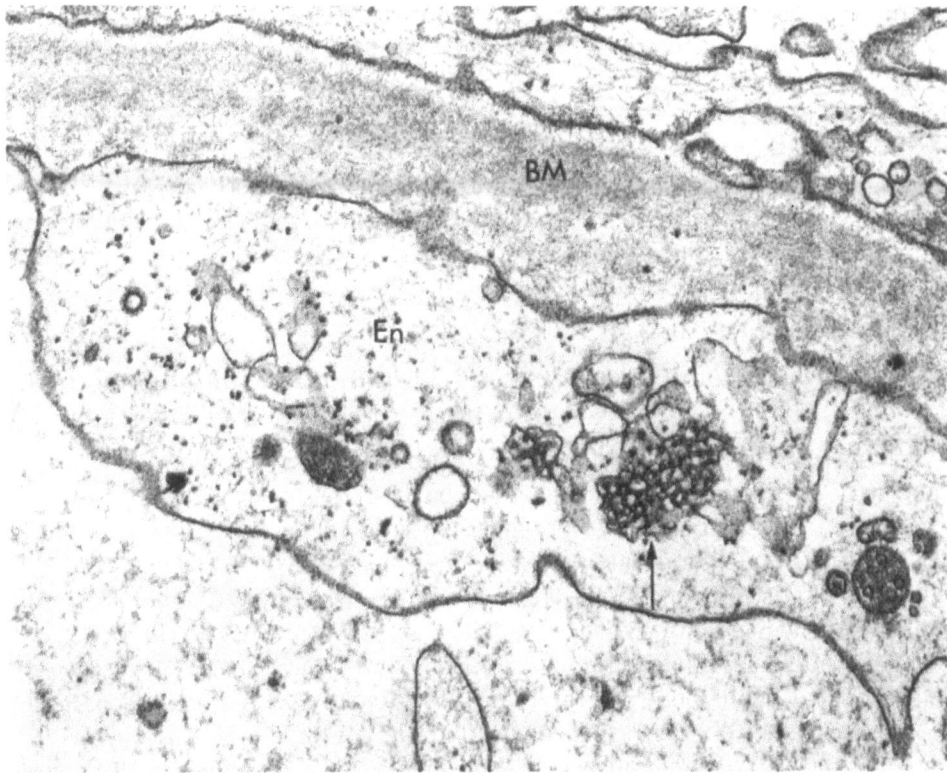

Fig. 18. Lupus nephritis. A myxovirus-like structure in an endothelial cell is indicated by an arrow. ×38850

BERRY, 1974). They are, however, not specific for lupus, having been demonstrated also in other renal diseases. Nevertheless, their prevalence in patients with systemic lupus erythematosus serves as a valuable adjunct in the diagnosis of this disease. Morphologically, the tubular structures resemble myxovirus particles, but are composed mainly of phospholipid and acid glycoprotein (SCHAFF et al., 1973). It is unlikely that they are of viral origin since they have been recently produced experimentally in cultured lymphocytes (POTHIER et al., 1973). They may be related to the synthesis of gamma globulin, or may represent a cell organelle formed in endothelial cells in response to injury.

Hematoxylin bodies, which are the only specific feature of systemic lupus erythematosus, have been described in electron microscopic investigations (COMERFORD and COHEN, 1967), but are difficult to recognize structurally.

There are several spontaneous diseases in animals which resemble human systemic lupus erythematosus and which are accompanied by glomerulonephritis. In dogs the disease is manifested by autoimmune hemolytic anemia, thrombocytopenia, and positive lupus preparation. The glomerular lesions include "wire-loops" and progressive inflammation and sclerosis leading to renal failure (LEWIS et al., 1965). In New Zealand mice, particularly in the hybrid NZB/W, deposits of gamma globulin and complement as well as DNA are seen along the glomerular basement membranes and in the mesangium. The animals have hemolytic anemia and die in renal failure (Bielschowsky et al., 1959). There are suggestions that the disease is induced or at least aggravated by viral infection or infections (Mellors et al., 1971; Tonietti et al., 1970). In the Aleutian mink the disease is definitely caused by virus (ADV) (Henson et al., 1962; Gorham et al., 1964) and is characterized by glomerulonephritis resembling lupus nephritis, by arteritis, and by plasma cell infiltrates in many organs.

2. Hemolytic Uremic Syndrome and Thrombotic Thrombocytopenic Purpura

Hemolytic uremic syndrome (HUS) and thrombotic thrombocytopenic purpura (TTP) are two diseases that have many clinical and laboratory features in common. They also produce similar histologic lesions in the kidney. Hemolytic uremic syndrome was first described by Gasser et al. (1955) in children but is also known to occur in adults. It is characterized by acute anemia of the hemolytic type with fragmented and distorted erythrocytes and evidence of hemolysis, by thrombocytopenia, and by acute renal insufficiency. Other organs in the body are rarely involved and then only to a mild degree. The main clinical manifestations of TTP are similar and also include hemolytic anemia and thrombocytopenia. Renal insufficiency, though, is rare and involvement of other organs, especially of the central nervous system, is very common. TTP occurs primarily in adults.

On histologic examination the kidney shows lesions in the glomeruli and in the arteries and arterioles. Tubules are involved only secondarily. This consists of patchy or more extensive necrosis and may be accompanied by necrosis of the glomeruli up to the point of extensive cortical necrosis.

The glomerular lesions are often subtle and may be minimal on light microscopy (Habib et al., 1967). In more severe cases thrombi may be present in the capillary lumina. The characteristic feature of the disease is found on electron microscopy. It consists of swelling and separation of the endothelium from the basement membrane (Vitsky et al., 1969) and sometimes focal destruction of the endothelial cells (Franklin et al., 1972). The subendothelial space becomes filled with pale, finely granular (Fig. 19), or sometimes finely fibrillar material occasionally with a suggestion of periodicity. This material stains strongly by immunofluorescence methods for fibrinogen or fibrin (Koffler and Paronetto, 1966). It varies in amount with the severity and duration of illness and tends to disappear with recovery but may persist for a considerable length of time. Mesangial cells may invade the subendothelial space and in more advanced cases mesangial matrix is laid down in a manner reminiscent of mesangiocapillary glomerulonephritis. Glomerular thrombi contain fibrin. They may cause complete obstruction and necrosis of the glomerulus and of the corresponding tubules.

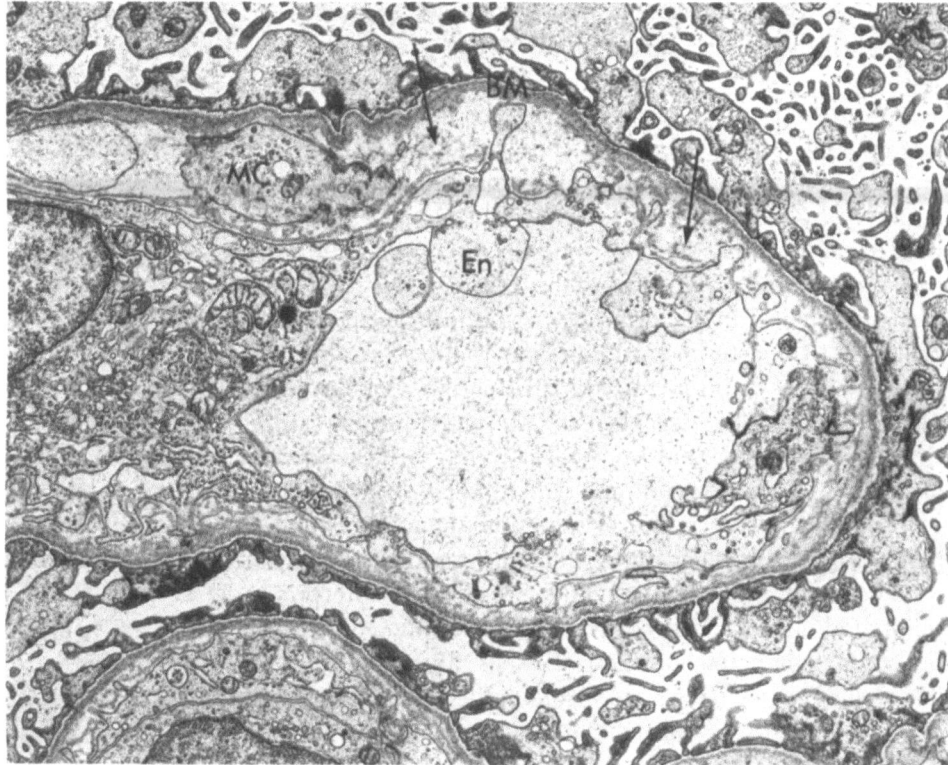

Fig. 19. Hemolytic uremic syndrome. The endothelium is separated from the basement membrane by very pale fluffy deposits (arrow) and cytoplasm of mesangial cells. ×6850

In addition to the endothelial detachment and capillary thrombosis, glomeruli may show other changes, some of which are recognizable on light microscopy. Fragmented red cells are noted in some cases. Cellular proliferation is rare in the early stage and may take the form of focal collections of polymorphonuclear leukocytes or of mononuclear cells, either endothelial or mesangial in origin. If the glomerular process does not resolve, a more striking, mainly mesangial proliferation occurs, simulating glomerulonephritis on light microscopy. However, on electron microscopy the presence of endothelial detachment and the characteristic granular or fibrillar pale material in the subendothelial spaces will establish the diagnosis. The arterial lesions involve arcuate and interlobular arteries and arterioles. These lesions are in many ways analogous to those in the glomerulus. There may be luminal thrombosis progressing to organization. The arterial walls in larger arteries show mucoid intimal swelling and fibrosis, and those of small arteries and arterioles, hyalinization and fibrinoid necrosis. In some cases electron microscopy reveals separation of the endothelium with accumulation of pale material in the subendothelial space in a manner closely reminiscent of the glomerular lesion. A very characteristic change is an aneurysm of the afferent arterioles at the point of entry into the glomerulus (Orbison, 1952). The aneurysm is frequently filled with thrombus, which may undergo "glomeruloid" organization (Umlas, 1972).

Progression of the glomerular lesions results in bland sclerosis with partial preservation of the lobular architecture. This process seems to ensue from organization of subendothelial and probably mesangial deposits. If a sufficient number of glomeruli are affected, permanent renal failure will ensue.

Thrombosis and organization will often result in permanent narrowing of the arterial lumina and consequent hypertension. This hypertension may attain malignant levels and lead to a variety of complications. In such cases fibrinoid necrosis of the arterioles and intimal swelling and fibrosis of the arteries may dominate the picture, and the distinction from primary malignant hypertension is often difficult even on the electron microscopic level, particularly since primary malignant hypertension may be accompanied by manifestations of hemolytic uremic syndrome (Linton et al., 1969).

The renal changes in TTP are similar in all histologic details but usually much milder. However aneurysms of afferent arterioles are not infrequent.

The hemolytic uremic syndrome is often interpreted as a form of disseminated intravascular coagulation (DIC) and compared with the experimental Shwartzman phenomenon (Erslev and Shapiro, 1971). While there are many similarities, there are also significant differences: In contrast to DIC, consumption of coagulation factors in hemolytic uremic syndrome is small and inconstant. In the Shwartzman reaction, glomerular capillaries become filled with fibrin exhibiting fibrillar structure with defined periodicity, and subendothelial deposits, if they occur, also consist of the same material. In hemolytic uremic syndrome, as has already been shown, the subendothelial deposits are usually granular or structureless, and do not stain for fibrin; intraluminal thrombi are relatively infrequent. There are suggestions that in hemolytic uremic syndrome the primary event is endothelial damage with secondary deposition of complete or incomplete coagulation products. However, it is possible that hemolytic uremic syndrome differs from DIC not so much in the initiating event as in the degree and speed, and perhaps, deviation of coagulation process from its usual pathway.

3. Radiation Nephritis

Accidental or deliberate exposure of the kidney to therapeutic radiation induces changes in the glomeruli, tubules and blood vessels whose severity varies with the dose and which tend to progress with time. On light microscopy tubules and arteries appear to be primarily affected. The glomerular changes, often interpreted as secondary or late, are manifested by progressive sclerosis with little or no cellular proliferation, by thickening of the capillary walls, and by increase of the mesangial matrix. There are very few data on the electron microscopic appearance of glomeruli in human radiation nephritis. One case was studied by Rosen et al. (1964), who found mesangial ingrowth

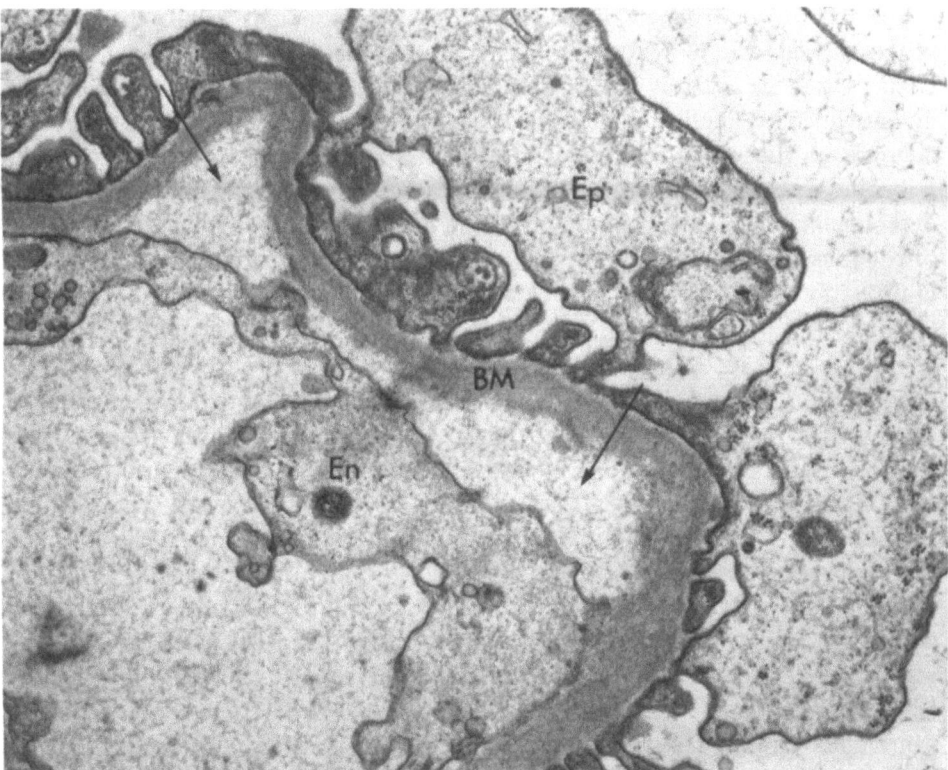

Fig. 20. Experimental radiation nephritis. Endothelium is detached from the basement membrane. The resulting space (arrows) is filled by fine protein precipitate of the same density as that in the capillary lumen. (Courtesy of Dr. A. MADRAZO.) ×21 350

between the endothelium and the basement membrane and deposition of a large amount of material apparently representing new basement membrane.

The explanation of these changes is provided by experimental studies that suggest that one of the earliest radiation effects (MADRAZO *et al.*, 1969, 1970) is detachment of the endothelium from the basement membrane of the glomerular capillaries (Fig. 20), and formation of new basement membrane by the detached endothelial cells. The space between the two basement membranes becomes filled by proliferating mesangium or by multiple layers of basement membrane. The glomerular mesangium shows slight cellular proliferation accompanied by lysis of the mesangial matrix. Later, mesangial sclerosis supervenes. Radiation also affects the glomerular cells, which show distortion of mitochondria, accumulation of vacuoles and lipid droplets, and nuclear pleomorphism. The cells either recover or regenerate and retain their ability to form intercellular material, i.e. basement membranes and mesangial matrix.

Tubular cells also undergo degeneration and become detached from their basement membranes. If severely affected, the cells disappear completely, leaving empty skeletons of basement membranes. If the damage is less severe, the recovering or regenerating cells form a new basement membrane and the space between the new and the old membrane becomes filled by collagenous tissue. Often recovery is incomplete, the tubules have an atrophic appearance and are lined by small cuboidal cells. The arterial lesions, consisting of extensive necrosis of the wall accompanied by thrombosis, usually appear late, contributing to the final destruction of the kidney. In the early stages only focal detachment of the endothelium from the arterial wall and some degeneration of the muscularis may be noted. The slow development of the vascular lesions is probably due to the low replication rate of their cells.

4. Hepatic Glomerulosclerosis

Hepatic glomerulosclerosis is defined as glomerular disease accompanying acute and chronic disturbances of the liver. Glomerular changes occur in liver cirrhosis (Bloodworth and Sommers, 1959) but also in acute viral hepatitis and in toxic liver damage (Sakaguchi et al., 1965a; Fisher and Perez-Stable, 1968). On light microscopy these changes are usually mild, but occasionally are severe enough to be described as glomerulonephritis (Fig. 21). In the mild cases the only prominent feature by light microscopy is thickening of the mesangial stalk with perhaps a suggestion of thickening of capillary walls. On electron microscopy several types of deposits may be observed in subepithelial spaces and the mesangium. One type is represented by fine osmiophilic granules 5–10 nm in diameter without a definite limiting membrane. A second type of deposit is amorphous and the third type consists of very dense (black) particles, rounded or irregular and measuring up to 100 nm in diameter. These particles are found mainly in the mesangial matrix.

In the more severe, particularly in the chronic cases, in addition to the deposits, there is an obvious increase in the amount of mesangial matrix (Fig. 21). The basement membranes of the capillaries also become thickened, though at this stage it is not always clear whether this thickening is due to the increase in the amount of basement membrane material or to organization of the previously laid down deposits. Quite often the mesangial matrix contains lamellated deposits of calcium.

With further progression of the disease the capillary wall becomes involved. This is manifested by considerable thickening and progressive irregularity of the basement membrane with focal indentations (notches) on the epithelial side and focal loss of foot processes. If the patient develops massive proteinuria or nephrotic syndrome, the loss of foot processes becomes diffuse.

Lesions of renal glomeruli often accompany experimentally induced liver disease. Ligation of the bile duct in the rat causes temporary jaundice and deposition of dense black particles 40–60 nm in diameter between the endothelium and the basement membrane, apparently within the lamina rara interna (Sakaguchi et al., 1965b). These granules are generally short lived and tend to disappear within 2–3 weeks. If the jaundice persists, moderate thickening of the capillary basement membranes, focal loss of foot processes, and some mesangial increase may be noted (Fig. 22).

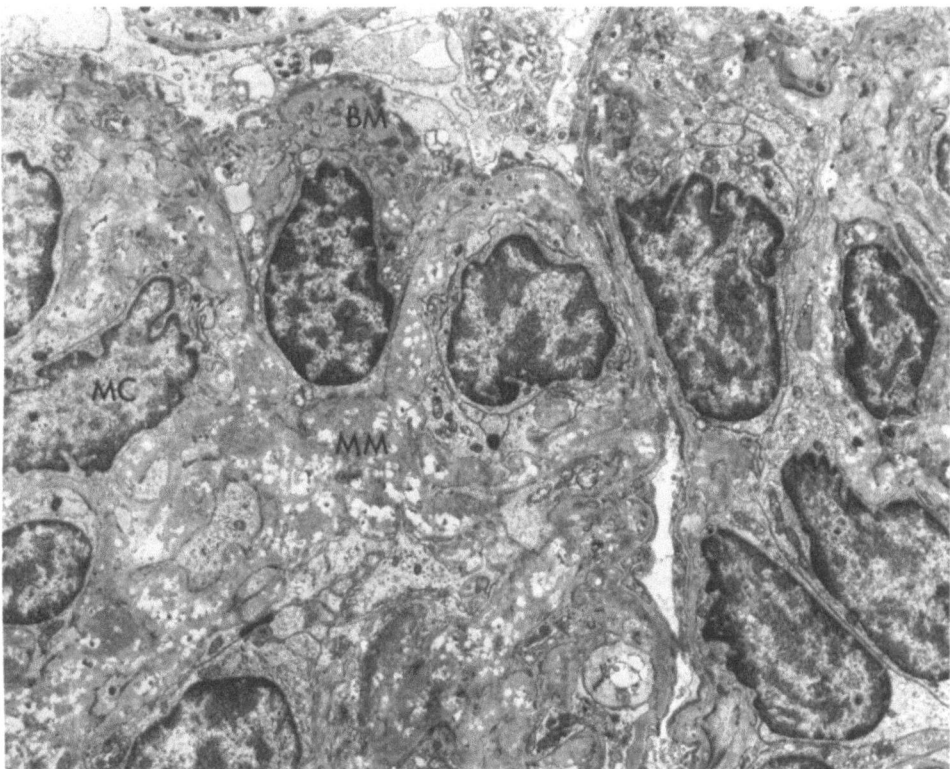

Fig. 21. Severe hepatic glomerulosclerosis. There is proliferation of mesangial cells and increase of mesangial matrix. Note marked "mottling" of the mesangial matrix. Many of the clear spaces contain small dark particles. ×4 500

In animals in which chronic liver disease has been induced by administration of carbon tetrachloride or of ethionine, glomeruli show progressive thickening of the mesangium and of the capillary basement membrane with loss of foot processes (SAKAGUCHI et al., 1964). This is accompanied by accumulation of amorphous proteinaceous material and of osmiophilic granules 5–10 nm in diameter between the endothelium and the basement membrane and in the mesangium. These deposits appear to undergo organization, thus adding to the thickening of the basement membrane and to the increase of the mesangial matrix.

5. Pre-eclamptic Nephropathy

The characteristic feature of pre-eclamptic nephropathy is an enlarged, bloodless glomerulus that shows little or no cellular proliferation. By light microscopy the cause of these changes is not easily discerned. However, electron microscopy clearly demonstrates two processes that are responsible for the obstruction of the capillaries and the thickening of the mesangium. One is a striking edema of endothelial and mesangial cells, accompanied by

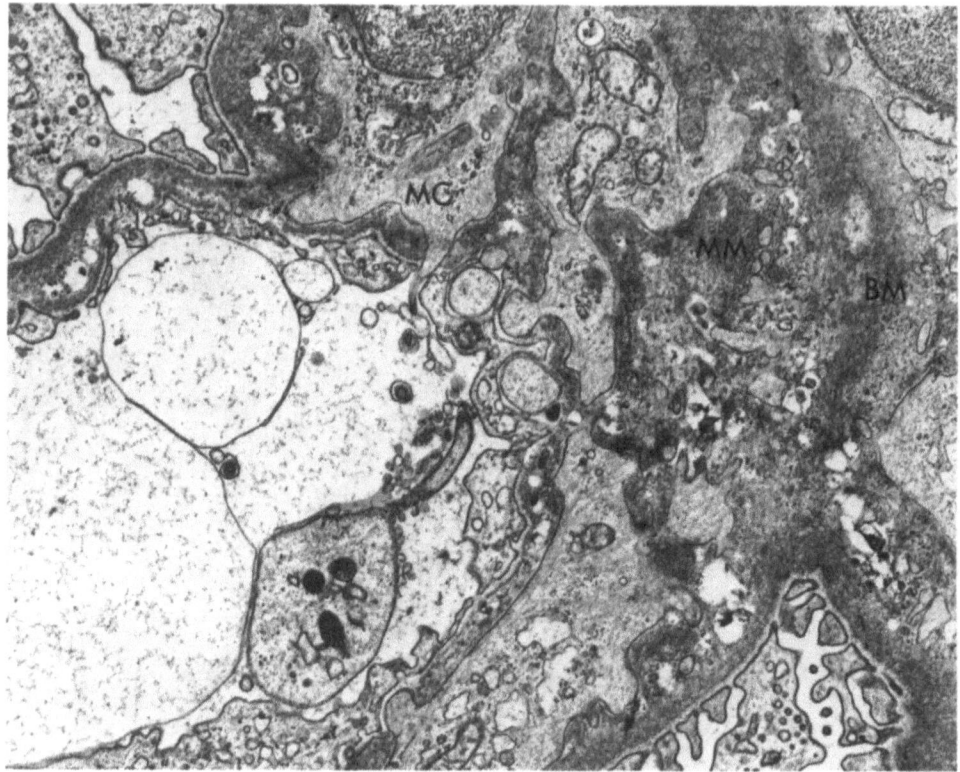

Fig. 22. Experimental bile duct ligation. There is focal proliferation of mesangium with many clear spaces in the matrix and dense particles. Note similarity to the human hepatic glomerulosclerosis. (Courtesy of Dr. H. Sakaguchi.) ×15 300

formation of intracytoplasmic vacuoles and intraluminal blebs (Spargo et al., 1959). Edema of the mesangial cells imparts a reticulated appearance to the mesangium. The second factor responsible for the narrowing of the capillary lumina is subendothelial and mesangial deposits (Mautner et al., 1962; Pirani et al., 1963; Faith and Trump, 1966) (Fig. 23). These tend to be finely granular and of moderate density, though some may be dark and coarse. A mixture of lighter and darker deposits may be found in the same capillary. The presence of deposits is usually associated with proteinuria though this is seldom severe enough to cause more than a focal loss of foot processes. By immunofluorescence the deposits consist mainly of fibrinogen or fibrinogen derivatives (Morris et al., 1964). Sometimes gamma globulins may also be present but inconstantly and in small amounts. The swollen endothelial and mesangial cells also contain material that has immunofluorescent properties of fibrinogen derivatives. No actual fibrin is found in pre-eclamptic nephropathy, but in eclampsia thrombi may occur in the glomerular capillaries. The subendothelial deposits are short-lived and usually disappear after the delivery with improvement in the patient's condition. The cellular edema may persist longer, occasionally for

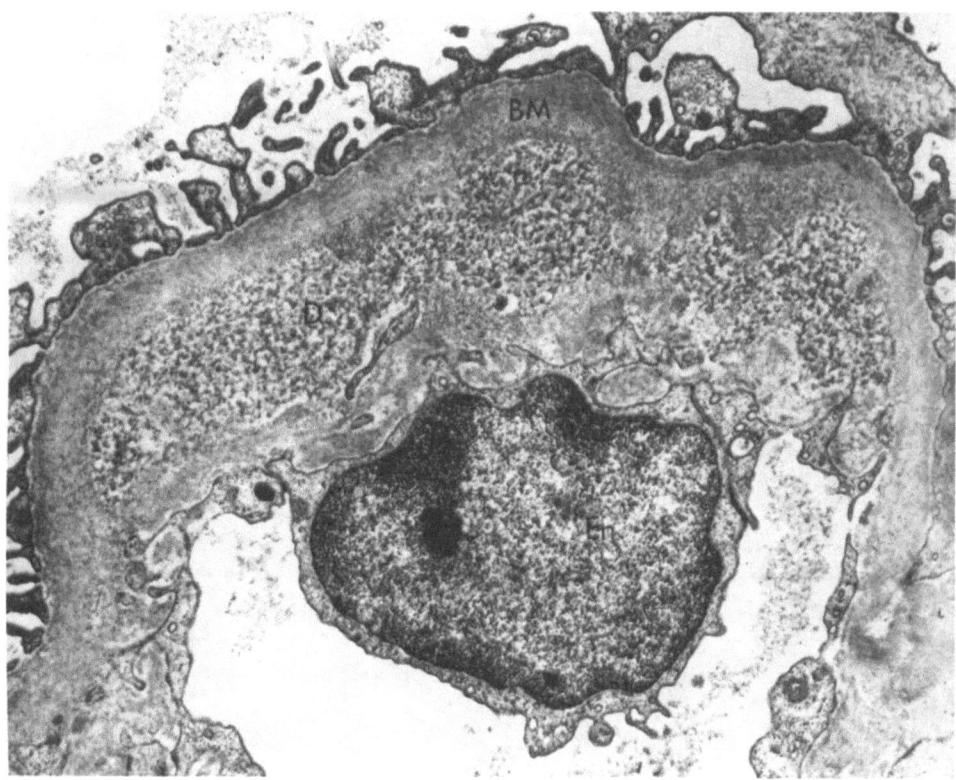

Fig. 23. Toxemia of pregnancy, resolving stage. The capillary lumen is patent, the endothelial cell is of approximately normal size. There is granular deposit in the overlying mesangial space. ×11600

months or years after the delivery. Pregnant sheep kept on low protein diet and actively exercised develop renal lesions similar to those of human pre-eclampsia (FERRIS *et al.*, 1969).

IV. Transplantation

Electron microscopy has served as an important aid in the analysis of glomerular lesions of transplanted kidneys, since on light microscopy, many of these lesions resemble various types of glomerulonephritis.

The changes in transplant-glomerulopathy have recently been described in great detail by ZOLLINGER *et al.* (1973) in this journal. We will therefore limit ourselves to a brief discussion. In general, our findings agree with those of ZOLLINGER'S.

The most striking ultrastructural change in glomeruli is the variable thickening of the lamina rara interna of the capillary basement membrane (HAMBURGER *et al.*, 1972; HULME *et al.*, 1972), which can take on extraordinary proportions in long-term survivors (BUSCH *et al.*, 1971) (Fig. 24). The thickening is due to subendothelial accumulation of electron lucent flocculent material,

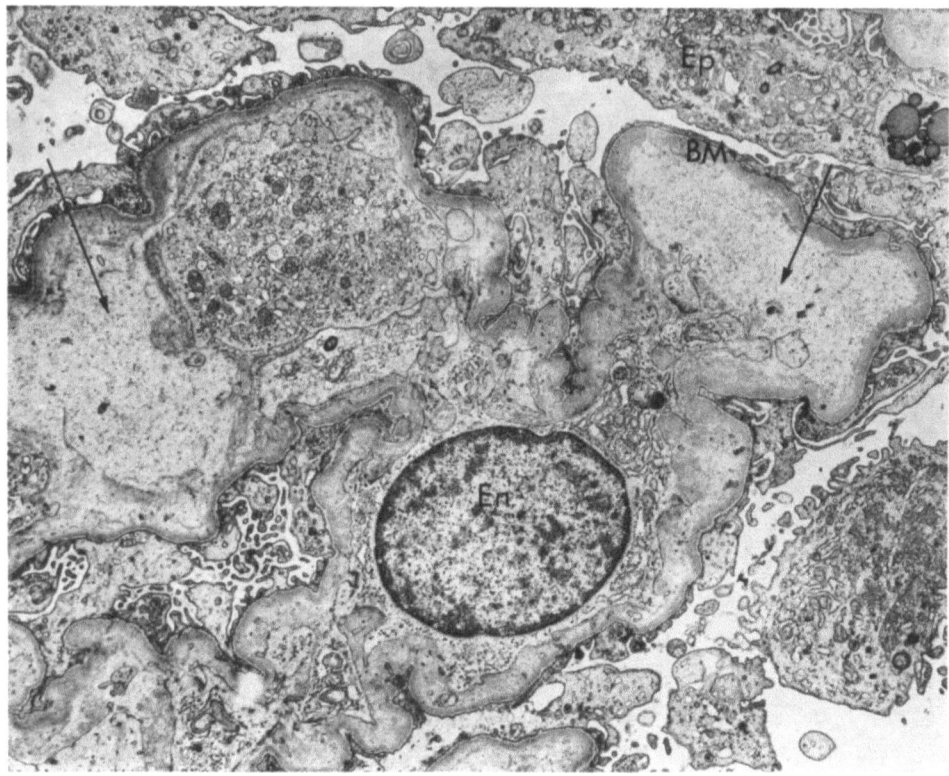

Fig. 24. Transplant glomerulopathy. Marked widening of the lamina rara interna (arrows), proliferation of endothelial cells and focal effacement of foot processes. ×4800

which may contain IgM, IgA, fibrin, and complement (Andres et al., 1970; Porter et al., 1968), as well as remnants of cytoplasmic structures. This process leads to marked narrowing of capillary lumina. Newly formed thin lamellae of basement membrane are sometimes present under the endothelium.

Electron dense deposits may be found in various locations along the basement membrane, and may, on occasion, be so numerous as to resemble membranous nephropathy (Olsen et al., 1974). Endothelial cells are usually swollen and vacuolated. The mesangium becomes slightly enlarged, and mesangial cell processes may extend into the subendothelial spaces. The podocytes show swelling and variable degrees of foot process loss.

Spherical particles (Burkholder et al., 1973) of various sizes may be present subepithelially or within the basement membrane (Rowlands et al., 1970; Olsen et al., 1974). It has been suggested that such particles represent herpes virus capsids (Busch et al., 1971), though this is doubted by other authors (Olsen et al., 1974).

The arteries and arterioles show marked intimal thickening, insudation of plasma elements into the wall, and narrowing of the lumina, causing additional ischemic changes in glomeruli.

The mononuclear cells infiltrating the interstitium and tubules have been identified electron microscopically (ROSENAU et al., 1969; HAMBURGER, 1972) as large lymphocytes with abundant cytoplasm, rough endoplasmic reticulum, many free ribosomes, but few other cell organelles.

Vascular and glomerular changes are believed to be due to primary damage of endothelial cells, possibly by humoral antibodies (ROWLANDS and BOSSEN, 1969). This damage facilitates penetration of plasma elements under the endothelium. The mononuclear cell infiltrate in the interstitial tissue is, on the other hand, the result of cellular immunity. Since almost all patients with renal transplants receive immunosuppressive drugs, the rejection changes are modified. Cellular immunity is markedly suppressed by steroids, but endothelial changes are only partly counteracted. ZOLLINGER et al. (1973) postulate that each individual patient reaches maximum rejection changes in about 5–12 months, and later remains stable; the degree of these changes varies from one patient to another. It has also been stated that there is a rough correlation between the degree of glomerular changes and HL-A-compatibility (HULME et al., 1972; ROWLANDS et al., 1970; ZOLLINGER et al., 1973).

References

ANDRES, G. A., ACCINNI, L., HSU, K., PENN, I., PORTER, K., RENDALL, J., SEEGAL, B., STARZL, T.: Human renal transplants. III. Immunopathologic studies. Lab. Invest. **22**, 588–604 (1970)

ANDRES, G. A., HSU, K. C., SEEGAL, B. C.: Immunoferritin technique for the identification of antigens by electron microscopy. In: Handbook of Experimental Immunology. Ed.: D. M. WEIR. Oxford, England: Blackwell Scientific Publications 1967

ANDRES, G. A., SEEGAL, B. C., HSU, K. C., ROTHENBERG, M. S., CHAPEAU, M. L.: Electron microscopic studies of experimental nephritis with ferritin-conjugated antibody. Localization of antigen-antibody complexes in rabbit glomeruli following repeated injections of bovine serum albumin. J. Exp. Med. **117**, 691–704 (1963)

ARAKAWA, M.: A scanning electron microscope study of the human glomerulus. Amer. J. Path. **64**, 457–466 (1971)

BARIETY, J., DRUET, P., LALIBERTE, F., SAPIN, C.: Glomerulonephritis with γ- and β1C-globulin deposits induced in rats by mercuric chloride. Amer. J. Path. **65**, 293–302 (1971)

BELL, E. T.: Lipoid nephrosis. Amer. J. Path. **5**, 587–622 (1929)

BEN-BASSAT, M., COHEN, L., ROSENFELD, J.: The glomerular basement membrane in the nail-patella syndrome. Arch. Path. **92**, 350–355 (1971)

BERGER, J., GALLE, P.: Depots denses au sein des membranes basales du rein. Presse Med. **71**, 2351–2354 (1963)

BERGER, J., HINGLAIS, N.: Les depots intercapillaries d'IgA-IgG. J. Urol. et de Neph. (Paris) **74**, 694–695 (1968)

BERMAN, L. B., MISRA, R. P.: Molecular nephrology (editorial). Amer. J. Med. **56**, 701–703 (1972)

BIELSCHOWSKY, M., HELYER, B. J., HOWIE, J. B.: Spontaneous haemolytic anemia in mice of the NZB/BL strain. Proc. U. Otago Med. Sch. **37**, 9–11 (1959)

BLOODWORTH, M. M. B., JR., SOMMERS, S. C.: "Cirrhotic glomerulosclerosis." A renal lesion associated with hepatic cirrhosis. Lab. Invest. **8**, 962–978 (1959)

BURKHOLDER, P. M., HYMAN, L. R., BARBER, T. A.: Extracellular clusters of spherical microparticles in glomeruli in human renal glomerular diseases. Lab. Invest. **28**, 415–425 (1973)

BUSCH, G. J., GALVANEK, E. G., REYNOLDS, E. S.: Human renal allografts. Analysis of lesions in long-term survivors. Human Path. **2**, 253–308 (1971)

Carroll, N., Crock, G. W., Funder, C. C., Green, C. R., Ham, K. N., Tange, J. D.: Glomerular epithelial cell lesions induced by N,N′-Diacetylbenzidine. Lab. Invest. **31**, 239–245 (1974)

Churg, J.: Electron microscopic aspects of renal pathology. In: Becker, E. L.: Structural Basis of Renal Disease, pp. 132–196. New York: Hoeber 1968

Churg, J., Grishman, E.: Ultrastructure of immune deposits in renal glomeruli. Ann. Int. Med. **76**, 479–486 (1972)

Churg, J., Grishman, E.: Application of thin sections to the problems of renal pathology. J. Mt. Sinai Hosp. **24**, 736–744 (1957)

Churg, J., Grishman, E.: Subacute glomerulonephritis. Amer. J. Path. **35**, 25–45 (1959)

Churg, J., Grishman, E., Goldstein, M. H., Yunis, S. L., Porush, J. G.: Idiopathic nephrotic syndrome in adults. A study and classification based on renal biopsies. New Eng. J. Med. **272**, 165–174 (1965)

Churg, J., Grishman, E., Mautner, W.: Nephrotoxic serum nephritis in the rat. Electron and light microscopic studies. Amer. J. Path. **37**, 729–749 (1960)

Churg, J., Habib, R., White, R. H. R.: Pathology of the nephrotic syndrome in children. A report for the international study of kidney disease in children. Lancet **1970 I**, 1299–1302

Churg, J., Mautner, W., Grishman, E., Eisner, G. M.: Structure of glomerular capillaries in proteinuria. Arch. Intern. Med. **109**, 97–115 (1962)

Churg, J., Morita, T., Suzuki, Y.: Glomerulonephritis with fibrin and crescent formation. In: Kincaid-Smith, P., Mathew, T. H., Becker, E. L.: Glomerulonephritis. Morphology, Natural History and Treatment, Part II, pp. 677–694. New York: John Wiley 1973

Churg, J., Sherman, R. L.: Pathologic characteristics of hereditary nephritis. Arch. Path. **95**, 374–379 (1973)

Comerford, F. R., Cohen, A. S.: The nephropathy of systemic lupus erythematosus. An assessment of clinical, light, and electron microscopic criteria. Medicine **46**, 425–473 (1967)

Dachs, S., Churg, J.: Iron nephropathy. Fed. Proc. **24**, 619 (1965)

Davies, D. R., Tighe, J. R., Jones, N. F., Brown, G. W.: Recurrent hematuria and mesangial IgA deposition. J. Clin. Path. **26**, 672–677 (1973)

Dixon, F. J.: Renal injury induced by antigen-antibody complexes and other immunologic means. Fed. Proc. **24**, 98–99 (1965)

Dixon, F. J., Feldman, J. D., Vasquez, J. J.: Experimental glomerulonephritis: The pathogenesis of a laboratory model resembling the spectrum of human glomerulonephritis. J. Exp. Med. **113**, 899–920 (1961)

Dixon, F. J., Wilson, C. B., Marquardt, H.: Experimental immunologic glomerulonephritis. In: Hamburger, J., Crosnier, J., Maxwell, M. H., Advances in Nephrology, Vol. 1, pp. 1–10. Chicago: Year Book Medical Publ. 1971

DuBois, E. L., Arterberry, J. D.: Etiology of discoid and systemic lupus erythematosus. In: Lupus Erythematosus, 2nd ed., p. 111. Ed.: E. L. DuBois. Los Angeles: Univ. of South. California Press 1974

Duffy, J. L., Cinque, T., Grishman, E., Churg, J.: Intraglomerular fibrin, platelet aggregation, and subendothelial deposits in lipoid nephrosis. J. Clin. Invest. **49**, 251–258 (1970)

Duffy, J. L., Letteri, J., Cinque, T., Hsu, P. P., Molho, L., Churg, J.: Renal vein thrombosis and the nephrotic syndrome. Amer. J. Med. **54**, 663–672 (1973)

Dujovne, I., Pollak, V. E., Pirani, C. L., Dillard, M. G.: The distribution and character of glomerular deposits in systemic lupus erythematosus. Kidney International **2**, 33–50 (1972)

Ehrenreich, T., Churg, J.: Pathology of membranous nephropathy. In: Pathology Annual 1968, Vol. 3, pp. 145–186. Ed.: S. C. Sommers. New York: Appleton-Century-Crofts 1968

Erslev, A. J., Shapiro, S. S.: In: Diseases of the Kidney, pp. 289–290. Eds.: M. E. Strauss and L. C. Welt. Boston: Little, Brown 1971

Fahr, Th.: Pathologische Anatomie des Morbus Brightii. In: Handbuch der speziellen pathologischen Anatomie und Histologie, Vol. VI, p. 232. Eds.: F. Henke und O. Lubarsch. Berlin: Springer 1925

FAITH, G. C., TRUMP, B. F.: The glomerular capillary wall in human kidney disease: Acute glomerulonephritis, systemic lupus erythematosus, and preeclampsia-eclampsia. Lab. Invest. **15**, 1682–1719 (1966)

FARQUHAR, M. G., VERNIER, R. L., GOOD, R. A.: An electron microscopic study of the glomerulus in nephrosis, glomerulonephritis, and lupus erythematosus. J. Exp. Med. **106**, 649–660 (1957)

FELDMAN, J. D., FISHER, E. R.: Renal lesions of aminonucleoside nephrosis as revealed by electron microscopy. Lab. Invest. **8**, 371–385 (1959)

FELDMAN, J. D., FISHER, E. R.: Chronic aminonucleoside proteinuria. Lab. Invest. **10**, 444–458 (1961)

FERRIS, T. F., HERDSON, P. B., DUNNILL, M. S., LEE, M. R.: Toxemia of pregnancy in sheep: A clinical physiological, and pathological study. J. Clin. Invest. **48**, 1643–1655 (1969)

FISHER, E. R., PEREZ-STABLE, E.: Cirrhotic (hepatic) lobular glomerulonephritis: Correlation of ultrastructural and clinical features. Amer. J. Path. **52**, 869–889 (1968)

FISHER, E. R., SHARKEY, D., PARDO, V., VUZEVSKI, V.: Experimental renal vein constriction. Its relation to renal lesions observed in human renal vein thrombosis and the nephrotic syndrome. Lab. Invest. **18**, 689–699 (1968)

FRANKLIN, W. A., SIMON, N. M., POTTER, E. W., KRUMLOVSKY, F. A.: The hemolytic-uremic syndrome. Arch. Path. **94**, 230–240 (1972)

GALLE, P., HINGLAIS, N., CROSNIER, J.: Recurrence of an original glomerular lesion in three renal allografts. Transplant. Proc. **3**, 368–370 (1971)

GASSER, V. C., GAUTIER, E., STECK, A., SIEBENMANN, R. E., OECHSLIN, R.: Hämolytisch-urämische Syndrome: Bilaterale Nierenrindennekrosen bei akuten erworbenen hämolytischen Anämien. Schweiz. Med. Wschr. **85**, 905–909 (1955)

GERMUTH, F. G., RODRIGUEZ, E.: Immune complex deposit and antibasement membrane disease. Boston: Little, Brown, 1973

GORHAM, J. R., LEADER, R. W., HENSON, J. B.: Experimental transmission of a virus causing hypergammaglobulinemia in mink: Sources and modes of infection. J. Infect. Dis. **114**, 341–345 (1964)

GRISHMAN, E., CHURG, J.: Focal glomerular sclerosis in nephrotic patients: An electron microscopic study of glomerular podocytes. Kidney International **7**, 111–122 (1975)

GRISHMAN, E., COHEN, S., SALOMON, M. I., CHURG, J.: Renal lesions in acute rheumatic fever. Amer. J. Path. **51**, 1045–1061 (1967)

GRISHMAN, E., PORUSH, J. G., LEE, S. L., CHURG, J.: Renal biopsies in lupus nephritis. Correlation of electron microscopic findings with clinical course. Nephron **10**, 25–36 (1973)

GRISHMAN, E., PORUSH, J. G., ROSEN, S. M., CHURG, J.: Lupus nephritis with organized deposits in the kidneys. Lab. Invest. **16**, 717–725 (1967)

GYORKEY, F., SINKOVICS, J., MIN, K. W., GYORKEY, P.: A morphologic study on the occurrence and distribution of structures resembling viral nucleocapsids in collagen diseases. Amer. J. Med. **53**, 148–158 (1972)

HABIB, R.: Focal glomerular sclerosis (editorial). Kidney International **4**, 355–361 (1973)

HABIB, R., KLEINKNECHT, C., GUBLER, M. C., LEVY, M.: Idiopathic membranoproliferative glomerulonephritis in children. Report of 105 cases. Clin. Nephrology **1**, 194–214 (1973)

HABIB, R., MATHIEW, H., ROYER, P.: Le syndrome hemolytique et uremique de l'enfant. Nephron **4**, 139–172 (1967)

HABIB, R., MICHIELSEN, P., DE MONTERA, H., HINGLAIS, N., GALLE, P., HAMBURGER, J.: Clinical and microscopic and electron microscopic data in the nephrotic syndrome of unknown origin. In: Ciba Foundation Symposium on Renal Biopsy, p. 70. Eds.: G. E. W. WOLSTENHOLME and M. P. CAMERON. London: Churchill 1961

HAMBURGER, J., CROSSIER, J., DORMONT, J., BACH, J.-F.: Renal Transplantation. Baltimore: Williams & Wilkins 1972

HAYSLETT, J. P., KASHGARIAN, M., BENSCH, K. G., SPARGO, B. H., FRIEDMAN, L. R., EPSTEIN, F. H.: Clinicopathologic correlations in the nephrotic syndrome due to primary renal disease. Medicine **52**, 93–120 (1973)

HAYSLETT, J. P., KRASSNER, L. S., BENSCH, K. G., KASHGARIAN, M., EPSTEIN, F. H.: Progression of "lipoid nephrosis" to renal insufficiency. New Engl. J. Med. **281**, 181–187 (1969)

HENSON, J. B., GORHAM, J. R., LEADER, R. W., WAGNER, B. M.: Experimental hyper-gammaglobulinemia in mink. J. Exp. Med. **116**, 357–364 (1962)

HEPTINSTALL, R. H.: The present status of focal glomerulonephritis. In: KINCAID SMITH, P., MATHEW, T. H., BECKER, E. L.: Glomerulonephritis. Morphology, Natural History and Treatment, Part I, pp. 287–300. New York: John Wiley 1973

HERMAN, R. C., PICKERING, R. J., MICHAEL, A. F., VERNIER, R. L., FISH, A. J., GEWURZ, H., GOOD, R. A.: Chronic glomerulonephritis associated with low serum complement activity (chronic hypocomplementemic glomerulonephritis). Medicine **49**, 207–226 (1970)

HEYMANN, W., HACKEL, D. B., HARWOOD, S., WILSON, S. G. F., HUNTER, J. L. P.: Production of nephrotic syndrome in rats by Freund's adjuvants and rat kidney suspensions. Proc. Soc. Exp. Biol. Med. **100**, 660–664 (1959)

HINGLAIS, N., GARCIA-TORRES, R., KLEINKNECHT, D.: Long-term prognosis in acute glomerulonephritis. The predictive value of early clinical and pathologic features observed in 65 patients. Amer. J. Med. **56**, 52–60 (1974)

HINGLAIS, N., GRUNFELD, J. P., BOIS, E.: Characteristic ultrastructural lesion of the glomerular basement membrane in progressive hereditary nephritis (Alport's syndrome). Lab. Invest. **27**, 473–487 (1972)

HOPPER, J., JR., RYAN, P., LEE, J. C., ROSENAU, W.: Lipoid nephrosis in 31 adult patients: Renal biopsy study by light, electron and fluorescent microscopy with experience in treatment. Medicine **49**, 321–341 (1970)

HORN, R. G., FAUCI, A. S., ROSENTHAL, A. S., WOLFF, S. M.: Renal biopsy pathology in Wegener's granulomatosis. Amer. J. Path. **74**, 423–440 (1974)

HULME, B., ANDREW, G., PORTER, K., OGDEN, D.: Human renal transplants. IV. Glomerular ultrastructure, macromolecular permeability, and hemodynamics. Lab. Invest. **26**, 2–10 (1972)

HYMAN, L. R., BURKHOLDER, P. M.: Focal sclerosing glomerulonephropathy with segmental hyalinosis. Lab. Invest. **28**, 533–544 (1973)

JAO, W., POLLAK, V. E., NORRIS, S. H., LEWY, P., PIRANI, C. L.: Lipoid nephrosis: An approach to the clinicopathologic analysis and dismemberment of idiopathic nephrotic syndrome with minimal glomerular changes. Medicine **52**, 445–468 (1973)

JENIS, E. H., SANDLER, P., HILL, G. S., KNEISER, M. R., JENSEN, G. E., ROSKES, S. D.: Glomerulonephritis with basement membrane dense deposits. Arch. Path. **97**, 84–91 (1974)

JOHNSTON, W. H., LATTA, H.: Acute focal glomerulonephritis in the rabbit induced by injection of *Saccharomyces cerevisiae*. An electron microscopic study. Lab. Invest. **26**, 741–754 (1972)

JONES, D. B.: Nephrotic glomerulonephritis. Amer. J. Path. **33**, 313–329 (1957)

KARNOVSKY, M. J., AINSWORTH, S. K.: The Structural Basis of Glomerular Filtration. In: Advances in Nephrology, Vol. 2. Eds.: J. HAMBURGER, J. CROSNIER, M. H. MAXWELL. Chicago: Year Book Medical Publ. 1972, pp. 35–60

KASHGARIAN, M., HAYSLETT, J. P., SIEGLE, N. J.: Lipoid nephrosis and focal sclerosis: distinct entities or spectrum of disease (editorial). Nephron **13**, 105–108 (1974)

KEFALIDES, N. A., FORSELL-KNOTT, L.: Structural changes in the protein and carbohydrate components of glomerular basement membrane in aminonucleoside nephrosis. Biochim. et biophys. acta **203**, 62–66 (1970)

KIMMELSTIEL, P., KIM, O. J., BERES, J.: Studies on renal biopsy specimens with the aid of the electron microscope. II. Glomerulonephritis and glomerulonephrosis. Amer. J. Clin. Path. **38**, 280–296 (1962)

KINCAID-SMITH, P.: The natural history and treatment of mesangiocapillary glomerulonephritis. In: Glomerulonephritis. Morphology, Natural History and Treatment, Part 1, pp. 591–609. Eds.: P. KINCAID-SMITH, T. H. MATHEW and E. L. BECKER. New York: John Wiley 1973

KLASSEN, J., ELWOOD, C., GROSSBERG, A. L., MILGROM, F., MONTES, M., SEPULVEDA, M., ANDRES, G. A.: Evolution of membranous nephropathy into anti-glomerular-basement-membrane glomerulonephritis. New Eng. J. Med. **290**, 1340–1344 (1974)

KLEMPERER, P., POLLACK, A. D., BAEHR, G.: Pathology of disseminated lupus erythematosus. Arch. Path. **32**, 569–631 (1941)

KOFFLER, D., AGNELLO, V., CARR, R. I., KUNKEL, H. G.: Variable patterns of immunoglobulin and complement deposition in the kidneys of patients with systemic lupus erythematosus. Amer. J. Path. **56**, 305–316 (1969)

KOFFLER, D., PARONETTO, F.: Fibrinogen deposition in acute renal failure. Amer. J. Path. **49**, 383–395 (1966)

KOFFLER, D., SCHUR, P. H., KUNKEL, H. G.: Immunological studies concerning the nephritis of systemic lupus erythematosus. J. Exp. Med. **126**, 607–624 (1967)

KURTZ, S. M.: The fine structure of the lamina densa. Lab. Invest. **10**, 1189–1208 (1961)

LANNIGAN, R., INSLEY, J.: Light and electron microscope appearances in renal biopsy material of recurrent hematuria in children. J. Clin. Path. **18**, 178–187 (1965)

LAVER, M. C., KINCAID-SMITH, P.: The natural history and treatment of membranous glomerulonephritis. In: Glomerulonephritis. Morphology, Natural History and Treatment, pp. 461–472. Eds.: P. KINCAID-SMITH,, T. H. MATHEW,, E. L. BECKER, New York: John Wiley 1973

LEWIS, R. M., SCHWARTZ, R., HENRY, W. B., JR.: Canine systemic lupus erythematosus. Blood **25**, 143–160 (1965)

LINTON, A. L., GAVRAS, H., GLEADLE, R. I., HUTCHISON, H. E., LAWSON, D. H., LEVER, A. F., MACADAM, R. F., McNICOL, G. P., ROBERTSON, J. I. S.: Microangiopathic haemolytic anemia and the pathogenesis of malignant hypertension. Lancet **1969 I**, 1277–1282

LÖHLEIN, M.: Über hämorrhagische Nierenaffektionen bei chronischer, ulzeröser Endocarditis. (Embolische nichteiterige Herdnephritis.) Med. Klin. Berl. **6**, 375 (1910)

MADRAZO, A., SUZUKI, Y., CHURG, J.: Radiation nephritis. Acute changes following high dose of radiation. Amer. J. Path. **54**, 507–528 (1969)

MADRAZO, A., SUZUKI, Y., CHURG, J.: Radiation nephritis. II. Chronic changes after high doses of radiation. Amer. J. Path. **61**, 37–56 (1970)

MAUTNER, W., CHURG, J., GRISHMAN, E., DACHS, S.: Preeclamptic nephropathy. Lab. Invest. **11**, 518–530 (1962)

McCLUSKEY, R. T.: Lupus Nephritis. In: Pathology Annual 1970, pp. 125–144. Ed.: S. C. SOMMERS. New York: Appleton-Century-Crofts 1970

McCOY, R. C., ABRAMOWSKY, C. R., TISHER, C. C.: IgA nephropathy. Amer. J. Path. **76**, 123–144 (1974)

McENERY, P. T., McADAMS, A. J., WEST, C. D.: Glomerular morphology, natural history and treatment of children with IgA-IgG mesangial nephropathy. In: Glomerulonephritis. Morphology, Natural History and Treatment, Part II, pp. 305–320. Eds.: P. KINCAID-SMITH, T. MATHEW, E. L. BECKER, New York: John Wiley 1973

McGOVERN, V. J.: Persistent nephrotic syndrome. A renal biopsy study. Aust. Ann. Med. **13**, 306–312 (1964)

MELLORS, R. C., OTEGA, L. G., HOLMAN, H. R.: Role of gamma globulins in pathogenesis of renal lesions in systemic lupus erythematosus and chronic membranous glomerulonephritis, with an observation on lupus cell reaction. J. Exp. Med. **106**, 191–202 (1957)

MELLORS, R. C., TOSHIKAZU, S., AOKI, T., HUEBNER, R. J., KRAWCZYNSKI, K.: Wildtype gross leukemia virus and the pathogenesis of the glomerulonephritis of New Zealand mice. J. exp. Med. **133**, 113–132 (1971)

MIN, K. W., GYORKEY, F., GYORKEY, P., YIUM, J. J., EKNOYAN, G.: The morphogenesis of glomerular crescents in rapidly progressive glomerulonephritis. Kidney International **5**, 47–56 (1974)

MORITA, T., LAUGHLIN, L. O., KAWANO, K., KIMMELSTIEL, P., SUZUKI, Y., CHURG, J.: Nail-patella syndrome. Light and electron microscopic studies of the kidney. Arch. Int. Med. **131**, 271–277 (1973b)

MORITA, T., SUZUKI, Y., CHURG, J.: Structure and development of the glomerular crescent. Amer. J. Path. **72**, 349–369 (1973a)

MORRIS, R. H., VASSALLI, P., BELLER, F. K., McCLUSKEY, R. T.: Immunofluorescent studies of renal biopsis in the diagnosis of toxemia of pregnancy. Obstet. Gynec. **24**, 32–46 (1964)

MOVAT, H. Z.: The fine structure of the glomerulus in membranous glomerulonephritis (lipoid nephrosis) in adults. Amer. J. Clin. Path. **32**, 109–127 (1959)

MUNK, F.: Pathologie und Klinik der Nephrosen, Nephritiden und Schrumpfnieren. Berlin-Wien: Urban & Schwarzenberg 1918

MURRAY, M., PIRIE, H. M., THOMPSON, H., JARRETT, W. F. H., WISEMAN, A.: Glomerulonephritis in a dog. A histological and electron microscopic study. Res. Vet. Science **2**, 493–495 (1971)

NAGI, A. H., ALEXANDER, F., LANNIGAN, R.: Light and electron-microscopical studies of focal glomerular sclerosis. J. Clin. Path. **24**, 846–850 (1971)

NARUSE, T., KITAMURA, K., MIYAKAWA, Y., SHIBATA, S.: Deposition of renal tubular epithelial antigen along the glomerular capillary walls of patients with membranous glomerulonephritis. J. Immunol. **110**, 1163–1166 (1973)

OKUMURA, K.: Induction of a disease resembling systemic lupus erythematosus in (57BL/GJ mice by prolonged immunization with egg albumin. Acta Path. Jap. **23**, 695–704 (1973)

OLSEN, S., BOHMAN, S-O, POSBORG-PATERSEN, V.: Ultrastructure of the glomerular basement membrane in long term renal allografts with transplant glomerular disease. Lab. Invest. **30**, 176–189 (1974)

ORBISON, J. L.: Morphology of thrombotic thrombocytopenic purpura with demonstrations of aneurysms. Amer. J. Path. **28**, 129–144 (1952)

PIRANI, C. L., POLLAK, V. E., LANNIGAN, R., FOLLI, G.: The renal glomerular lesions of pre-eclampsia: Electron microscopic studies. Amer. J. Obstet. Gynec. **87**, 1047–1070 (1963)

PORTER, K., ANDRES, G., CALDER, M., DOSSETOR, J., HSU, J., RENDALL, K., SEEGAL, J., STARZL, T.: Human renal transplants. II. Immunofluorescent and immunoferritin studies. Lab. Invest. **18**, 159–171 (1968)

POTHIER, L., UZMAN, B. G., KASAC, M. M., SAITO, H., ADAMS, R. A.: Immunoglobulin synthesis and tubular arrays in the endoplasmic reticulum in transplanted human tumors of lymphoid origin. Lab. Invest. **29**, 607–613 (1973)

RICH, A. R.: A hitherto undescribed vulnerability of the juxtamedullary glomeruli in the lipoid nephrosis. Bull. Johns Hopkins Hosp. **100**, 173–186 (1957)

RICHET, G., FILLASTRE, J-P., MOREL-MAROGER, L., BARIETY, J.: Change from diffuse proliferative to membranous glomerulonephritis: Serial biopsies in four cases. Kidney International **5**, 57–71 (1974)

ROBACK, S. A., HERMAN, R. C., HOYER, J., GOOD, R. A.: Wegener's granulomatosis in a child: Observations on pathogenesis and treatment. Amer. J. Dis. Child. **118**, 608–614 (1969)

ROSEN, S., SWERDLOW, M. A., MUEHRCKE, R. C., PIRANI, C. L.: Radiation nephritis. Light and electron microscopic observations. Amer. J. Clin. Path. **41**, 487–502 (1964)

ROSENAU, W., LEE, J. C., NAJARIAN, J. S.: A light, fluorescence, and electron microscopic study of functioning human renal transplants. Surg. Gyn. Obst. **128**, 62–76 (1969)

ROWLANDS, D. T., BOSSEN, E. H.: Immunological mechanisms of allograft rejection. Arch. Intern. Med. **123**, 491–500 (1969)

ROWLANDS, D. T., BURKHOLDER, P. M., BOSSEN, E. H., LIN, H. H.: Renal allografts in HL-A matched recipients. Amer. J. Path. **61**, 177–210 (1970)

RUMPELT, H. R., THOENES, W.: Focal sclerosing glomerulopathy (glomerulonephritis)—diffuse process. Klin. Wochenschr. **50**, 1143–1146 (1972)

SAKAGUCHI, H., DACHS, S., GRISHMAN, E., CHURG, J.: Renal glomerulus in obstructive jaundice. Arch. Path. **79**, 512–517 (1965b)

SAKAGUCHI, H., DACHS, S., GRISHMAN, E., PARONETTO, F., SALOMON, M., CHURG, J.: Hepatic glomerulosclerosis. An electron microscopic study of renal biopsies in liver diseases. Lab. Invest. **14**, 533–545 (1965a)

SAKAGUCHI, H., DACHS, S., MAUTNER, W., GRISHMAN, E., CHURG, J.: Renal glomerular lesions after administration of carbon tetrachloride and ethionine. Lab. Invest. **13**, 1418–1426 (1964)

SCHAFF, Z., BARRY, D. W., GRIMLEY, P. M.: Cytochemistry of tubulo-reticular structures in lymphocytes from patients with systemic lupus erythematosus and in cultured human lymphoid cells. Comparison to a paramyxovirus. Lab. Invest. **29**, 577–586 (1973)

SCOTT, R. C., HURVITZ, A. I., EHRENREICH, T., DERR, J. W.: Idiopathic membranous glomerulonephritis in a cat. J. Amer. Animal Hosp. Assoc. In publication

SHIBATA, S., SAKAGUCHI, H., NAGASAWA, T., NARUSE, T.: Nephritogenic glycoprotein. II. Experimental production of membraneus glomerulonephritis in rats by a single injection of homologous renal glycopeptide. Lab. Invest. **27**, 457–465 (1972)

SIMON, G. T., CHATELANAT, F.: Ultrastructure of the normal and pathological glomerulus. In: The Kidney, Vol. I. Ed.: C. ROUILLER, pp. 262–349. New York: Academic Press 1969

SINGER, D. B., HILL, L. L., ROSENBERG, H. S., MARSHALL, J., SWENSON, R.: Recurrent hematuria in childhood. New Engl. J. Med. **279**, 7–12 (1968)

SPARGO, B., McCARTNEY, C. P., WINEMILLER, R.: Glomerular capillary endotheliosis in toxemia of pregnancy. A.M.A. Arch. Path. **68**, 593–599 (1959)

SPEAR, G. S., SLUSSER, R. J.: Alport's syndrome emphasizing electron microscopic studies of the glomerulus. Amer. J. Path. **69**, 213–224 (1972)

STRIKER, G. E., CUTLER, R. E., HUANG, T. W., BENDITT, E. P.: Renal failure, glomerulo-nephritis and glomerular epithelial cell hyperplasia. In: Glomerulonephritis. Morphology, Natural History and Treatment, Part II, pp. 657–675. Eds.: P. KINCAID-SMITH, T. H. MATHEW, E. L. BECKER. New York: John Wiley 1973

TONIETTI, G., OLDSTONE, M. B. A., DIXON, F. J.: The effect of induced chronic viral infections on the immunologic diseases of New Zealand mice. J. Exp. Med. **132**, 89–109 (1970)

TRUMP, B. F., BENDITT, E. P.: Electron microscopic studies of human renal disease: Observations of normal visceral glomerular epithelium and its modification in disease. Lab. Invest. **11**, 753–781 (1963)

UMLAS, J.: Glomeruloid structures in thrombotic thrombocytopenic purpura, glomerulo-nephritis and disseminated intravascular coagulation. Human Path. **3**, 437–441 (1972)

URIZAR, R. E., MICHAEL, A., SISSON, S., VERNIER, R. L.: Anaphylactoid purpura. II. Immunofluorescent and electron microscopic studies of the glomerular lesions. Lab. Invest. **19**, 437–450 (1968)

VAN DE PUTTE, L. B. A., DE LA RIVIERE, G. B., VAN BREDA VRIESMAN, P. J. C.: Recurrent or persistent hematuria. Sign of mesangial immuno-complex deposition. New Engl. J. Med. **290**, 1165–1170 (1974)

VITSKY, B. H., SUZUKI, Y., STRAUSS, L., CHURG, J.: The hemolytic-uremic syndrome: A study of renal pathologic alterations. Amer. J. Path. **57**, 627–647 (1969)

WEST, C. D., McADAMS, A. J., McCONVILLE, J. M., DAVIS, N. C., HOLLAND, N. H.: Hypocomplementemic and normocomplementemic persistent (chronic) glomerulo-nephritis: clinical and pathologic characteristics. J. Pediatrics **67**, 1089–1112 (1965)

WOOD, C.: Crystalline phospholipid deposits in renal glomeruli in glomerulonephritis (Abstr.). Amer. J. Path. **66**, 59a (1972)

ZOLLINGER, H. V.: Niere und ableitende Harnwege. In: W. DOERR, E. UEHLINGER, Spezielle pathologische Anatomie, Band 3, S. 366. Berlin-Heidelberg-New York: Springer 1966

ZOLLINGER, H. V., MOPPERT, J., THIEL, G., ROHR, H.-P.: Morphology and pathogenesis of glomerulopathy in cadaver kidney allografts treated with antilymphocyteglobulin. Clinical, light, electron and immunofluorescent optic examinations. Current Topics in Pathology **57**, 1–48 (1973)

Institute of Pathology, University of Tübingen, Federal Republic of Germany
(Director: Prof. Dr. A. Bohle)

The Morphologic Course of Different Glomerulonephritides (Examination of Repeat Biopsies in 264 Patients) *

Heide Fischbach

With 25 Figures

Contents

I. Introduction 155

II. Material and Methods 156

III. Results 157
    1. Minimal Changes Without Nephrotic Syndrome 158
    2. Minimal Changes With Nephrotic Syndrome 160
    3. Focal Sclerosing Glomerulonephritis 162
    4. Perimembranous Glomerulonephritis 166
    5. Membranoproliferative Glomerulonephritis 170
    6. Endocapillary (Acute) Glomerulonephritis 172
    7. Mesangioproliferative Glomerulonephritis 176
    8. Mesangioproliferative Glomerulonephritis With Focal Crescents 181
    9. Rapidly Progressive Glomerulonephritis 182
        a) Mesangioproliferative Glomerulonephritis With Diffuse Crescents . . . 183
        b) Necrotizing Glomerulonephritis 186

IV. Discussion 186
    1. Morphologic Course of Untreated Patients 187
    2. Morphologic Course of Treated Patients 190
    3. Influence of Noninflammatory Lesions on Morphologic Course 190
    4. Which Glomerulonephritides Lead to Renal Atrophy or Renal Insufficiency? 195

V. Summary 196

Acknowledgments 197

References 197

I. Introduction

Since the renal biopsy was first introduced by Iversen and Brun (1951), it has been possible not only to gain morphologic information at autopsy but also to observe the active morphologic course of glomerulonephritis. So far, however, only occasional observations on the morphologic course of the glomerulonephritides have been published. It seems, therefore, justifiable to report on our 264 cases with follow-up biopsies, although. Our case material is, of course, insufficient for the purpose of making absolute conclusions.

* Supported by the Deutsche Forschungsgemeinschaft.

The present paper attempts to describe the morphologic course of the glomerulonephritides and to compare it with the clinical course. The following questions will be discussed:

1. What is the course of glomerulonephritides without therapy?
2. What influence has therapy on the morphologic course?
3. Which factors of a noninflammatory kind lead to changes in the course?
4. Which forms of glomerulonephritis produce renal insufficiency?

II. Material and Methods

Since 1964, about 3 000 renal biopsies and surgically removed kidneys with inflammatory diseases have been sent from all parts of the Federal Republic and West Berlin to the Institute of Pathology at Tübingen, for histologic examination. Among these biopsies were 333 repeat biopsies. Sixty-nine of these serial biopsies could not be used for the following reasons: In 30 cases the biopsy material did not contain enough glomeruli to make a diagnosis. In 10 patients the intervals between biopsies were too short. In 12 patients we did not get sufficient data on the clinical course. In 10 cases additional complications occurred, such as malignant nephrosclerosis, amyloidosis, diabetes mellitus, or renal tuberculosis. Seven biopsies could not be classified morphologically. Out of the remaining 264 patients, 222 underwent renal biopsy twice, 36 three times, 4 four times, 1 five times and 1 six times. The interval between the first and the last renal biopsy had to be at least 6 months. This did not concern patients with endocapillary (acute) glomerulonephritis, with mesangioproliferative glomerulonephritis with focal crescents, and with rapidly progressive glomerulonephritis, or when the patients died of the renal disease.

The biopsy material was sent to us fixed in 4% formalin. After the usual embedding in paraffin, 3–4 μ sections were stained according to the Masson-Goldner method and the PAS reaction was performed. Further stains like HE, EvG, nonspecific esterase reaction, and the fibrin stain according to Ladewig, were made when needed. If problems arose with regard to the basement membrane structure, as, for instance, the occurrence of deposits or so-called splitting, the paraffin material was deparaffinized, fixed again in 2% osmium acid, and embedded in metacrylat. From these plexiglass blocks 0.5–1 μ semithin sections were produced with a Reichert ultramicrotome. Silver impregnation was performed according to MOVAT (1961). Semithin sections were made in 136 cases. If the diagnosis was not clear, the plexiglass blocks were cut and then examined under the electron microscope. After uranyl- and lead salt staining, six cases were studied with the electron microscope (Elmiskop I [Siemens]).

For judgment of the morphologic course, each biopsy had to contain a sufficient number of glomeruli. The quantity of glomeruli that was needed differed according to the forms of glomerulonephritis. For the study of an endocapillary (acute) glomerulonephritis, 5 glomeruli were sufficient, because this disease involves all glomeruli equally. In the other glomerulonephritis forms at least 10 glomeruli were necessary. This number was, however, unsatisfactory when focal changes and end-stage kidneys occurred in the study.

The degree of severity of the disease was measured by the proliferation of the cells of glomeruli, by the extent of possible hyalinosis, and by basement membrane lesions.

The counting of cells in silver-impregnated semithin sections was not feasible because of the relatively small quantity of glomeruli in these particular biopsies.

Evaluation of the clinical course was made possible from the clinical data received at the time of biopsy. To evaluate the data we followed the methods proposed by RENNER et al. (1969): We classified as improvement or deterioration changes of clearance data by more than 15 ml/min, of proteinuria by more than 50% of the initial value, of total serum protein by more than 1 g/100 ml, of arterial blood pressure by more than 20 mm Hg, as well as the increase or decrease of hematuria. As the function of the kidney is best demonstrated by clearance data, the greatest importance was attached to these factors. When clearance data was missing, BUN or creatinine in serum, which were always given, were compared.

Diagnosis of a nephrotic syndrome was made if there was: gross proteinuria with edema, albumin in serum (i.s.) ≤ 2 g%, or cholesterol ≥ 300 mg%. Hypertension was diagnosed in adults when the blood pressure reached a systolic value above 150 mm Hg or a diastolic value above 100 mm Hg and, in children, when the blood pressure exceeded 135 mm Hg or 95 mm Hg respectively.

If patients were treated with drugs, the immunsuppressive and/or cytotoxic therapy was considered the most significant. Only with hesitation was indomethacin therapy preferred to steroid therapy. A patient, for instance, treated with steroids, indomethacin, and azathioprine, was classified as "immunsuppressive and/or cytotoxic therapy."

Among our 264 biopsies no two patients with the same glomerular disease received identical therapy. To describe the individual courses of the 264 patients would be impossible. Thus, we divided the patients into the following therapy groups: symptomatic treatment, steroid therapy only, indomethacin therapy, and immunsuppressive and/or cytotoxic therapy. When necessary, patients of all groups were given diuretics, antibiotics, and antihypertension or anabolic drugs. Pure heparin therapy was tried in one patient and heparin in combination with cyclophosphamide in two others.

III. Results

The classification of our 264 biopsies into the glomerulonephritis forms and therapy groups is shown in Table 1.

Table 1. Frequency of glomerulonephritis forms and their treatment

Glomerulonephritis form	No.	Therapy				
		Without therapy	Steroids	Indomethacin	Immunosuppressives	Heparin
Minimal changes without nephrotic syndrome	32	15	4	8	5	0
Minimal changes with nephrotic syndrome	21	0	14	1	6	0
Focal sclerosing glomerulonephritis	38	8	7	9	14	0
Perimembranous glomerulonephritis	34	6	6	6	16	0
Membranoproliferative glomerulonephritis	20	3	3	8	6	0
Endocapillary (acute) glomerulonephritis	13	1	0	0	11	1
Mesangioproliferative glomerulonephritis	72	22	10	14	26	0
Mesangioproliferative glomerulonephritis with focal crescents	14	5	3	0	6	0
Mesangioproliferative glomerulonephritis with diffuse crescents	11	5	2	0	2	2
Necrotizing glomerulonephritis	9	4	2	0	3	0

1. Minimal Changes Without Nephrotic Syndrome

In this glomerulonephritis form, with the light microscope, only slight changes can be discerned which scarcely differ from normal. When counting the cells in silver impregnated semithin section, Wehner et al. (1974) could verify a proliferation of mesangial cells.

The minimal changes without nephrotic syndrome may occur either as a stage of healing of an endocapillary (acute) glomerulonephritis or of a mesangioproliferative glomerulonephritis or it may occur without any pre-existing illness.

We classified 32 serial biopsies of 17 male and 15 female patients from 3–49 years of age. It was known that one patient suffered from an acute poststreptococcal nephritis several years before. Before the first renal symptoms appeared, 3 patients had had a virus influenza. One patient exhibited pathologic urine findings two weeks after tonsillitis. Two patients maintained a proteinuria after the end of pregnancy. The remaining 25 patients had no pre-existing or simultaneous illness.

As first symptom occurred:

Proteinuria	15 patients
Lidedema in the morning	4 patients
Microscopic hematuria	6 patients
Macroscopic hematuria	4 patients
Back pain	2 patients
Acute poststreptococcal nephritis	1 patient

The intervals between initial symptoms and first biopsy were:

0–6 months	14 patients
7–24 months	14 patients
>24 months	4 patients

On the average, we received the last biopsy 18.7 (6–35) months after the first. From 29 patients we obtained two biopsies and from 3 patients three biopsies for examination. Fifteen patients were untreated, 4 were treated with steroids, eight with indomethacin, and 5 with immunsuppressives or cytotoxics. Table 2 shows the effects of the various therapies.

Table 2. Clinical and morphologic results of therapy in minimal changes without nephrotic syndrome ($+$ = improved; $\emptyset$ = unchanged; $-$ = deteriorated)

Therapy	No.	Clinical course			Morphologic course		
		$+$	$\emptyset$	$-$	$+$	$\emptyset$	$-$
Without therapy	15	3	12	0	0	14	1
Steroids	4	3	1	0	0	4	0
Indomethacin	8	2	3	3	0	5	3
Immunsuppressives or cytotoxics	5	2	2	1	0	3	2

In the histologic conclusion it has to be remembered that the involved glomeruli look normal by light microscopy, so that morphologic improvement is not possible. Furthermore, hypertensive glomerular lesions occurred in two patients under treatment with indomethacin, with blood pressures of 160/100 mm Hg, and 150/105 mm Hg, respectively while on antihypertensive therapy. In these biopsies several glomeruli were concentrically sclerosed. In further glomeruli there was a moderate mesangial widening without a notable increase in cells. In other glomeruli several lobules were hyalinized and, adhesions with Bowman's capsule were found, mostly near the hilum. The arterioles showed clearly a hyalinosis of the wall. In four cases proliferation of the intercapillary cells increased, so that the last biopsy produced a mesangioproliferative glomerulonephritis.

Tubular lesions in the sense of an acute renal failure were not observed.

2. Minimal Changes With Nephrotic Syndrome

This glomerulonephritis, which is associated with a nephrotic syndrome often encountered in children, was called lipoid nephrosis by Volhard and Fahr (1914). By light microscopy the glomeruli seem to be normal. Only by counting the cells could Wehner et al. (1971) verify an increase in intercapillary cells. On the basis of the normal findings with light microscopy, the disease was referred to by Habib et al. (1961) "minimal changes." With the electron microscope, Farquhar et al. (1957) observed fusion of the foot processes of the epithelial cells, provided that the biopsy material was being examined during a nephrotic syndrome. Bohle et al. (1969) called this disease an acute membranous glomerulonephritis or a minimal proliferative intercapillary glomerulonephritis with nephrotic syndrome.

Among the 21 patients with this glomerulonephritis were 7 children. Fourteen patients were male and 7 female. In one patient the nephrotic syndrome occurred during radiation therapy for lymphogranulomatosis. In all the other patients no pre-existing or simultaneous illness was known.

In all cases the onset of the acute disease was marked by severe edema. Only one patient had an associated hematuria. The intervals between the first symptoms and the first biopsy were:

0–6 months	12 patients
7–24 months	2 patients
>24 months	7 patients

On the average, the last biopsy was obtained 24.7 (6–63) months after the first. From 16 patients we got two, from 3 patients three, and from 2 patients four renal biopsies for examination. All patients were treated with drugs. Steroids were administered to 14 patients, continuously or during relapses. Indomethacin was prescribed for 1 patient and immunosuppressives or cytotoxics to 6 patients. Table 3 shows the effects of the various therapies.

Table 3. Clinical and morphologic results of therapy in minimal changes with nephrotic syndrome ($+$ = improved; $\emptyset$ = unchanged; $-$ = deteriorated)

Therapy	No.	Clinical course			Morphologic course		
		$+$	$\emptyset$	$-$	$+$	$\emptyset$	$-$
Without therapy	0						
Steroids	14	5	7	2	0	12	2
Indomethacin	1	0	1	0	0	1	0
Immunsuppressives or cytotoxics	6	4	1	1	0	5	1

With the light microscope a morphologic improvement cannot be verified, because the involved glomeruli cannot be distinguished from normal glomeruli. This applies equally to minimal changes without nephrotic syndrome and to minimal changes with nephrotic syndrome (Figs. 1 and 2).

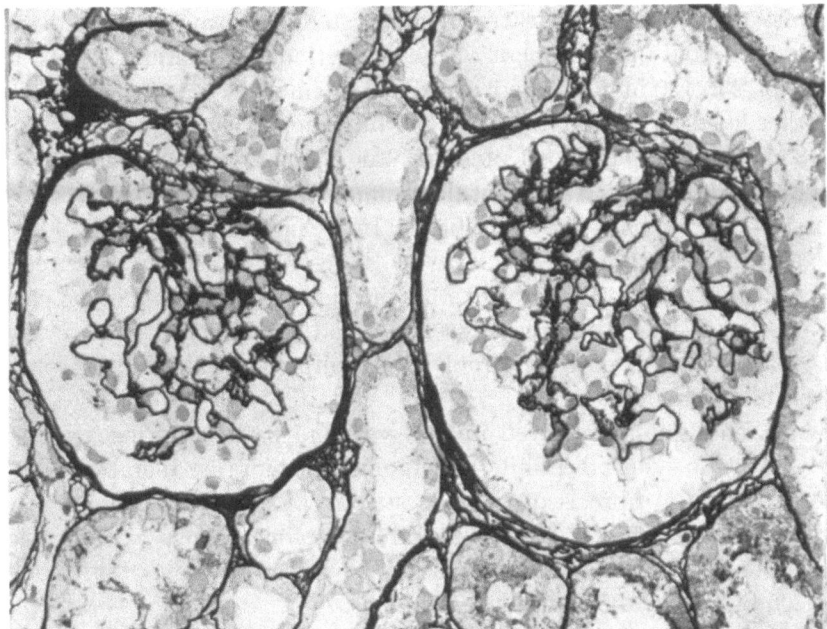

Fig. 1. Minimal changes with nephrotic syndrome. First biopsy in 13-year-old male. Clinical data: 2 years frequent relapsing nephrotic syndrome; proteinuria: 10 g/day, RBC neg., BP 165/100 mm Hg, creatinine clearance 105 ml/min. Plexiglass-embedded, silver impregnation, 375:1

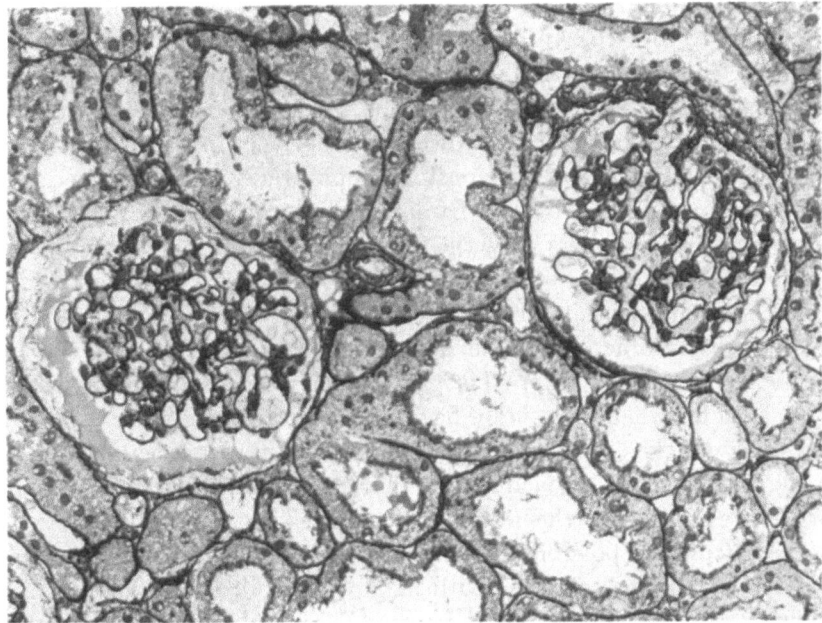

Fig. 2. Minimal changes. Fourth biopsy 3 years after first one (Fig. 1). Clinical data: With azathioprine therapy the nephrotic syndrome disappeared; proteinuria: none, RBC neg., BP 130/80 mm Hg, creatinine clearance 113 ml/min. Plexiglass-embedded, silver impregnation, 250:1

While on continuous treatment with steroids, two patients developed hypertension, and diminishment of renal function. One patient with a hypertension of 240/120 mm Hg died of uremia 15 months after the first biopsy. The other lived for 13 months after the first biopsy; her creatinine-clearance was 38 ml/min, and her blood pressure was 170/110 mm Hg under antihypertensive chemotherapy. The typical minimal glomerular lesions occurred in the first biopsies of both patients (Fig. 3). In the last biopsies severe glomerular and vascular hypertensive lesions were seen (Fig. 4) which obscured completely the inflammatory alterations. In the glomeruli there appeared capillary wall aneurysms with thromboses, a mesangial widening without a clear increase of cells, PAS-positive droplets in epithelial cells, and a concentric sclerosis of Bowman's capsule.

Acute renal failure occurred in a 55-year old patient during a recurrence of the nephrotic syndrome while undergoing azathioprine therapy. This renal failure led to focal fibrosis of the interstitium and to focal tubular atrophy. The glomeruli in these areas, having in the second biopsy exhibited lesions only due to a fibrosis of Bowman's capsule and to a slight "tuft collapse" were completely hyalinized in later biopsies.

3. Focal Sclerosing Glomerulonephritis

This disease variant of the persistent nephrotic syndrome was named focal sclerosing glomerulonephritis by McGovern (1964). He distinguished it with slight variation from the nephrotic syndrome as having a more unfavorable prognosis. Fahr (1925) had already pointed out such variations in cases of prolonged lipoid nephrosis. Rich (1957) noted the occurrence of segmental hyalinosis in the corticomedullary junction in children who died after a continuous nephrotic syndrome. The disease is marked clinically by a therapy-resistant proteinuria or by a persistent nephrotic syndrome. There is also usually a microscopic hematuria. By light microscopy some of the glomeruli look unchanged while others show the following variations, which are restricted to the lobules: adhesions of the abnormal lobules with Bowman's capsule, swelling and lipoid deposits in the endothelial cells, slight proliferation of the mesangial cells, sporadic droplike deposits of PAS-positive material in the epithelial cells (Fig. 5). Later this glomerulus segment becomes hyalinized (Fig. 6). The abnormalities usually begin at the corticomedullary junction and worsen fairly quickly. The disease can lead to renal insufficiency.

In renal biopsies it often happens that the juxtamedullary cortical area is not affected although the number of glomeruli is sufficient. Diagnosis is therefore not always possible at the onset of the disease. The morphologist must diagnose minimal changes with nephrotic syndrome. Thus, in 12 cases from our study only in the second set of biopsies was the focally sclerosed character of the disease verified by means of proven focuses.

In 38 patients aged 10–60 years could the morphologic course be followed. Twenty-four patients were male and 14 patients were female.

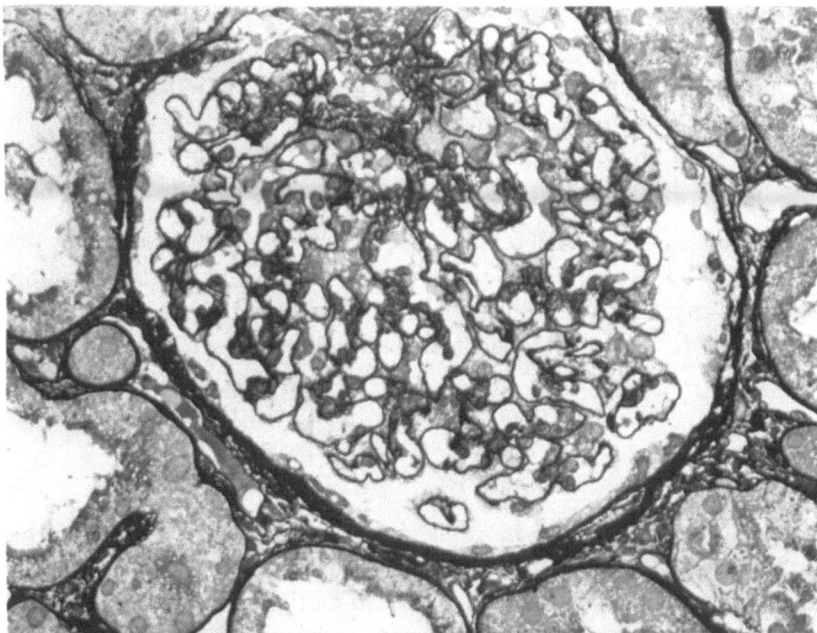

Fig. 3. Minimal changes with nephrotic syndrome. First biopsy in 43-year-old male. Clinical data: Nephrotic syndrome; proteinuria: $20^0/_{00}$, RBC: neg., BP 150/80 mm Hg, BUN 35 mg %. Plexiglass-embedded, silver impregnation, 350:1

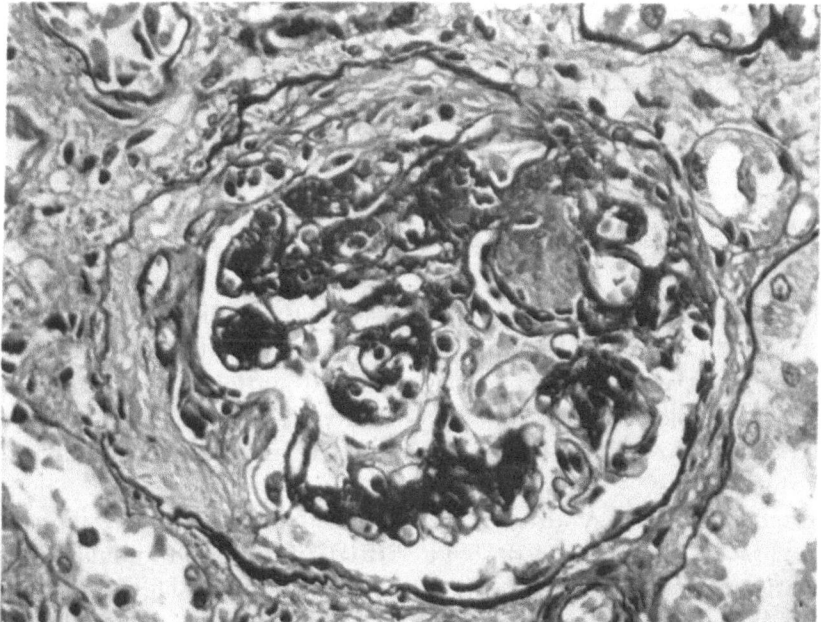

Fig. 4. Severe glomerular and vascular hypertensive lesions obscure the minimal changes. Autopsy of kidney 15 months after first biopsy (Fig. 3). Clinical data: Steroid-resistant nephrotic syndrome, proteinuria: 60 g/day, RBC: neg., BP 240/120 mm Hg, death by uremia. Paraffin-embedded, PAS-reaction, 255:1

Pre-existing or simultaneous illnesses as they were noted were:

Tonsillitis	2 patients
"Acute" glomerulonephritis	2 patients
Infectious episodes	1 patient
Lymphogranulomatosis	2 patients
Endocarditis	1 patient

Of the remaining 30 patients no pre-existing or simultaneous illnesses were known. In the case of 16 patients proteinuria was an incidental finding. In the case of 22 patients the disease began suddenly with a nephrotic syndrome.

The intervals between the occurrence of the first symptoms and the first biopsy was:

0–6 months	14 patients
7–24 months	10 patients
>24 months	14 patients

On the average, the last biopsies were received 21.6 (2–96) months after the first. From 29 patients we obtained two biopsies, from 8 patients three and from 1 patient four biopsies for examination. Eight patients were untreated, 7 were treated with steroids, 9 with indomethacin, and 14 with immunsuppressives or cytotoxics. The effects of therapy are shown in Table 4.

Table 4. Clinical and morphologic results of therapy in focal sclerosing glomerulonephritis ($+$ = improved; $\emptyset$ = unchanged; $-$ = deteriorated)

Therapy	No.	Clinical course			Morphologic course		
		$+$	$\emptyset$	$-$	$+$	$\emptyset$	$-$
Without therapy	8	1	2	5	0	3	5
Steroids	7	3	4	0	0	2	5
Indomethacin	9	1	6	2	0	5	4
Immunsuppressives or cytotoxics	14	4	4	6	0	2	12

There was a striking discrepancy between the clinical and the morphologic course during chemotherapy. In the case of 17 patients the proteinuria decreased, whereas glomerular lesions remained stationary or increased.

In the renal biopsies of 17 patients with hypertension the additional hypertensive glomerular lesions could not be clearly differentiated from the inflammatory lesions.

During a nephrotic syndrome, 5 patients had an acute renal failure which, in the case of 4 patients, led to interstitial fibrosis and tubular atrophy. Two patients died of uremia 2 months after the beginning of the disease, and 2 patients were chronically dialyzed. Simultaneously, glomerular lesions appeared with a retraction of the glomerular tuft to the hilum (BURCK et al., 1967), and a "tuft collapse" occurred, that is, the basement membrane of the glomerular capillaries appeared pleated. Later, such glomeruli hyalinized.

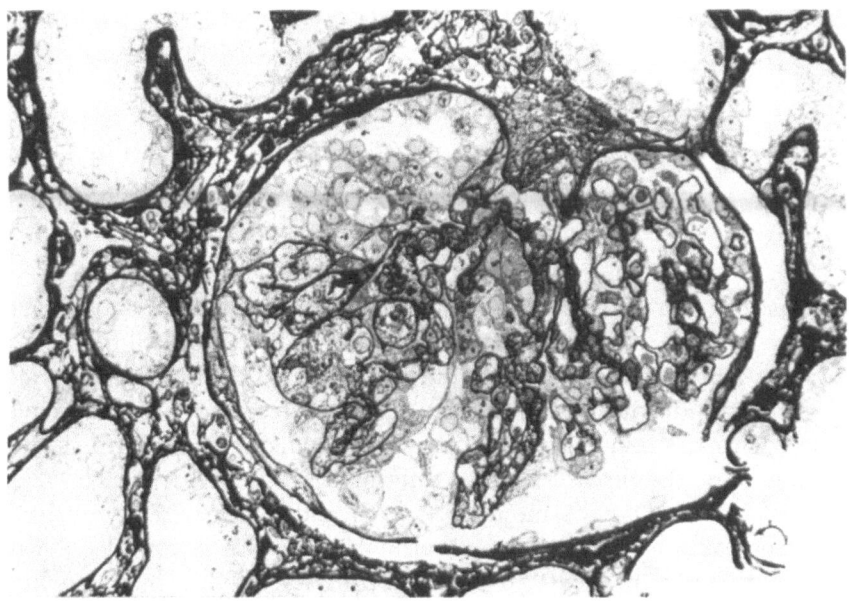

Fig. 5. Focal sclerosing glomerulonephritis. First biopsy in 53-year-old male. Clinical data: For 2 months nephrotic syndrome, at times acute renal failure, BP 160/110 mm Hg. Plexiglass-embedded, silver impregnation, 375:1

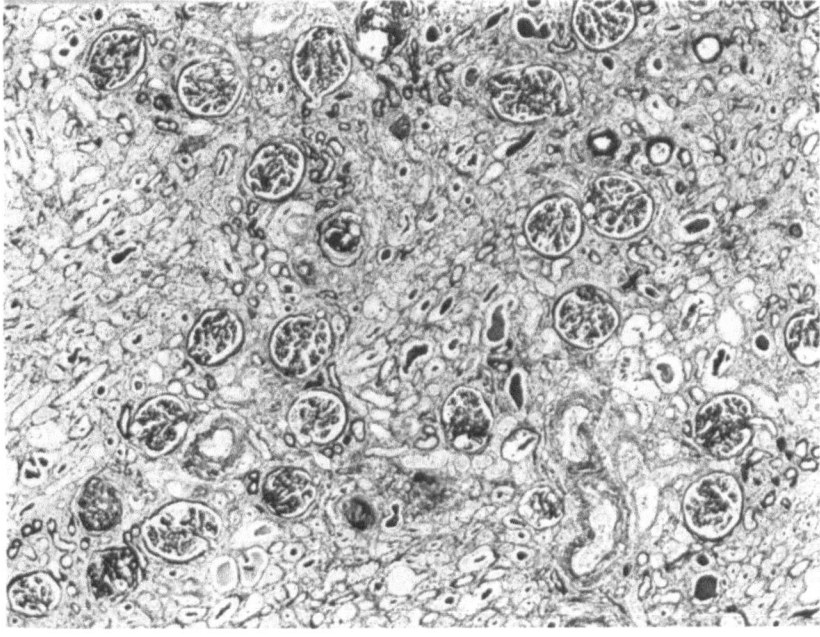

Fig. 6. Focal sclerosing glomerulonephritis with persistent acute renal failure. Autopsy of kidney 1 year after first biopsy (Fig. 5). Clinical data: Anuria for 1 year, BP moderately elevated, treatment with indomethacin. Paraffin-embedded, PAS-reaction, 55:1

Table 5. *The morphologic course in focal sclerosing glomerulonephritis relative to the onset ($+$ = improved; $\emptyset$ = unchanged; $-$ = deteriorated)*

	No.	$+$	$\emptyset$	$-$
Acute onset of illness	22	0	4	18
Gradual onset of illness	16	0	8	8

In the case of 12 patients the disease led to a shrinking of the renal parenchyma and thus to renal insufficiency (creatinine-clearance ≤ 40 ml/min). In 4 of these 12 patients the disease began gradually. Even in the first biopsy, 7 months to 22 years after diagnosis of the kidney disease, a decrease of renal parenchyma was noted. In the remaining 8 patients onset a nephrotic syndrome brought on a sudden of the disease. At the time of the last biopsy which was after 2 (two patients), 3, and 5 months, 3, 4, 8, and 9 years, respectively, renal insufficiency was observed. If the morphologic course is considered without regard to therapy, it seems to be important for the prognosis to know if the onset of the disease was sudden or gradual (Table 5).

When the onset was gradual, the morphologic lesions remained stationary in 8 cases out of 16, whereas the glomerular lesions increased in 18 cases out of 22 when the disease began with a nephrotic syndrome.

4. Perimembranous Glomerulonephritis

In 1957, Jones described basement membrane lesions of the glomerular capillaries as having spikelike basement membrane protuberances during renal disease with a nephrotic syndrome. He mainly observed adults. In keeping with Bell (1946), he called this "membranous glomerulonephritis". French authors called this disease "extramembranous glomerulonephritis" (Habib et al., 1961). Bohle (1964) introduced the term "perimembranous glomerulonephritis".

Ehrenreich and Churg (1968) divided the development of perimembranous glomerulonephritis into four stages. In stage I, in only a few capillary areas are immunoglobulin deposits and basement membrane protuberances discernible (Fig. 7). The disease is more easily recognized at this early stage by using immunohistologic methods instead of the light microscope. Granular deposits of IgG and β_{1C} complement in the basement membrane are always seen Stage II is characterized by spikes seen diffusely over all capillary walls. These spikes are protuberances of the basement membrane and grow out between the immune deposits. After some time (the period varies), stage II basement membrane lesions reach stage III (Fig. 8), during which the deposits are completely incorporated by the basement membrane. The subendothelial surface of the basement membrane here is generally quite smooth. In a further stage the deposits or incorporations can appear washed out; the basement

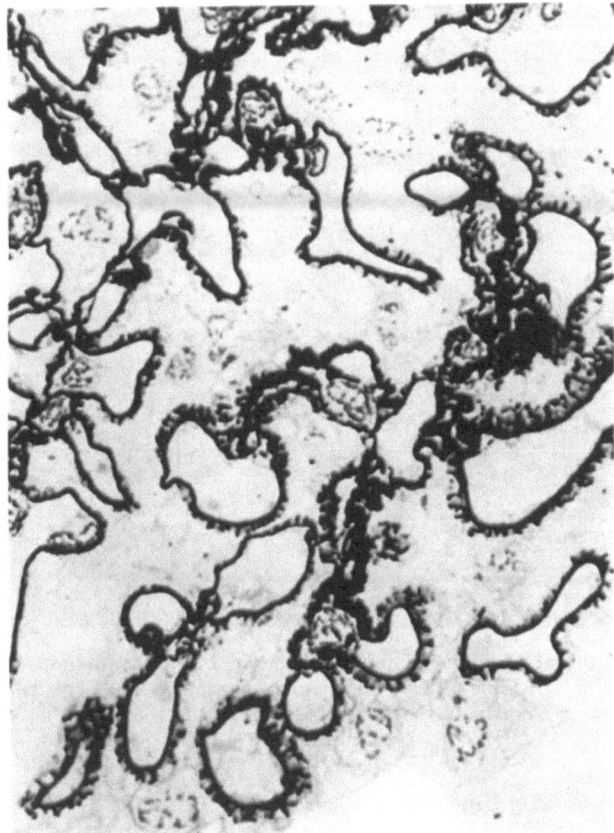

Fig. 7. Perimembranous glomerulonephritis, stage I. First biopsy in 39-year-old male. Clinical data: Nephrotic syndrome; proteinuria: 6 g/day, RBC: +, BP 120/90 mm Hg, creatinine-clearance: normal. Plexiglass-embedded, silver impregnation, 1150:1

membrane then looks like links in a chain (stage IV). This division into stages refers only to the lesions in the basement membrane without regards to the complete findings in the kidneys. In evaluating the morphologic findings, we chose, therefore, the division into stages as practiced by EHRENREICH and CHURG only as a basis not exclusive of other criteria.

We were able to examine several renal biopsies from 22 male and 12 female patients who had perimembranous glomerulonephritis. In only 3 patients were pre-existing or simultaneous illnesses noted: two patients had tonsillitis, and one patient had proteinuria after treatment with D-Penicillamin, which had been used because of severe rheumatoid arthritis.

Nineteen patients stated that the onset of their disease was sudden, 17 patients had generalisid edema, of sudden onset, and 2 patients had macroscopic hematuria. In 15 patients the disease began gradually. As initials symptoms 13 patients presented with lid- or ankle edema, and 2 patients complained of back pain.

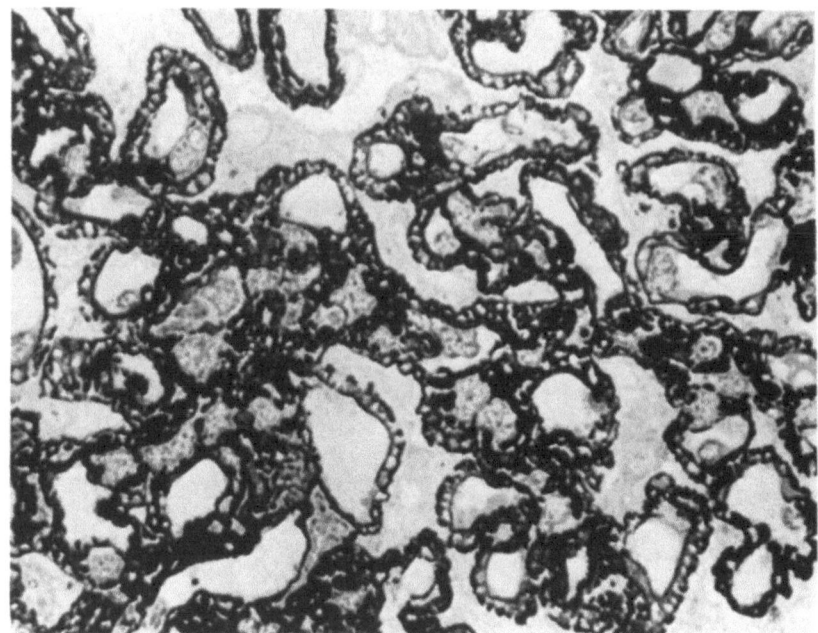

Fig. 8. Perimembranous glomerulonephritis, stage III. Second biopsy 13 months after the first one (Fig. 7). Clinical data: Proteinuria: trace, RBC: neg., BP 125/90 mm Hg, creatinine-clearance: normal, treatment with steroide. Plexiglass-embedded, silver impregnation, 1150:1

The interval between initial symptoms and first biopsy was:

0–6 months	15 patients
7–24 months	17 patients
>24 months	2 patients

On the average, the last biopsy was received 28.7 (2–83) months after the first. From 26 patients we obtained two biopsies, from 7 patients three, and from 1 patient five biopsies for examination. Six patients were untreated, 6 patients were administered steroids, 6 were given indomethacin, and 16 were treated with immunsuppressives or cytotoxics. The effects of therapy are shown in Table 6.

Table 6. Clinical and morphologic results of therapy in perimembranous glomerulonephritis (+ = improved; Ø = unchanged; — = deteriorated)

Therapy	No.	Clinical course			Morphologic course		
		+	Ø	—	+	Ø	—
Without therapy	6	0	3	3	0	4	2
Steroids	6	3	3	0	1	1	4
Indomethacin	6	1	3	2	1	2	3
Immunsuppressives or cytotoxics	16	10	3	3	3	3	10

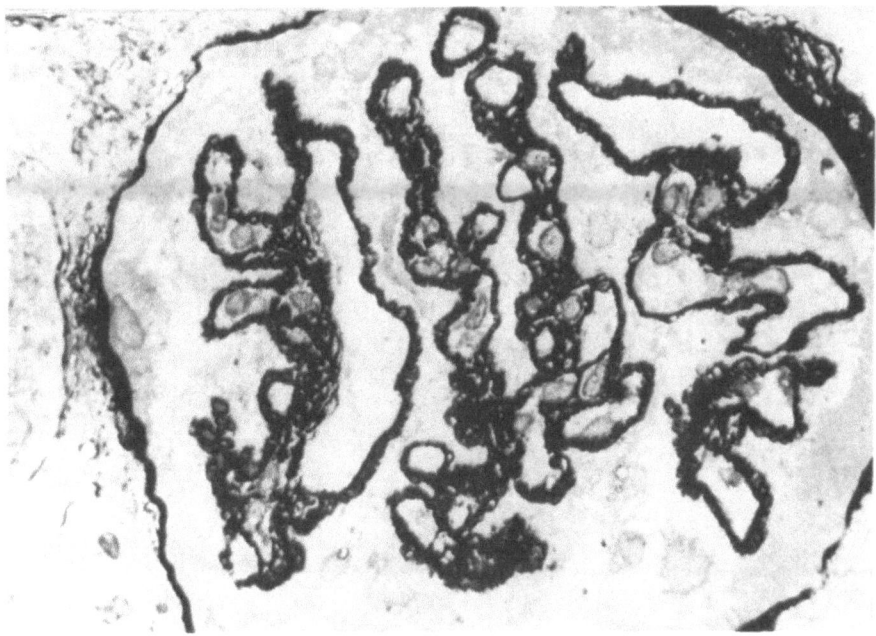

Fig. 9. Perimembranous glomerulonephritis, stage II–III. First biopsy in 36-year-old female. Clinical data: Proteinuria 6 g/day, RBC: +, BP 120/80 mm Hg, creatinine-clearance 110 ml/min. Plexiglass-embedded, silver impregnation, 940:1

The difference was notable between the clinical and morphologic courses in 21 out of the 34 patients. In 11 patients who had been treated with drugs, the clinical findings showed improvement whereas the morphologic findings revealed either a stationary condition (4 patients) or a deteriorated one (7 patients), as can be seen in Figs. 7 and 8.

In 8 patients the clinical symptoms remained unchanged; in the biopsy material of 6 patients deterioration was noted, and in 2 patients the glomerular lesions were decreased. In 2 patients the morphologic findings were unchanged despite a deterioration of clinical findings.

In 5 patients with improved morphologic findings (Table 6) we observed a transition from stages II–III to stage IV. This may be regarded as a beginning of a healing proces; as at the same time the basement membrane was not only split but on the whole had become more "slim" (Figs. 9 and 10) and hyalinization in these biopsies was not seen.

Such improvements were observed in all therapy groups. Because we have thus far studied only a few untreated patients (6 of 34), we can not now attribute such these improvements to the therapy applied. It may be that untreated patients improve spontaneously. We have not seen yet complete healing of perimembranous glomerulonephritis like that described by BARIÉTY *et al.* (1968) in two patients after combined steroid and cytotoxic therapy. Although 10 out of 18 patients had a temporary hypertension and the rest a persistent hypertension, we were only able to verify glomerular hyper-

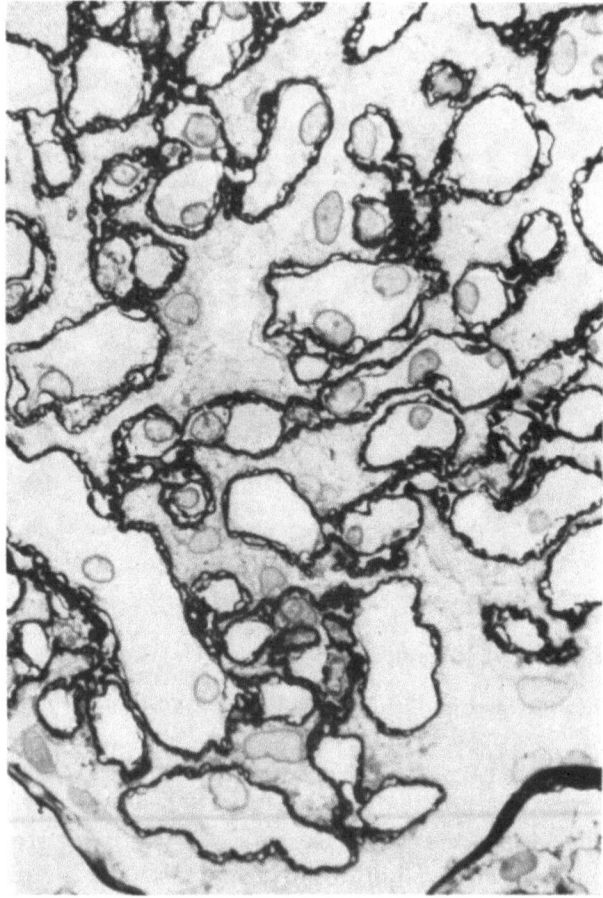

Fig. 10. Perimembranous glomerulonephritis, stage IV. Second biopsy 29 months after the first one (Fig. 9). Clinical data: Proteinuria: trace, RBC: neg., BP 120/80 mm Hg, creatinine-clearance 139 ml/min, treatment with azathioprine. Plexiglass-embedded, silver impregnation, 940:1

tensive lesions in one patient. This patient had an acute renal failure during a nephrotic syndrome and developed hypertension during the anuric period. The patient died 2 months later from duodenal ulcer hemorrhage after steriod treatment during persistent acute renal failure and continuous hypertension. In the remaining 33 patients with perimembranous glomerulonephritis, no tubular lesions in the sense of ischemic tubular lesions were noted.

5. Membranoproliferative Glomerulonephritis

This disease, first described by ROYER *et al.* (1962) in 3 children, may occur in 3 histologic forms. In the simple and lobular forms, protein—consisting mainly of β_{1C} complement—is deposited between basement membrane and endothelial cells. Thus, the endothelial cells are separated from the basement membrane and a new formation of basement membrane and mesangial cells interpose between the protein depots and the endothelial cells. An irregular splitting of the basement membrane is simulated, especially when the protein depots disappear. The differential diagnosis between membranoproliferative glomerulonephritis in this histologic pattern, on the one hand, and stage IV perimembranous glomerulonephritis, on the other, may be difficult (MOREL-MAROGER et al., 1972). Simultaneously with changes in the basement membrane, a proliferation of mesangial cells develops, which is sometimes diffuse (simple form), or sometimes concentrated in the lobule centers (lobular form). The third histologic pattern of membranoproliferative glomerulonephritis (dense deposits) was described for the first time by BERGER and GALLE in 1963. The protein deposits, located in the basement membrane, thus cause the width of the membrane to vary irregularly. The impregnation of the basement membrane with silver salts in the semithin section is only partially feasible. In this form, as well, the intercapillary cells proliferate. Since the three histologic patterns can be found in the same kidney and side by side in one glomerulus (BOHLE et al., 1974), we have come to the conclusion that a differentiation is not significant.

In some patients a hypocomplementemia occurred coincidentally with precipitation of β_{1C} complement (WEST et al., 1965). We examined biopsies of 20 patients exhibiting membranoproliferative glomerulonephritis. The patients were 14–52 years old, 12 males and 8 females. We encountered the simple form of the membranoproliferative glomerulonephritis in 15 patients, the lobular form in 3 patients, and the dense-deposit form in 2 patients. In one case the disease began after tonsillitis. Two patients had glomerulonephritis along with disseminated lupus erythematosus. Among the remaining 17 patients no pre-existing or simultaneous illness was known.

The first symptoms were as follows:

Nephrotic syndrome	9 patients
Ankle edema	4 patients
Proteinuria	6 patients
Microscopic hematuria	1 patient

The intervals between initial symptoms and the first biopsies were:

0–6 months	8 patients
7–24 months	5 patients
>24 months	7 patients

On the average, the last biopsy was received 24.0 (8–53) months after the first. From 16 patients we obtained 2, and from 3 patients we obtained three biopsies for examination. Three patients were untreated, 3 were treated with steroids, 8 with indomethacin, and 6 with immunsuppressives or cytotoxics. Table 7 shows the results of therapies.

Table 7. Clinical and morphologic results of therapy in membranoproliferative glomerulonephritis (+ = improved; ∅ = unchanged; − = deteriorated)

Therapy	No.	Clinical course			Morphologic course		
		+	∅	−	+	∅	−
Without therapy	3	0	1	2	0	1	2
Steroids	3	1	1	1	0	1	2
Indomethacin	8	2	1	5	0	1	7
Immunsuppressives or cytotoxics	6	4	0	2	4	0	2

Table 8. The influence of hypertension on the morphologic course in membranoproliferative glomerulonephritis (+ = improved; ∅ = unchanged; − = deteriorated)

	No.	+	∅	−
Normotensive patients	6	3	2	1
Hypertensive patients	14	1	1	12

In membranoproliferative glomerulonephritis differences between the clinical and the morphologic courses can again often be observed. In 26% of cases the clinical symptoms improved while the morphologic findings remained unchanged or deteriorated. The aggravating influence of hypertension on the morphologic course is shown in Table 8.

It is difficult to differentiate in membranoproliferative glomerulonephritis between hypertensive glomerular lesions and inflammatory changes, since even without additional hypertensive lesions, segmental hyalinosis and adhesions between the glomerular tuft and Bowman's capsule occur.

In 8 patients tubular lesions were also encountered with focal tubular atrophy and interstitial fibrosis, and in some cases were found after a clinically verified acute renal failure during a nephrotic syndrome. At first the glomeruli in these areas were well preserved; in later stages they hyalinized.

One patient, who had had a dense-deposit form, exhibited a special morphologic course: In the first biopsy, the basement membrane was thickened in a ribbonlike pattern (Fig. 11), and the deposits were dense in the electron microscope. In the third biopsy, 29 months later, these deposits had almost completely disappeared (Fig. 12), and the basement membrane was irregular with double contours, but in part appearing absolutely normal.

6. Endocapillary (Acute) Glomerulonephritis

This glomerulonephritis characteristically occurs after streptococcal infections. The typical clinical symptoms are hematuria, proteinuria, edema, oliguria, and hypertension. Morphologically, during the first 3–4 weeks of the disease, a marked proliferation of all three cell forms of the glomerular capillary loops is seen. The capillary lumina are often closed because of the proliferated and swollen endothelial cells (Fig. 13). In the lumina there are usually a

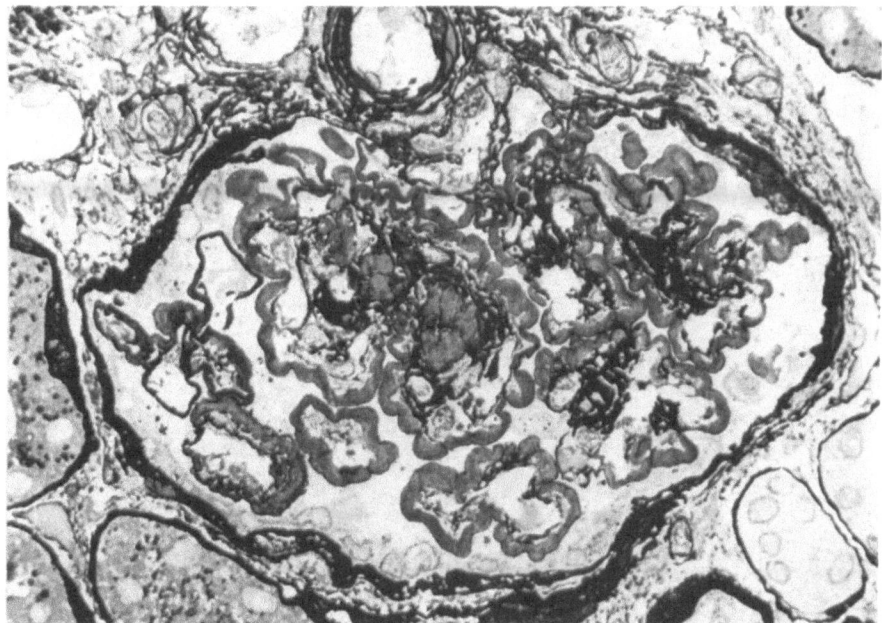

Fig. 11. Membranoproliferative glomerulonephritis, Berger-Galle-type First biopsy in 32-year-old male. Clinical data: Proteinuria: 1.8 g/day, RBC: ++, BP 150/100 mm Hg, inulin clearance 88 ml/min. Plexiglass-embedded, silver impregnation, 590:1

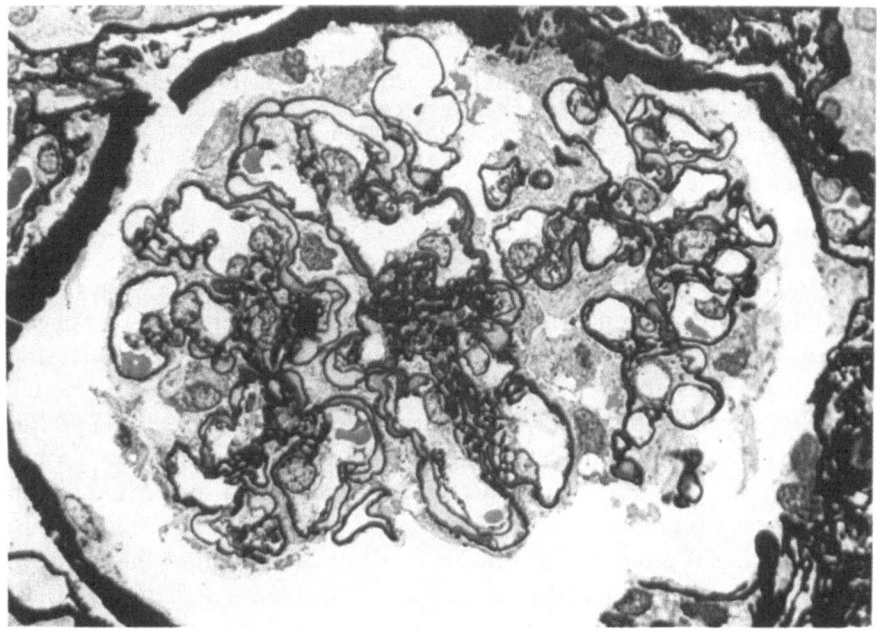

Fig. 12. Membranoproliferative glomerulonephritis. Third biopsy 29 months after the first one (Fig. 11). Clinical data: Proteinuria 0.3 g/day, RBC: +, BP 160/110 mm inulin clearance 81 ml/min, treatment with azathioprine. Plexiglass-embedded, silver impregnation, 590:1

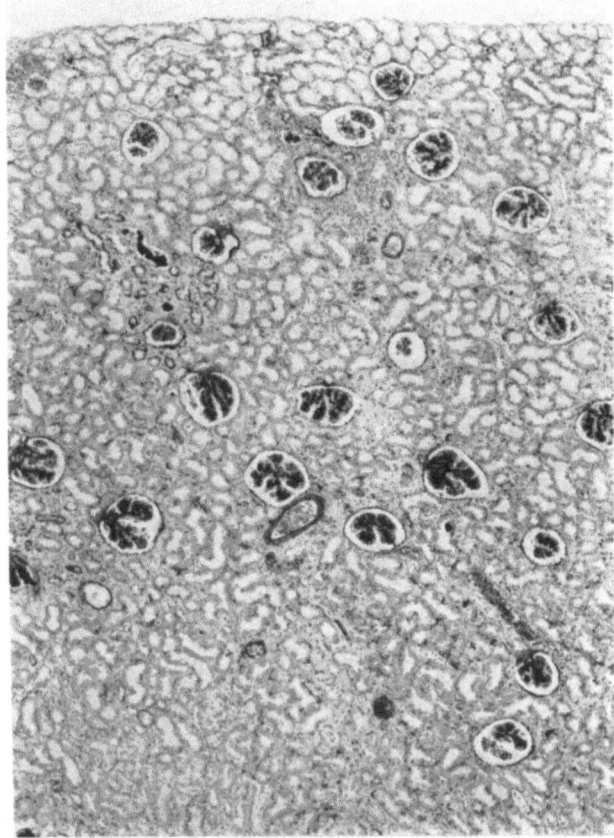

Fig. 13. Endocapillary (acute) glomerulonephritis. First biopsy in 28-year-old male. Clinical data: Acute onset with edema 14 days previously, proteinuria: 11 g/day, RBC: +, BP 165/110 mm Hg, inulin clearance 22.2 ml/min. Plexiglass-embedded, silver impregnation, 1150:1

striking number of granulocytes. On the epithelial side of the basement membrane the so-called humps in the semithin sections can be seen (Fig. 13). These humps are immuno-complex deposits and are reported to appear in this form only in acute serum-sickness nephritis (KIMMELSTIEL et al., 1967). The epithelial cells act as phagocytes on the humps which usually disappear after a 6 week period. Moreover, in all initial biopsies we encountered proliferation of the capsule epithelial cells in 10–30% of the glomeruli. These proliferations were mostly restricted to one sector of Bowman's capsule. Approximately 4–10 weeks later, proliferation of endothelial and epithelial cells decreased, whereas mesangial proliferation continued. Clear lobulation of the glomerulus then became evident (Fig. 14). At this time, we observed here and there a so-called splitting of the basement membrane, which was not found in later biopsies. Clinically, there was at this time usually no or slight reduction of renal function. In many cases a microscopic hematuria and a proteinuria persisted, and the blood pressure was usually normal. Since the clinical features

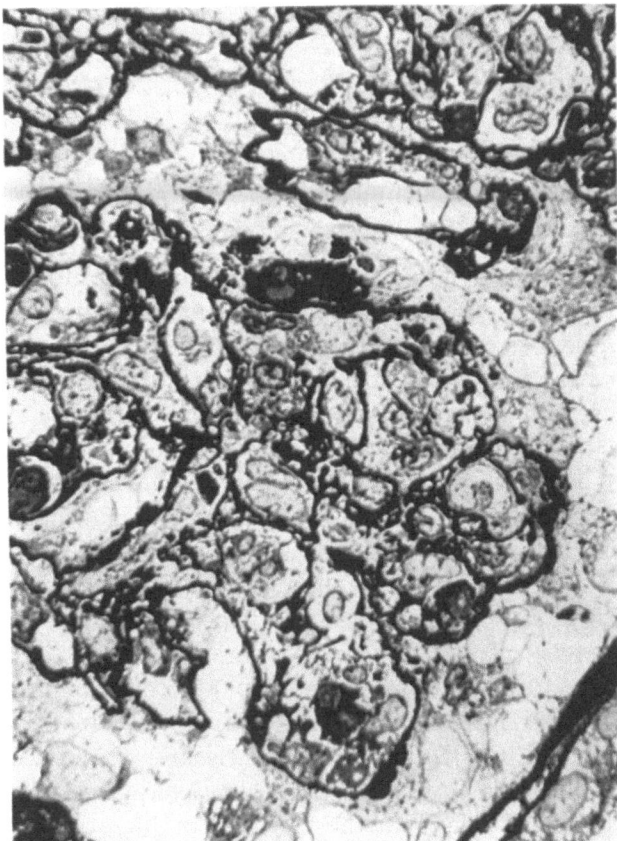

Fig. 14. Endocapillary (acute) glomerulonephritis in remission. Autopsy of kidney of 21-year-old female. Clinical data: 9 months previously endocapillary (acute) glomerulo-nephritis (histologically verified); before death no proteinuria, no retention, normal BP. Death from bronchopneumonia under treatment with azathioprine. Paraffin-embedded, PAS-reaction, 42:1

of endocapillary (acute) glomerulonephritis are clear and the course is known to be favorable, a pathologist was rarely required for diagnosis and course control. Therefore, we examined only 13 repeat biopsies of 10 male and 3 female patients aged 14–57 years.

The following disorders pre-existed:

Tonsillitis	5 patients
Sore throat	1 patient
Bronchial pneumonia	1 patient
Virus infection	1 patient
Secondarily infected mycosis of the feet	1 patient

In 4 cases no pre-existing disorders were known.

The first symptoms were:

Generalized edema	5 patients
Oliguria	2 patients
Anuria	1 patient
Macroscopic hematuria	3 patients
Proteinuria as on incidental finding	1 patient
Weakness and thirst	1 patient

The intervals between initial symptoms and first biopsies were 14–60 days. The last biopsies were received 6 weeks to 33 months after the first.

Renal biopsies were performed in 9 patients twice, in 2 patients three times, in 1 patient four times and in 1 patient six times. All patients were given penicillin, and 12 patients were also given azathioprine or cytotoxics. One of these patients was treated with cyclophosphamide combined with heparin. We could find no difference between the morphologic courses in the untreated patients and the one treated with immunsuppressives and/or cytotoxics. The recovery time in all cases was about the same as those investigated in repeat biopsies by Feldman et al. (1966), Jennings and Earle (1961), Michael et al. (1966), Neustein and Davis (1965), Okuda et al. (1970), Strunk et al. (1964), Travis et al. (1973), and White (1964). Within about 6 months, in the 10 patients whose morphologic course improved, the renal function was nearly normal (creatinine clearance ≥ 80 ml/min) and blood pressure was normal. Only a slight proteinuria and a microscopic hematuria persisted. Morphologically we still found, however, a clear proliferation of mesangial cells. It was clear that the degree of proliferation depended on the timing of the biopsy. In the biopsies, which were performed again 15 and 33 months later in 2 patients, a minimal abnormality in glomerular structure was noted.

In 3 patients the morphologic course was complicated by tubular lesions (Fig. 15). Besides the glomerular lesions typical of endocapillary glomerulonephritis, the proximal tubular epithelium was somewhat swollen or low. We saw a larger number of mitoses in the regenerating epithelium cells and also birefringent (oxalate) crystals lying in the tubular lumina. These tubular lesions are similar to those observed in acute renal failure (Bohle et al., 1964; Schubert, 1968). In those patients with oligo- or anuria at the beginning of the disease, the second biopsy was performed 1, 3, and 4 months later. All patients exhibited in more than 50% of glomeruli a diffuse or more segmental proliferation of the cells of Bowman's capsule (Fig. 16). At the same time, following persistent tubular lesions, a focal interstitial fibrosis occurred. This process is identical with that described by Schubert in 1971 concerning persistent acute renal failure.

7. Mesangioproliferative Glomerulonephritis

This form was called subchronic glomerulonephritis by Volhard and Fahr (1914). Wehner et al. (1969) classified it among the postacute proliferative glomerulonephritides. Since 1970 (Churg et al.), "mesangioproliferative glomerulonephritis" has been used. This form comprises at least two etiologically

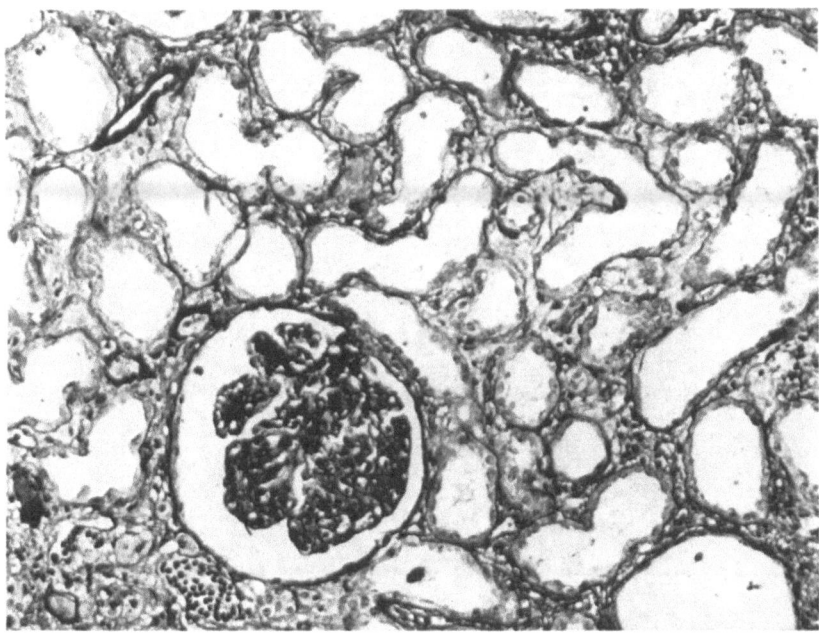

Fig. 15. Endocapillary (acute) glomerulonephritis with acute renal failure. First biopsy in 57-year-old male. Clinical data: Oliguria, proteinuria: $8^0/_{00}$, RBC: +, BP 180/100 mm Hg, creatinine in serum: 18.0 mg %. Paraffin-embedded, Masson-Goldner stain, 170:1

different types of glomerulonephritis which, morphologically, cannot be separated. On the one hand are glomerulonephritides that show a state of healing after endocapillary (acute) glomerulonephritis. On the other is the large group of mesangioproliferative glomerulonephritides that are discovered mostly by chance without signs of pre-existing poststreptococcal nephritis. The expression "mesangioproliferative" is, therefore, the most neutral one, as it is only descriptive. It implies neither a preliminary acute occurrence nor progression to a stage of chronic renal insufficiency.

In the glomeruli, a diffuse increase of intercapillary cells is noted and the mesangium is increased, varying according to the degree of severity. Adhesions may occur between the capillary tuft and Bowman's capsule. We have studied 72 cases—46 males and 26 females—aged 2–62 years. In 16 patients an acute poststreptococcal nephritis occurred within 2 years before the first biopsy; 7 had nonspecific viral respiratory tract infection prior to showing urine abnormalities; and in 49 patients no pre-existing or simultaneous illnesses were known.

The disease began with the following initial symptoms:

Acute poststreptococcal nephritis	16 patients
Proteinuria	27 patients
Edema	9 patients
Nephrotic syndrome	2 patients
Hypertension, headache, dizziness	8 patients
Microscopic hematuria	4 patients
Macroscopic hematuria	5 patients
Nonspecific symptoms	3 patients

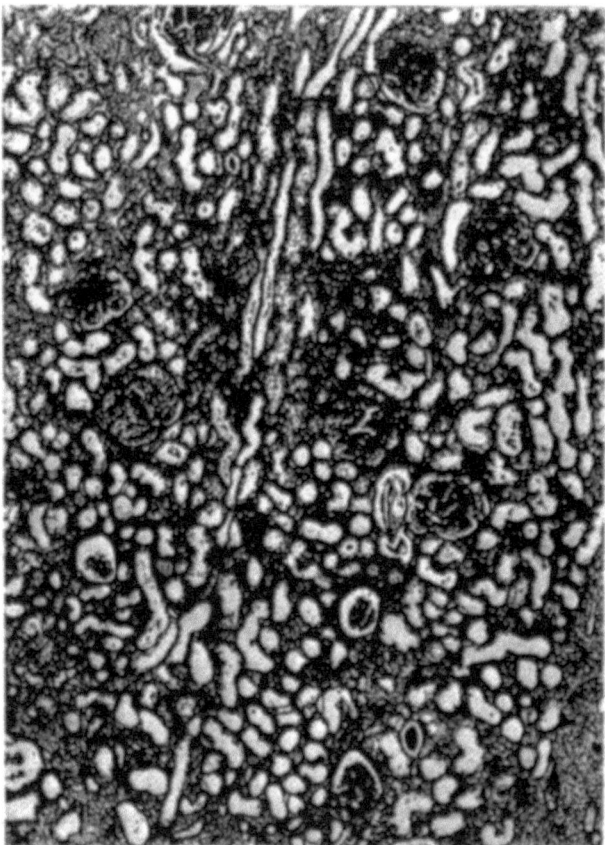

Fig. 16. Mesangioproliferative glomerulonephritis with focal crescents after endocapillary (acute) glomerulonephritis with acute renal failure. Second biopsy 4 months after the first one (Fig. 15). Clinical data: Proteinuria: $3^0/_{00}$, RBC: $+++$, BP 210/120 mm Hg, creatinin in serum: 2 mg %, treatment with azathioprine. Paraffin-embedded, PAS-reaction, 55:1

The intervals between the first symptoms and the first biopsy were:

0–6 months	36 patients
7–24 months	17 patients
>24 months	19 patients

On the average, we received the last biopsy 22.5 (6–122) months after the first one. From 61 patients we received two, from 10 patients three, and from 1 patient we obtained four biopsies for examination. Twenty-two patients were untreated, 10 received steroids, 14 were treated with indomethacin, and 26 with immunsuppressives or cytotoxics. Table 9 shows effects of therapy.

It can be seen that therapy had no influence neither on the clinical nor on the morphologic course.

Different courses were, however, shown in patients with pre-existent post-streptococcal nephritis, as against those without such history (Table 10).

Table 9. Clinical and morphologic results of therapy in mesangioproliferative glomerulonephritis ($+$ =improved; $\emptyset$ = unchanged; $-$ =deteriorated)

Therapy	No.	Clinical course			Morphologic course		
		$+$	$\emptyset$	$-$	$+$	$\emptyset$	$-$
Without therapy	22	8	11	3	7	9	6
Steroids	10	4	2	4	2	4	4
Indomethacin	14	6	6	2	2	11	1
Immunsuppressives or cytotoxics	26	9	13	4	3	13	10

Table 10. The morphologic course in mesangioproliferative glomerulonephritis ($+$ =im-
proved; $\emptyset$ = unchanged; $-$ =deteriorated)

	No.	$+$	$\emptyset$	$-$
Acute onset in the last 2 years after streptococcal infection	16	11	4	1
Without previous streptococcal infection	56	3	33	20

Sixteen patients had had a pre-existing poststreptococcal nephritis. In 11 the morphologic as well as the clinical findings had improved by the time of the last biopsy. The proliferation of the mesangial cells clearly decreased. The finding in the last biopsy corresponded to a minimal change without nephrotic syndrome. In two other patients the glomerular changes remained stationary for 6 months and 8 months, respectively. In two other patients, in the period of 2 and 7 years, respectively, the mesangial proliferation clearly decreased. In one of the two, however, many glomeruli were hyalinized and in the other patient, glomerular hypertensive lesions occurred occasionally. Both courses were, therefore, classified as "unchanged". After the acute phase had passed, one patient gradually developed a malignant hypertension. Because of this therapy-resistant hypertension a bilateral nephrectomy was necessary 4 years after the first biopsy. In these kidneys severe glomerular and vascular hypertensive lesions were superimposed on the former inflammatory glomerular lesions. In 3 out of the 56 patients without acute pre-existing illness, the proliferation of the mesangial cells decreased clearly over a period of 8, 10, and 15 months. One of these patients was untreated, 1 patient treated with indomethacin, and 1 with azathioprine. In 33 patients without a preliminary poststreptococcal nephritis, the morphologic findings remained the same; in 20 patients, the findings in the last biopsies revealed a state of deterioration as opposed to those in the first biopsies.

The influence of hypertension on the morphologic course is shown in Table 11.

Among the 21 patients with a morphologic deterioration, only 5 showed an increase in mesangial proliferation. In 1 patient focal scars occurred in the glomeruli. Development of hypertensive lesions, in 15 cases proved to further aggravate the conditions had (Figs. 17 and 18). The following statistics were

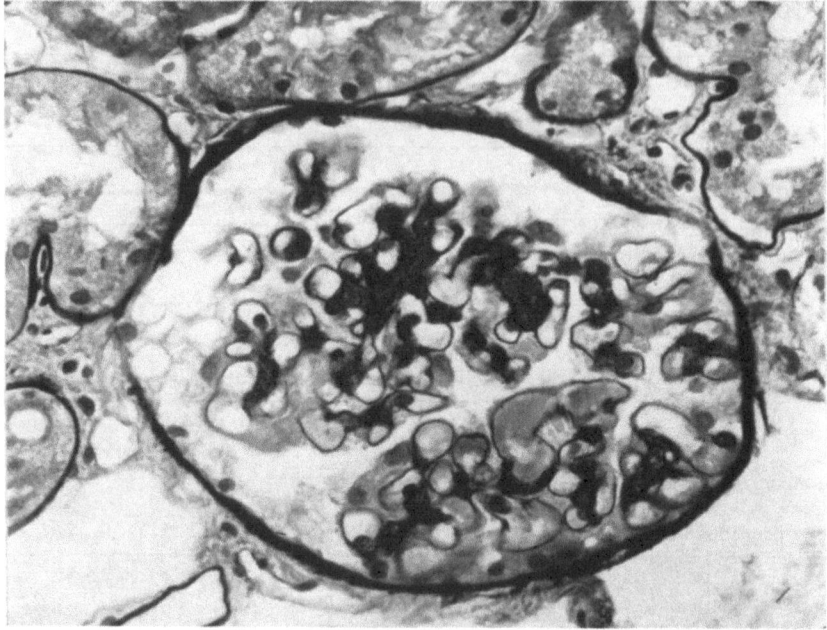

Fig. 17. Mesangioproliferative glomerulonephritis. First biopsy in 34-year-old male. Clinical data: Proteinuria: trace, RBC: +, BP 160/110 mm Hg, creatinine in serum: 1.0 mg %. Paraffin-embedded, PAS-reaction, 460:1

Table 11. The influence of hypertension on the morphologic course in mesangioproliferative glomerulonephritis (+ = improved; ∅ = unchanged; — = deteriorated)

	No.	+	∅	—
Normotensive patients	42	13	23	6
Hypertensive patients	30	1	14	15

compiled when the average blood pressure was determined at the time of the last biopsy:

Morphologically improved	$124.3 \pm 11.1/77.5 \pm 11.9$ mm Hg
Morphologically unchanged	$139.6 \pm 23.9/89.2 \pm 14.2$ mm Hg
Morphologically deteriorated	$154.5 \pm 28.5/97.0 \pm 13.5$ mm Hg

Of the 72 patients with mesangioproliferative glomerulonephritis only 8 had a loss of renal parenchyma with a corresponding reduction of renal function (found in 2 patients in the first biopsy, in 6 patients in the last biopsy). All these patients were hypertensive and exhibited severe glomerular and vascular hypertensive lesions. In our particular study a mesangioproliferative glomerulonephritis did not turn into a chronic renal failure without this additional damage.

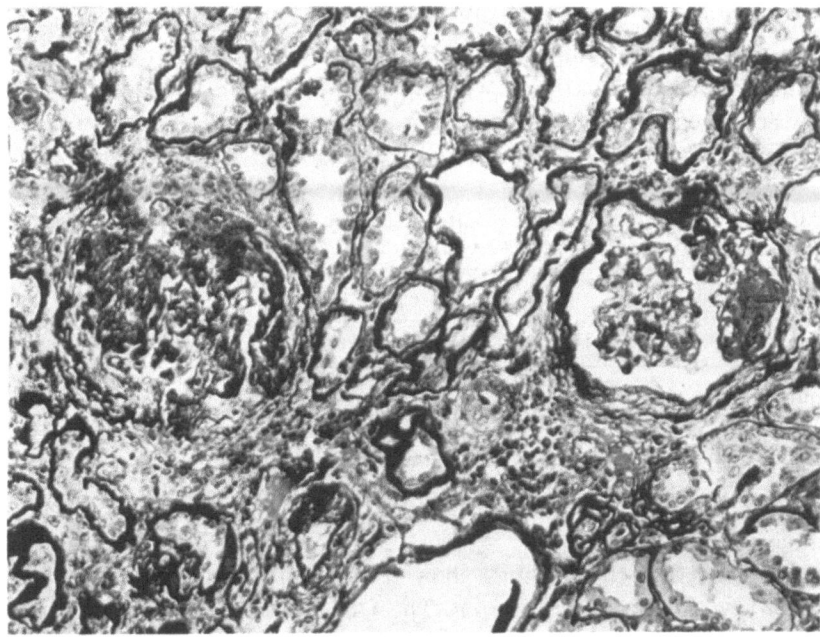

Fig. 18. Mesangioproliferative glomerulonephritis with glomerular hypertensive lesions. Third biopsy 3 years after the first one (Fig. 17). Clinical data: Proteinuria: 3 g/day, RBC: +, BP 150/110 mm Hg (with antihypertension therapy), creatinine in serum: 1.4 mg %. Paraffin-embedded, PAS-reaction, 195:1

8. Mesangioproliferative Glomerulonephritis With Focal Crescents

In this form, described by Habib (1970), the morphologic findings show a mesangial hypercellularity with increase of mesangial area, extensive adhesions between glomerular tuft and Bowman's capsule, and segmental crescents. This form had earlier been classified as rapidly progressive. Habib (1972) separated types I and II, mesangioproliferative glomerulonephritis with focal crescents, from type III, rapidly progressive glomerulonephritis. We examined 14 repeat biopsies of 8 male and 6 female patients aged 5–73 years.

The following pre-existing or simultaneous illnesses were observed:

Schönlein-Henoch's purpura	3 patients
Poststreptococcal nephritis	1 patient
Disseminated lupus erythematosus	1 patient
Upper respiratory infection	1 patient
"Rheumatism"	1 patient
Leg ulcer	1 patient

In 6 patients no pre-existing or simultaneous illness was known. The intervals between the first symptoms and the first biopsies were:

0–6 months	12 patients
6–8 months	1 patient
3 years	1 patient

On the average, we received the last biopsy 10.2 (2–39) months after the first. From 12 patients we obtained two, and from 2 patients 3 biopsies for examination. Five patients were untreated, 3 were treated with steroids, and 6 were given immunsuppressives or cytotoxics. Table 12 shows the effects of therapy.

Table 12. Clinical and morphologic results of therapy in mesangioproliferative glomerulo-nephritis with focal crescents (+ = improved; Ø = unchanged; – = deteriorated)

Therapy	No.	Clinical course			Morphologic course		
		+	Ø	–	+	Ø	–
Without therapy	5	2	1	2	0	3	2
Steroids	3	2	1	0	0	2	1
Immunsuppressives or cytotoxics	6	2	1	3	2	0	4

Morphologically, the findings showed an improvement in 2 patients who had been treated with azathioprine. The focal crescents were mostly fibrosed. In the glomeruli, only a marked mesangial hypercellularity was noted.

In 5 patients the glomerular lesions remained stationary for 6, 14, 15, 18, and 29 months. Apart from scarred lesions we also encountered glomeruli with fresh focal crescents. The mesangium exhibited in the last biopsy a clear but variable increase in cells. In addition, there were many adhesions between the glomerular tuft and Bowman's capsule.

Seven patients exhibited in their last biopsy a steady increase of the glomerular lesions. Many glomeruli were partly or completely hyalinized, and the renal parenchyma was shrunken. Due to persistent acute renal failure in two cases, tubular atrophy and an interstitial fibrosis occurred (Figs. 19 and 20). The glomeruli in these biopsies were almost completely damaged. Both patients died of uremia 2 and 3 months after the first biopsy.

9. Rapidly Progressive Glomerulonephritis

Rapidly progressive glomerulonephritis was named "peracute" or "sub-acute" by VOLHARD and FAHR (1914). ELLIS (1942) called this form "rapidly progressive", because it leads to death from uremia within a few months. With light microscopy most of the glomeruli (more than 50%) show diffuse crescents. The glomerular tuft may display a rather extreme proliferation of glomerular cells (mesangioproliferative glomerulonephritis with diffuse crescents) or it may be necrotizing (necrotizing glomerulonephritis).

Some cases reveal a periglomerulitis with infiltrates of monocytes, lymphocytes, plasma cells, and sporadically located granulocytes. In almost every case, tubular lesions and resulting acute renal failure is evident. Vascular changes are not found in rapidly progressive glomerulonephritis, though they may occur later on in patients who have been dialyzed for a longer time.

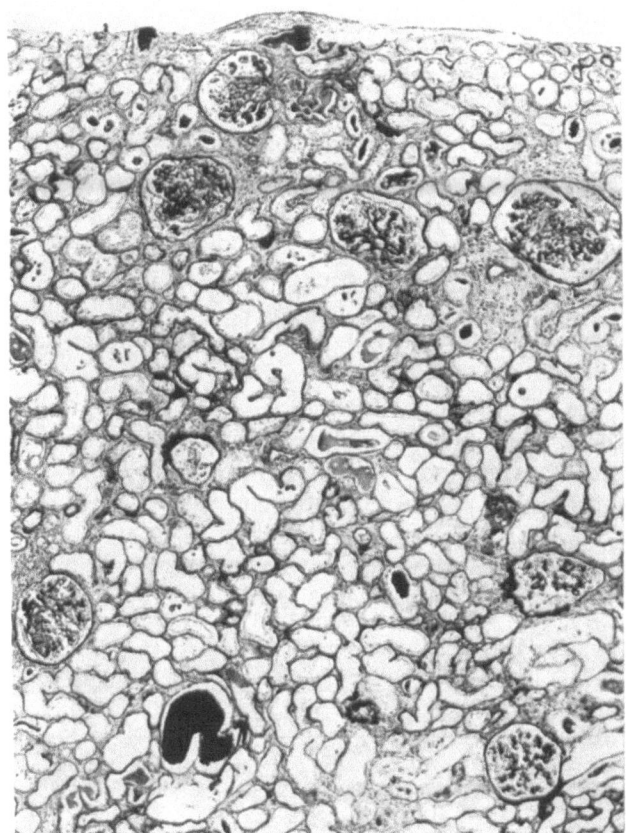

Fig. 19. Mesangioproliferative glomerulonephritis with focal crescents and with acute renal failure. First biopsy in 56-year-old female. Clinical data: Proteinuria: trace, RBC: (+), BP 160/100 mm Hg, creatinine in serum: 15.1 mg %. Paraffin-embedded, PAS-reaction, 70:1

a) Mesangioproliferative Glomerulonephritis With Diffuse Crescents

Ten male and 1 female patients aged 16–62 years exhibited this form. The following pre-existing or simultaneous illnesses were observed:

Goodpasture's syndrome	3 patients
Allergic vasculitis	4 patients
Tonsillitis	1 patient

In 3 patients no pre-existing or simultaneous illnesses were known. The intervals between initial symptoms and the first biopsy were:

<1 month	6 patients
1–6 months	4 patients
9 months	1 patient

On the average, we received the last biopsy 3.6 (0,5–10) months after the first. From 8 patients we obtained 2 and from 3 patients 3 biopsies for

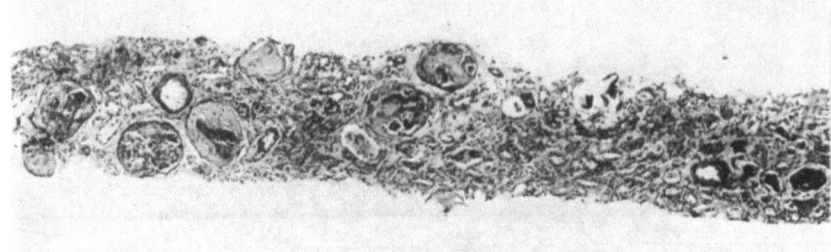

Fig. 20. Mesangioproliferative glomerulonephritis with focal crescents and with persistent acute renal failure. Second biopsy 2 months after the first one (Fig. 19). Clinical data: For 2 months anuria, BP 120/70 mm Hg. Paraffin-embedded, PAS-reaction, 55:1

examination. Five patients were untreated, 2 were given steroids, 2 were treated with azathioprine, and 2 with heparin. The following effects of therapies were discovered (Table 13):

Table 13. Clinical and morphologic results of the therapy in mesangioproliferative glomerulonephritis with diffuse crescents ($+$ =improved; $\emptyset$ =unchanged; $-$ =deteriorated)

Therapy	No.	Clinical course			Morphological course		
		$+$	$\emptyset$	$-$	$+$	$\emptyset$	$-$
Without therapy	5	2	1	2	1	2	2
Steroids	2	1	0	1	1	0	1
Azathioprine	2	0	1	1	0	1	1
Heparin	2	1	0	1	1	0	1

Independent of the different therapies (steroids, azathioprine, heparin), the morphologic lesions in the patients with Goodpasture's syndrome pro‐gressed to a stage of total scarring of all glomeruli.

Mesangioproliferative glomerulonephritis with diffuse crescents seems, how‐ever, to show a more favorable course in patients with allergic diseases. Thus, in a 46-year-old patient with dermatitis herpetiformis treated with heparin, fibrosis of some of the crescents with re-epithelialization of the tuft-facing side occurred as well as a complete disappearance of some of the cres‐cents (Figs. 21 and 22). In 2 other patients with allergic disease, the morpho‐logic findings remained to a large extent the same for 1 and 2 months in one case or improved after 26 months in the other.

In 84% of all the glomeruli of a 16-year-old patient we found crescents after a tonsillitis. These crescents covered the complete circumference of Bowman's capsule. In the semithin section, "humps" were to be seen as evidence of a poststreptococcal etiology. In the second biopsy 3 months later, the patient no longer showed crescents. The glomerular lesions were those of a moderate mesangioproliferative glomerulonephritis.

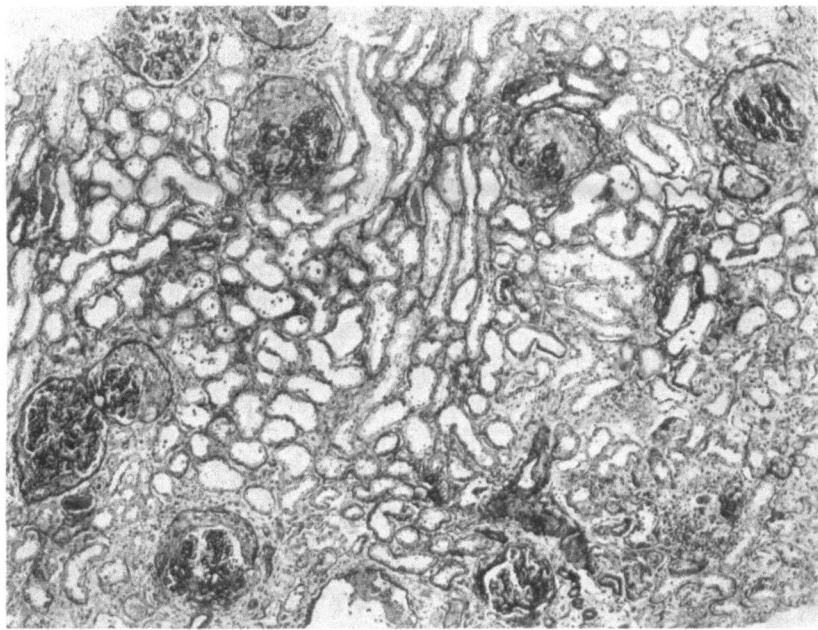

Fig. 21. Mesangioproliferative glomerulonephritis with diffuse crescents. First biopsy in 46-year-old male. Clinical data: Proteinuria: $2^0/_{00}$, RBC: macroscopic, BP 140/90 mm Hg, creatinine in serum: 4.8 mg %. Paraffin-embedded, PAS-reaction, 55:1

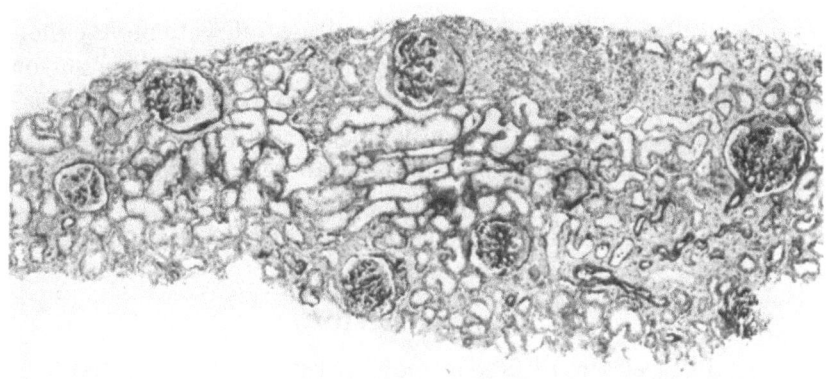

Fig. 22. Mesangioproliferative glomerulonephritis with diffuse crescents. Second biopsy 3 months after the first one (Fig. 21). Clinical data: Proteinuria $0.5^0/_{00}$, RBC: neg., BP 150/90 mm Hg, creatinine in serum: 1.8 mg %, treatment with heparin. Paraffin-embedded, PAS-reaction, 42:1

The disease in the remaining patients led to total scarring of all glomeruli found in the last biopsy.

Ischemic tubular lesions of different degrees of severity were seen in the renal tissue of all patients except the 1 patient with poststreptococcal nephritis.

b) Necrotizing Glomerulonephritis

In this form of rapidly progressive glomerulonephritis, the necrosis predominates from the beginning of the disease (Fig. 23). The structure of the glomerulus is almost completely destroyed. The crescents are not as diffuse or numerous as those found in the mesangioproliferative form. Periglomerulitis is often observed in the necrotizing from, although it is not always found in all kidneys. In the course of the disease the glomeruli become scarred (Fig. 24). Late stages of necrotizing glomerulonephritis cannot be distinguished from late stages of mesangioproliferative glomerulonephritis with diffuse crescents.

We examined nine biopsies of 5 male and 4 female patients aged 16–46 years. In 2 patients the glomerulonephritis occurred with Goodpasture's syndrome, and in 2 with Wegener's granulomatosis. Of the remaining 5 patients no pre-existing or simultaneous illnesses were known.

The intervals between initial symptoms and first biopsies were less than 1 month in the case of 7 patients, 6 weeks in the case of 1 patient, and 4 months in the case of another.

We obtained the second biopsy, on the average, 3.1 months (0.5–10) months after the first one. From all patients we received renal tissue twice for examination. Four patients were untreated, 2 patients were administered steroids, 3 were treated with azathioprine.

All patients either died or were chronically dialyzed. One patient with Goodpasture's syndrome showed some improvement and went 1 month without dialysis.

Morphologically, we found in the last biopsy of all patients the glomeruli totally scarred (Fig. 24). The hyalinized glomeruli were partially surrounded by round cells and were phagocytosed so that after prolonged dialysis, only a small number of glomeruli apparently existed in the kidney.

We could observe this periglomerulitis in all cases of this group, that is, not only in the patients with Wegener's granulomatosis.

All biopsies displayed the morphologic signs of an acute renal failure.

IV. Discussion

Since renal biopsies were first introduced by Iversen and Brun (1951), it has been possible to examine renal tissue with the light microscope, immunfluorescent techniques, and with the electron microscope, and thus to correlate clinical symptoms with morphologic changes. Hence, it has been possible to take note of early changes histologically and to describe not only the clinical but also the morphologic course by means of serial biopsies. As a result of biopsy studies, the former classification of the glomerulonephritides, which was based on clinical symptoms and autopsy findings (Volhard, 1918; Ellis, 1942), became largely ineffectual inasmuch as all symptoms are encountered, more or less frequently, in all forms of glomerulonephritis (Kincaid-Smith, 1967; Bohle et al., 1969; Wehner et al., 1969; Habib, 1970).

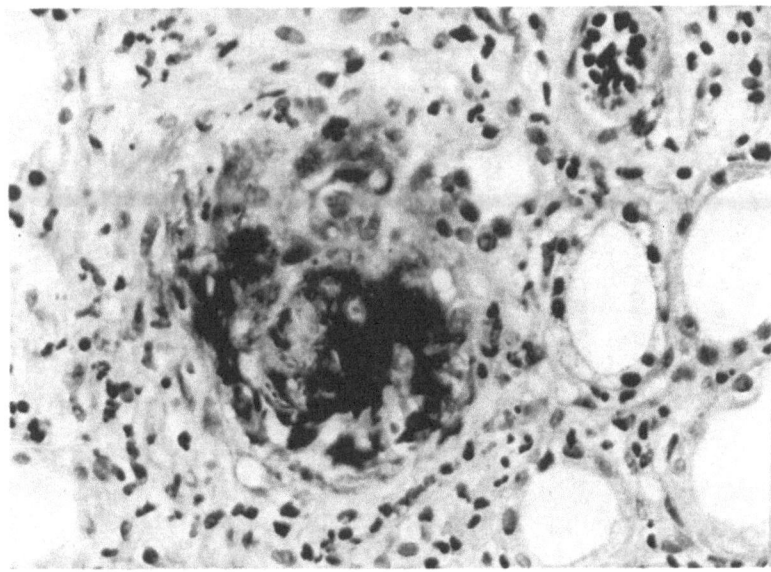

Fig. 23. Necrotising glomerulonephritis. First biopsy in 20-year-old female. Clinical data: Proteinuria: trace, RBC: macroscopic, BP 140/80 mm Hg, creatinine in serum: 7.7 mg%. Paraffin-embedded, Masson-Goldner stain, 375:1

In 1950, FARNSWORTH reported on the influence of corticosteroids on the nephrotic syndrome. Since CHASIS *et al.* (1949) published for the first time a report on the treatment of nephrotic-syndrome children with a nitrogen mustard therapy, attempts have been made to treat glomerulonephritis with immunsuppressives and/or cytotoxics, the rationale being that an immunologic reaction, in the sense of an antigen-antibody reaction, could play an important role pathogenically in glomerulonephritis (MASUGI, 1934). Moreover, since 1967, indomethacin therapy (MICHIELSEN and LAMBERT), and, since 1966, heparin therapy, based on the experiments of VASSALLI and McCLUSKEY (1964), have become common in some forms (SHIRES *et al.*, 1966).

It is, therefore, not surprising that there are few reports of untreated cases that have been biopsied. Since 1951, patients with histologically verified renal lesions have been treated with drugs, and cannot be compared with those before 1951 who have not been treated. One further difficulty arises when comparing our results with those of other authors who have only performed one diagnostic biopsy, that is, a divergence between the clinical and morphologic courses, especially in patients treated with drugs.

1. Morphologic Course of Untreated Patients

The morphologically controlled untreated cases which have been published so far are shown in Table 14.

Table 14 shows that those cases with minimal changes without nephrotic syndrome have a good prognosis even without chemotherapy. In the minimal-

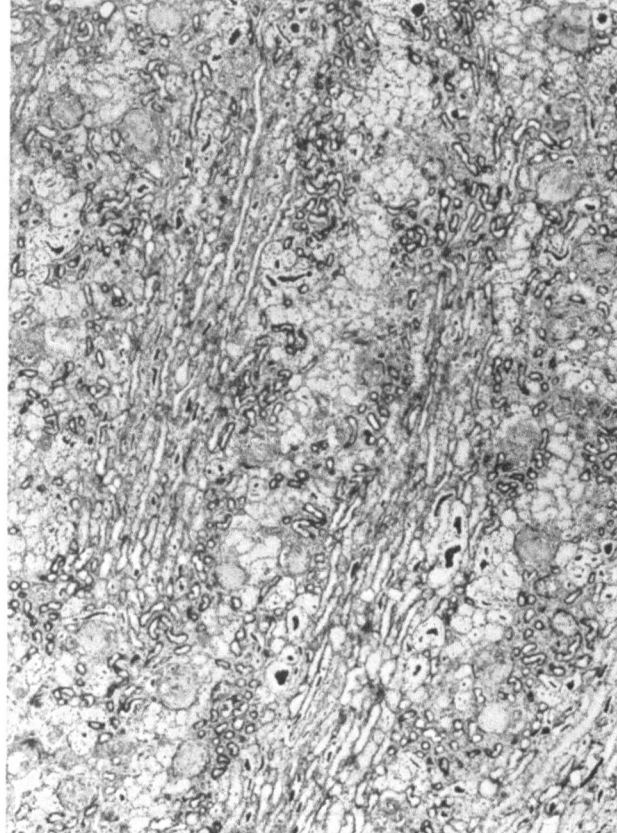

Fig. 24. End-stage kidney after necrotizing glomerulonephritis. Nephrectomy 10 months after first biopsy (Fig. 23). Clinical data: Dialysis since onset of illness, BP moderately elevated. Paraffin-embedded, PAS-reaction, 42:1

changes category, the nephrotic syndrome will increase the chance of complications (acute renal failure, hypertension, infections). Since the clinicians who sent us the biopsy material did not deny treatment to a patient with this disease, we saw no untreated cases.

Focal sclerosing glomerulonephritis usually leads to renal insufficiency and has, therefore, a bad prognosis (Table 14).

In most cases of perimembranous glomerulonephritis the disease progresses slowly. On the other hand, membranoproliferative glomerulonephritis leads in a shorter time to chronic renal failure with loss of renal parenchyma. Acute endocapillary (acute) glomerulonephritis has a good prognosis as long as no complications occur.

Quite a good prognosis, too, is the case with the mesangioproliferative glomerulonephritis; however, this form is often complicated by hypertension which clearly leads to a deteriorating morphologic course.

Mesangioproliferative glomerulonephritis with focal crescents has a more favorable prognosis than that with diffuse crescents. However, a restitutio

Table 14. Morphologic course of glomerulonephritis in untreated patients (+ =improved; ∅ = unchanged; − =deteriorated)

Authors	No.	Morphological course		
		+	∅	−
Minimal changes without nephrotic syndrome:				
Levy et al. (1973)	3	0	3	0
Our cases	15	0	14	1
Focal sclerosing glomerulonephritis:				
Hyman et al. (1973)	3	0	0	3
Our cases	8	0	3	5
Perimembranous glomerulonephritis				
Forland et al. (1969)	2	0	1	1
Franklin et al. (1973)	2	0	0	2
Our cases	6	0	4	2
Membranoproliferative glomerulonephritis:				
Burkholder et al. (1970)	2	1	0	1
Herdman et al. (1970)	11	0	11	0
Kincaid-Smith (1972)	13	0	0	13
Our cases	3	0	1	2
Endocapillary (acute) glomerulonephritis:				
Feldman et al. (1966)	2	2	0	0
Jennings et al. (1961)	12	7	5	0
Michael et al. (1966)	4	4	0	0
Okuda et al. (1970)	5	3	2	0
Strunk et al. (1964)	1	1	0	0
Travis et al. (1973)	57	52	2	3
Wegmann et al. (1973)	1	1	0	0
White (1964)	3	0	2	1
Our case	1	1	0	0
Mesangioproliferative glomerulonephritis:				
Our cases	22	7	9	6
Mesangioproliferative glomerulonephritis with focal crescents:				
Our cases	5	0	3	2
Mesangioproliferative glomerulonephritis with diffuse crescents:				
Forland et al. (1966)	3	0	0	3
Leonard et al. (1970)	6	1	3	2
Wegmann et al. (1973)	1	1	0	0
Our cases	5	1	2	2
Necrotising glomerulonephritis:				
Leonard et al. (1970)	1	0	0	1
Our cases	4	0	0	4

ad integrum is not possible in the former, and in most cases this form, over a more prolonged period, will lead to chronic renal failure. In mesangio-proliferative glomerulonephritis with diffuse crescents only the poststreptococcal form has a favorable prognosis similar to that of endocapillary (acute) glomerulonephritis (Reichel *et al.*, 1974), but this form occurs very rarely.

The prognosis of the necrotizing glomerulonephritis is fatal.

2. Morphologic Course of Treated Patients

More reports are available on morphologically controlled courses of individual glomerulonephritis forms under treatment with steroids, indomethacin, azathioprine, cytotoxics, and heparin than on untreated cases, although the number of patients is usually small. In Table 15, we have endeavored to categorize the research that has been published thus far and our findings relating to observations of morphologic courses under treatment.

A morphologic improvement in two cases of perimembranous glomerulonephritis has been described by Olbing *et al.* (1973) after steroid therapy, and two more cases have been reported by Bariéty *et al.* (1969) after combined steroid and cytotoxic treatment. Cade *et al.* (1971) observed in mesangioproliferative glomerulonephritis a reduction in proliferation after heparin therapy (Table 15). Especially good results with anticoagulant in membranoproliferative glomerulonephritis and in rapidly progressive glomerulonephritis were reported by Kincaid-Smith *et al.* (1968, 1970, 1972). After indomethacin therapy, Michielsen *et al.* (1969) verified an improvement of the morphologic findings in 6 patients with mesangioproliferative glomerulonephritis (Table 15). The rest of the morphologic improvements listed in Table 15 were not explicitly attributed by the authors to the therapy used.

In none of the forms we were able to note an influence of the therapy on the morphologic course although the clinical improvement was indisputable. In some patients under treatment, paradoxically, a clinical cure coincide with progression of the morphologic lesions. On the other hand, in an increasing number of publications, attention has been drawn to the risks of long-term therapy with steroids and cytotoxics. Thus, Blake *et al.* (1970) pointed out that more patients died from side-effects due to steroids (hypertension, ulcer bleeding, apoplexy) than from renal insufficiency. The same warning was expressed in the Report by the Medical Research Council in 1971. In the case of two children being treated with cytotoxics for nephrotic syndrome, one contracted measles (Meadow *et al.*, 1969) and the other varicella (Scheinmann *et al.*, 1971) which both proved fatal. Spermiogenesis (Miller, 1971) and ovarian function (Miller *et al.*, 1971) are influenced as well. Jensen (1967) pointed out chromosomal changes due to azathioprine therapy.

So far, no side-effects of indomethacin have been found.

3. Influence of Noninflammatory Lesions on Morphologic Course

The prognosis may worsen considerably if tubular lesions occur in addition to glomerular lesions. The nephrotic syndrome with a reduction of intravascular blood volume predisposes to acute renal failure. Thus, the severity

Table 15. Morphologic course of Glomerulonephritides in treated patients (st = steroids; i = indomethacin; a = azathioprine; c = cytotoxics; h = heparin. + = improved; ∅ = unchanged; − = deteriorated)

Authors	No.	Therapy	Morphologic course		
			+	∅	−
Minimal changes without nephrotic syndrome:					
Our cases	17	st, i, a, c	0	12	5
Minimal changes with nephrotic syndrome:					
Folli et al. (1958)	1	st	0	1	0
Habib et al. (1971)	17	unknown	0	9	8
Hardwicke et al. (1967)	7	st	0	7	0
Hopper et al. (1970)	11	st, a	0	11	0
Our cases	21	st, i, a, c	0	18	3
Focal sclerosing glomerulonephritis:					
Habib et al. (1971)	2	unknown	0	2	0
Hyman et al. (1973)	12	st, a, c	0	0	12
Levy et al. (1973)	2	unknown	0	0	2
McIntosh et al. (1972)	2	st + a	1	0	1
Our cases	30	st, i, a, c	0	9	21
Perimembranous glomerulonephritis:					
Bariéty et al. (1968)	2	st + c	2	0	0
Chan et al. (1966)	4	st	0	4	0
Forland et al. (1969)	8	st	1	2	5
Franklin et al. (1973)	14	st	0	3	11
Gluck et al. (1973)	11	unknown	2	4	5
Habib et al. (1971)	4	unknown	0	4	0
Hardwicke et al. (1967)	5	st	0	0	0
Olbing et al. (1973)	2	st	2	0	0
Our cases	28	st, i, a, c	5	6	17
Membranoproliferative glomerulonephritis:					
v. Acker et al. (1970)	7	st	0	0	7
Bariéty et al. (1971)	21	st, a, c	2	18	1
Burkholder et al. (1970)	3	st + a	1	2	0
Cameron et al. (1970)	12	st, a, c,	0	12	0
Fries et al. (1968)	6	a	0	6	0
Habib et al. (1971)	11	unknown	0	11	0
Herdman et al. (1970)	11	st, a, h	0	11	0
Holland et al. (1972)	5	st, a, h	1	0	4
Kincaid-Smith (1972)	16	c + h	5	9	2
McIntosh et al. (1972)	3	st, i, a	3	0	0
Our cases	17	st, i, a, c	4	2	11
Endocapillary (acute) glomerulonephritis:					
Jennings et al. (1961)	1	st	1	0	0
Kincaid-Smith et al. (1970)	2	h	2	0	0
McIntosh et al. (1972)	9	st + a	6	3	0
Travis et al. (1973)	3	st, a	0	0	3
White et al. (1966)	1	st + a	0	0	1
Our cases	12	a, c, h	9	0	3

Table 15 (continued)

Authors	No.	Therapy	Morphologic course		
			+	Ø	−
Mesangioproliferative glomerulonephritis:					
BOOTH *et al.* (1970)	7	a, c	0	7	0
CADE *et al.* (1971)	8	h	8	0	0
FREEDMAN *et al.* (1970)	6	h	2	1	3
FRIES *et al.* (1968)	3	a	1	1	1
HARDWICKE *et al.* (1967)	13	st	0	13	0
KRUMHAAR *et al.* (1971)	15	st	0	11	4
MICHIELSEN *et al.* (1969)	7	i	6	1	0
QUIRIN *et al.* (1971)	19	i	0	9	10
WHITE *et al.* (1966)	7	a, c	2	4	1
Our cases	50	st, i, a, c	7	28	15
Mesangioproliferative glomerulonephritis with focal crescents:					
Our cases	9	st, a, c	2	2	5
Mesangioproliferative glomerulonephritis with diffuse crescents:					
BERLYNE *et al.* (1964)	6	st	0	0	6
KINCAID-SMITH *et al.* (1968)	1	h	1	0	0
KINCAID-SMITH *et al.* (1970)	1	h+c	1	0	0
Our cases	7	st, a, c, h	2	1	4
Necrotizing glomerulonephritis:					
LEONARD *et al.* (1970)	3	st	0	2	1
Our cases	5	st, a	0	0	5

of the proteinuria does not necessarily determine the occurrence of an acute renal failure. Only one patient had a renal failure in addition to an existing minimal-changes lesion with a proteinuria of 10 g/day. This led to focal interstitial fibrosis, tubular atrophy, and to hyalinosis of glomeruli. Another patient, however, with a massive proteinuria of 80 g/day did not suffer from an acute renal failure.

In cases of focal sclerosing glomerulonephritis we observed an acute renal failure with the corresponding tubular lesions in 5 patients with proteinuria of 10–30 g/day. Only 1 patient completely recovered from the tubular lesions. The other 4 patients exhibited, after 2–12 months an extensive tubular atrophy (Fig. 6) and a diffuse interstitial fibrosis. Besides the inflammatory lesions the glomeruli showed a "collapse of capillary walls" (Fig. 6) or were completely hyalinized. In the hyalinized glomeruli of one patient there was the striking presence of marked calcium deposits.

Among the 34 patients with perimembranous glomerulonephritis, only 1 patient had renal failure during a nephrotic syndrome. Severe hypertension also developed at the same time.

In 8 out of 20 patients with membranoproliferative glomerulonephritis and a persistent nephrotic syndrome, ischemic tubular lesions could be detected and found to aggravate the morphologic condition. Interstitial fibrosis occurred with tubular atrophy as well as with hyalinosis of glomeruli. The clinical course and the prognosis of membranoproliferative glomerulonephritis varies according to whether a nephrotic syndrome develops, as described by CAMERON et al. (1973).

The good prognosis of endocapillary (acute) glomerulonephritis worsens considerably if, an acute renal failure occurs. Further investigations should answer whether a diffuse or focal extracapillaty proliferation occurs (Figs. 15 and 16); whether there is a connection between the existence of crescents and the acute renal failure; and whether it was accidental that in our three cases such courses developed.

We could not observe additional ischemic lesions in any of the 72 patients with mesangioproliferative glomerulonephritis.

Both patients who died from a mesangioproliferative glomerulonephritis with focal crescents had suffered for a longer period from an acute renal failure which had led to tubular atrophy (Figs. 21 and 22). This tubular destruction resulted in scarring of the related glomeruli. Acute renal failure occurs in most cases of rapidly progressive glomerulonephritis. It has little influence on the glomerular lesions as improvement is only possible in quite exceptional cases.

The impact of hypertension on the prognosis of glomerulonephritis was first pointed out by ELLIS (1942). He called the combination of glomerulo-nephritis with hypertension a "circulus vitiosus". According to MEYER et al. (1973), the glomerular hypertensive lesions may develop directly if the elevated blood pressure directly affects the glomerular capillaries. The indirect hyper-tensive lesions occur when glomerular flow is reduced due to constriction of the preglomerular vessels. The direct glomerular lesions are characterized (according to MEYER et al., 1973) by the following-aneurysmal widening of the capillary wall with thrombotic material within these aneurysms (Fig. 4), partly focal, partly diffuse mesangium widening, focal damage to glomerular lobules, and PAS-positive inclusions in the epithelial cells. The indirect glomerular lesions occur as a result of deficient blood flow after constriction of preglomerular vessels due to arterio- and arteriolosclerosis, or as a con-sequence of an obliterating endarteriitis (FAHR). The typical lesions in the glomerulus are characterized by the collapse of loops, scars mostly in the hilar region, and adhesions of individual lobule areas, and the special type of damage to the glomeruli. The collapse of loops coincides with a widening of the glomerular capillary wall. This widening is, however, misleading due to a pleating of the basement membrane which is only detectable in the semithin section. In the scarred glomeruli the clearly PAS-positive loop con-volute is surrounded by only slightly colored lamellas.

It is possible to produce in rats similar glomerular lesions as observed in man through hypertension resulting from unilateral constriction of the renal artery in the contralateral unconstricted kidney (HELMCHEN, 1973). In Fig. 25 epithelial cell droplets can be seen in the lower glomerulus. In the glomerulus to the right a capillary wall aneurysm is present. In the glomerulus

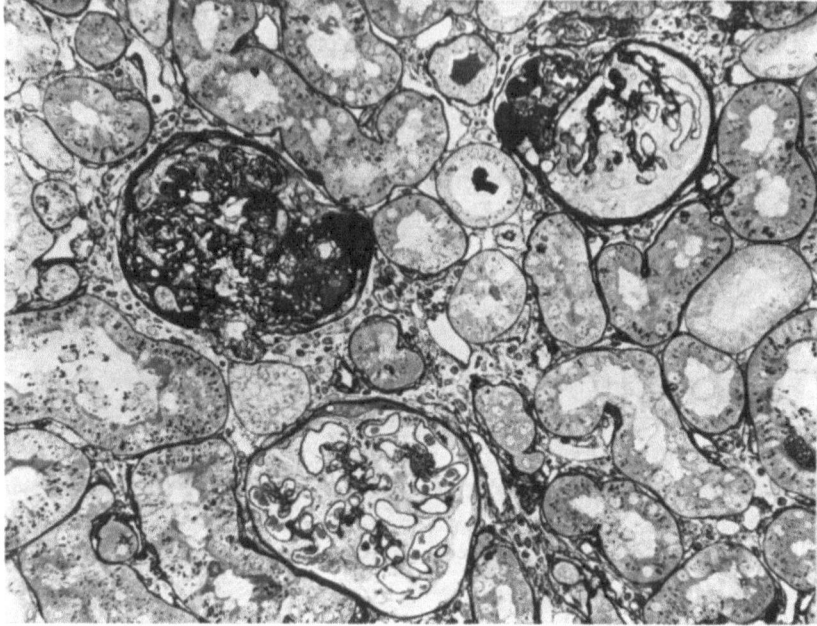

Fig. 25. Rat kidney. Hypertensive glomerulopathy in the unclamped kidney from clamping the centralateral renal artery. Duration of hypertension 8 months. Plexiglass-embedded, silver impregnation, 275:1. (I am grateful to Priv.-Doz. Dr. U. Helmchen for this material)

to the left beside the aneurysm, the mesangium has widened as well as the basement membrane. The kidney, however, protected from the raised blood pressure by the clamp, does not exhibit glomerular or vascular lesions.

The hypertensive lesions reported above thus occur independently of pre-existing inflammatory glomerular lesions. Direct as well as indirect hypertensive glomerular lesions are seen in the same kidney side by side, as is shown in Fig. 18. The left glomerulus is indirectly damaged (collapse of loops), and the right one is directly damaged (thrombosed capillary wall aneurysm). The morphologic differentiation between primary inflammatory and hypertensive glomerular lesions is not always possible in advanced stages of renal damage, but is possible through repeat biopsies. The frequency of hypertension depends on the particular glomerulonephritis.

In the minimal-changes form without nephrotic syndrome, hypertension is rare (2 out of 32 patients). If hypertension does exist, it can lead to a more serious progression of the kidney disease which, otherwise, would take a relatively harmless course. Both our patients with minimal changes with nephrotic syndrome, who exhibited a renal insufficiency, had also glomerular lesions due to hypertension (Figs. 3 and 4). These lesions completely obscured this minimal changes form. Without a preceding biopsy it would have been impossible to diagnose the original disease.

In the cases of focal sclerosing glomerulonephritis, 17 out of 28 patients had hypertension. In this form, differentiation between inflammatory and hypertensive lesions is particularly difficult, because the final stages with hyalinosis in single loops and adhesions are very similar. It may be possible to differentiate by localizing the lesions in the glomerulus. Inflammatory lesions are distinctly peripheral while hypertensive ones are nearer to the hilum. In the whole kidney inflammatory lesions are juxtamedullary and hypertensive ones are diffuse.

In perimembranous glomerulonephritis hypertensive glomerular lesions only rarely occur in addition to inflammatory lesions, although hypertension is often noted. The influence of a hypertension on the prognosis of the membranoproliferative glomerulonephritis was pointed out by v. ACKER et al. (1970) and HERDMAN et al. (1970). They held that therapy with steroids or with azathioprine and heparin would not show any success, but the course would depend on blood pressure values. Our results (Table 8) confirm their observation. So far we have not observed hypertensive glomerular lesions in the endocapillary (acute) glomerulonephritis, although short term hypertension often occurred in the cases. Hypertension in mesangioproliferative glomerulonephritis clearly worsens the morphologic course. So far, we have not observed a mesangioproliferative glomerulonephritis that led to chronic renal failure without the existence of additional glomerular and vascular hypertensive lesions. Mesangioproliferative glomerulonephritis with focal or diffuse crescents and necrotizing glomerulonephritis exhibit such severe lesions that the prognosis is likely may to be very little affected by hypertensive lesions.

4. Which Glomerulonephritides Lead to Renal Atrophy or Renal Insufficiency?

All rapidly progressive glomerulonephritides lead to rapid chronic renal failure without necessarily renal atrophy.

In the cases of focal sclerosing glomerulonephritis, perimembranous glomerulonephritis, membranoproliferative glomerulonephritis, as well as in cases of mesangioproliferative glomerulonephritis with focal crescents, it can be expected that after varying periods of time chronic renal failure will appear without additional damaging factors.

In consequence of additional hypertensive lesions, 8 out of 72 patients with mesangioproliferative glomerulonephritis developed renal insufficiency.

As a result of a concomitant acute renal failure in 3 patients with endocapillary (acute) glomerulonephritis, the character of the glomerular disease changed. A mesangioproliferative glomerulonephritis with diffuse or focal crescents appeared and led to a less of renal parenchyma 3, 9, and 10 months after onset of the disease. Table 16 gives the number of patients, and states how long after the onset of their disease the individual forms led to chronic renal failure.

Table 16. Frequency of chronic renal insufficiency in Glomerulonephritides

Form of glomerulonephritis	Chronic renal failure/ total No. patients	Time after onset
Minimal changes with nephrotic syndrome	2/21	13, 15 months
Focal sclerosing glomerulonephritis	12/38	2, 2, 3, 5 months 2, 3, 4, 8, 9, 11, 22, 24 years
Perimembranous glomerulonephritis	5/34	2 months, 2, 3, 4, 6 years
Membranoproliferative glomerulonephritis	7/20	1, 2, 2, 4, 7, 8, 11 years
Endocapillary (acute) glomerulonephritis	3/13	3, 9, 10 months
Mesangioproliferative glomerulonephritis	8/72	2, 3, 4, 4, 5, 5, 5, 6 years
Mesangioproliferative glomerulonephritis with focal crescents	7/14	2, 3, 8, 11, 16, 22, 39 months
Rapidly progressive glomerulonephritis	17/20	from the beginning

V. Summary

By means of 264 repeat biopsies in kidneys of patients with glomerulonephritis, an attempt has been made to describe the morphologic course of the individual forms, and to compare it with the clinical course.

The mild glomerular lesions in the minimal-changes form without nephrotic syndrome usually remain unchanged, and the prognosis is good.

The morphologic course of the minimal-changes form with nephrotic syndrome appears similarly unchanged. In this form, however, the incidence of complications (acute renal failure, hypertension, infection) is increased due to the nephrotic syndrome. Focal sclerosing glomerulonephritis, perimembranous glomerulonephritis, and membranoproliferative glomerulonephritis are glomerular diseases which progress slowly, leading usually to renal insufficiency.

In the case of endocapillary (acute) glomerulonephritis, the morphologic healing lags behind clinical improvement by several months. The prognosis is much worse when an acute renal failure occurs as well. In three patients with such a complication a transition to mesangioproliferative glomerulonephritis with focal or diffuse crescents was observed. Three, 9, and 10 months later a loss of renal parenchyma had occurred.

Mesangioproliferative glomerulonephritis may develop after an acute endocapillary glomerulonephritis or without any pre-existing illness. Morphologically, it is not possible to distinguish between the two types. The prognosis is good as long as no hypertension complicates the condition.

The prognosis of mesangioproliferative glomerulonephritis with focal crescents is certainly better than this form with diffuse crescents. In most cases the inflammatory process advances and leads to loss of renal parenchyma months or years later. Apart from very rare exceptions the rapidly progressive glomerulonephritis soon leads to renal insufficiency.

We have not noted any influence of treatment with steroids, indomethacin immunsuppressives, or cytotoxics on the morphologic course.

As soon as the glomerulonephritis is complicated by the occurrence of hypertension or acute renal failure, the prognosis rapidly worsens. Hypertension may change the morphologic findings completely since glomerular and vascular hypertensive lesions can obscure the primary inflammatory pattern.

An acute renal failure persisting for a longer time may lead to tubular atrophy with interstitial fibrosis and hyalinosis of glomeruli. Moreover, in the the case of such a chronic deficiency of blood flow, a collapse of the glomerular capillary wall may occur which also leads to the scarring of glomeruli.

After varying periods of time, renal insufficiency occurs as a consequence of the rapidly progressive, focal sclerosing, perimembranous, and membranoproliferative glomerulonephritis, and mesangioproliferative glomerulonephritis with focal crescents. All other forms, based on our experience, only lead to loss of renal parenchyma or to renal insufficiency if noninflammatory additional injury occurs as is the case with hypertension and acute renal failure.

Acknowledgments

I should like to thank Prof. Dr. A. BOHLE for the use of material and for stimulating discussion in the preparation of this work.

For the clinical data I should like to thank colleagues from the Medical Clinics of Freiburg (Prof. Dr. KLUTHE), München (Prof. Dr. EDEL), Göttingen (Prof. Dr. SCHELER), Bonn (Dr. FROTSCHER), Augsburg (Prof. Dr. RENNER), Heesen (Dr. RINSCHE), Münster (Prof. Dr. LOSSE), Tübingen (PD Dr. BUNDSCHU), Stuttgart (Dr. STREICHER), Mainz (Prof. Dr. STRAUB), Freiburg (PD Dr. HOPPE-SEYLER), Berlin (Dr. HÖFER), Köln (Prof. Dr. SIEBERTH, Prof. Dr. RENNER), Erlangen (Prof. Dr. DEMLING), Fulda (Prof. Dr. NIETH), Karlsruhe (Prof. Dr. SCHIRMEISTER), Bremen (Dr. POTJAN), Neuwied (Prof. Dr. HUBER), Marl (Dr. BÜRGEL), Erbach (Dr. KOPP), Sigmaringen (Dr. AMANN), Essen (Prof. Dr. BOCK), Giessen (Prof. Dr. SCHÜTTERLE), Mannheim (Prof. Dr. STRAUCH), Darmstadt (Prof. Dr. FUCHS), and Passau (Dr. FISCHER).

I am grateful for the excellent technical assistance of Mrs. F. SCHULZ, Mrs. D. BECK, and Miss E. FINGER.

For the English translation I should like to thank Mrs. K. SCHMIDT and Dr. G. NEILD.

References

ACKER, K. J. V., BRANDE, J. V. D., VINCKE, H.: Membranous-proliferative glomerulonephritis. Helv. paediat. Acta **25**, 204–218 (1970)

BARIÉTY, J., DRUET, PH., LOIRAT, PH., LAGRUE, G.: Les Glomérulonéphrites Pariétoprolifératives. Étude Histopathologique en Microscopie optique, électronique et en immunohistochimie de 49 cas. Corrélations anatomocliniques. Path. Biol. **19**, 259–283 (1971)

BARIÉTY, J., SAMARCQ, P., LAGRUE, G., FRITEL, D., MILLIEZ, P.: Évolution ultrastructurale favorable de deux cas de Glomérulopathies primitives à dépots ExtraMembranoux diffus. Presse méd. **76**, 2179–2182 (1968)

Bell, E. T.: Renal Diseases. Philadelphia: Lea and Febiger 1946

Berger, J., Galle, P.: Dépôts denses au sein des membranes basales du rein. Étude en microscopies optique et électronique. Presse méd. **71**, 2351–2354 (1963)

Berlyne, G. M., Baker, S. B.: Acute anuric glomerulonephritis. Quart. J. Med. **33**, 105–115 (1964)

Black, D. A. K., Rose, G., Brewer, D. B.: Controlled Trial of Prednisone in Adult Patients with the Nephrotic Syndrome. Brit. Med. J. (1970), **3**, 421–426

Bohle, A.: Neue pathologisch-anatomische Befunde bei glomerulären Nierenkrankheiten. Dtsch. med. J. **15**, 372–379 (1964)

Bohle, A., Buchborn, E., Edel, H. H., Renner, E., Wehner, H.: Zur pathologischen Anatomie und Klinik der Glomerulonephritis. I. Die akuten und perakuten Glomerulonephritiden. Klin. Wschr. **47**, 733–742 (1969)

Bohle, A., Gärtner, H. V., Fischbach, H., Bock, K. D., Edel, H. H., Frotscher, U., Kluthe, R., Mönninghoff, W., Scheler, F.: The Morphological and Clinical Features of Membranoproliferative Glomerulonephritis in Adults. Virch. Arch. A **363**, 213–224 (1974)

Bohle, A., Jahnecke, J.: Vergleichende histometrische Untersuchungen an bioptisch und autoptisch gewonnenem Nierengewebe mit normaler Funktion und bei akutem Nierenversagen. Klin. Wschr. **42**, 1–12 (1964)

Booth, L. J., Aber, G. M.: Immunosuppressive Therapy in Adults with Proliferative Glomerulonephritis. Controlled Trial. Lancet **1970 II**, 1010–1013

Burck, H. Ch., Gayer, J.: Chronopathologie des akuten Nierenversagens. Zugleich ein Beitrag zur Vita reducta. Virch. Arch. **340**, 276–288 (1966)

Burkholder, P. M., Marchand, A., Krueger, R. P.: Mixed Membranous and Proliferative Glomerulonephritis. A Correlative Light, Immunofluorescence and Electron Microscope Study. Lab. Invest. **23**, 459–479 (1970)

Cade, J. R., de Quesada, A. M., Shires, D. L., Levin, D. M., Hackett, R. L., Spooner, G. R., Schlein, E. M., Pickering, M. J., Holcomb, A.: The Effect of Long Term High Dose Heparin Treatment on the Course of Chronic Proliferative Glomerulonephritis. Nephron **8**, 68–70 (1971)

Cameron, J. S., Glasgow, E. F., Ogg, C. S., White, R. H.: Membranoproliferative Glomerulonephritis and Persistent Hypocomplementaemia. Brit. Med. J. **1970**, **4**, 7–14

Cameron, J. S., Ogg, C. S., White, R. H. R., Glasgow, E. F.: The clinical features and prognosis of patients with normocomplementemic mesangiocapillary glomerulonephritis. Clin. Nephrol. **1**, 8–13 (1973)

Chan, W. C., Tsao, Y. C.: Diffuse membranous glomerulonephritis in children. J. Clin. Path. **19**, 464–469 (1966)

Chasis, H., Goldring, W., Baldwin, D. S.: Effect of Febrile Plasma, Typhoid Vaccine and Nitrogen Mustard on Renal Manifestations of Human Glomerulonephritis. Proc. Soc. Exp. Biol. (N.Y.) **71**, 565–567 (1949)

Churg, J., Habib, R., White, R. H. R.: Pathology of the Nephrotic Syndrome in Children. A Report for the International Study of Kidney Disease in Children. Lancet **1970 I**, 1299–1302

Ehrenreich, T., Churg, J.: Pathology of Membranous Nephropathy. Path. Ann. **3**, 145–186 (1968)

Ellis, A.: Natural history of Bright's disease: Clinical, histological and experimental observations. Lancet **1942 I**, 1–7

Fahr, Th.: Pathologische Anatomie des Morbus Brightii. In: Handbuch der speziellen pathologischen Anatomie und Histologie (Hrsg. F. Henke and O. Lubarsch,) 6. Bd., 1. Teil, pp. 156–472. Berlin: Springer 1925

Farnsworth, E. D.: Metabolic changes associated with administration of adrenocorticotrophin in the nephrotic syndrome. Proc. Soc. Exp. Biol. (N.Y.) **74**, 60 (1950)

Farquhar, M. G., Vernier, R. L., Good, R. A.: Electronmicroscope of the glomerulus in nephrosis, glomerulonephritis and lupus erythematosus. J. Exp. Med. **106**, 649–660 (1957)

Feldman, J. D., Mardiney, M. R., Shuler, S. E.: Immunology and morphology of acute poststreptococcal glomerulonephritis. Lab. Invest. **15**, 283–301 (1966)

FOLLI, G., POLLAK, V. E., REID, R. T. W., PIRANI, C. L., KARK, R. M.: Electronmicroscopic Studies of Reversible Glomerular Lesions in the Adult Nephrotic Syndrome. Ann. Intern. Med. **49**, 775–795 (1958)

FORLAND, M., JONES, R. E., EASTERLING, R. E., FORRESTER, R. H.: Clinical and renal biopsy observations on oliguric glomerulonephritis. J. Chron. Dis. **19**, 163–177 (1966)

FORLAND, M., SPARGO, B. H.: Clinicopathological Correlations in Idiopathic Nephrotic Syndrome with Membranous Nephropathy. Nephron **6**, 498–525 (1969)

FRANKLIN, W. A., JENNINGS, R. B., EARLE, D. P.: Membranous glomerulonephritis: Long-term serial observations on clinical course and morphology. Kidney Intern. **4**, 36–56 (1973)

FREEDMAN, P., MEISTER, H. P., DE LA PAZ, A., RONAGHY, H.: The clinical, functional, and histologic response to heparin in chronic renal disease. Invest. Urol. **7**, 398–409 (1970)

FRIES, D., BRUNA-BLANC, N., BANSILLON, ZECH, P., TOUBOUL, P., CANARELLI, G., TRAEGER, J.: Traitement des glomérulonéphrites primitives prolifératives par l'azathioprine. J. Urol. Néphrol. **74**, 1012–1021 (1968)

GLUCK, M. C., GALLO, G., LOWENSTEIN, J., BALDWIN, D. S.: Membranous glomerulonephritis. Evolution of Clinical and Pathologic Features. Ann. Intern. Med. **78**, 1–12 (1973)

HABIB, R.: Classification anatomique des néphropathies glomérulaire. Pädiat. Fortbild.-kurse **28**, 3–47 (1970)

HABIB, R.: Classification of glomerulopathies. Presented at Meeting of Arb. Gem. pädiat. Nephrol. Heidelberg, November 1972

HABIB, R., KLEINKNECHT, C.: The primary nephrotic syndrome of childhood. Classification and clinicopathologic study of 406 cases. Path. Ann. **6**, 417–474 (1971)

HABIB, R., MICHIELSEN, P., DE MONTERA, E., HINGLAIS, N., GALLE, P., HAMBURGER, J.: Clinical, microscopic and electron microscopic data in the nephrotic syndrome of unknown origin. In: Ciba Foundation Symposium on Renal Biopsy (eds. G. E. W. WOLSTENHOLME and M. P. CAMERON). London: Churchill, 1961

HARDWICKE, J., BLAINEY, J. D., BREWER, D. B., SOOTHILL, J. F.: The Nephrotic Syndrome. In: Proc. 3rd Int. Congr. Nephrol. Washington. Vol. II, pp. 69–82. Basel and New York: Karger, 1966

HELMCHEN, U.: Der relative Reninismus als ein pathogenetisches Prinzip der renalen Hypertonie. Tübingen: Hab.-Schrift, 1973

HERDMAN, R. C., EDSON, J. R., PICKERING, R. J., FISH, A. J., MARKER, ST., GOOD, R. A.: Anticoagulants in renal disease in children. Amer. J. Dis. Child. **119**, 27–35 (1970)

HERDMAN, R. C., MICHAEL, A. F., GOOD, R. A.: Immunosuppressive and Anticoagulant Therapy of Renal Disease. In: Proc. 4th Int. Congr. Nephrol. Stockholm, Vol. III, pp. 62–71. Basel, München and New York: Karger, 1970

HERDMAN, R. C., PICKERING, R. J., MICHAEL, A. F., VERNIER, R. L., FISH, A. J., GEWURZ, H., GOOD, R. A.: Chronic Glomerulonephritis Associated with Low Serum Complement Activity (Chronic Hypocomplementemic Glomerulonephritis). Medicine (Baltimore) **49**, 207–226 (1970)

HOLLAND, N. H., BENNETT, N. M.: Hypocomplementemic (Membranoproliferative) Glomerulonephritis. Amer. J. Dis. Child. **123**, 439–445 (1972)

HOPPER, J., RYAN, P., LEE, J. C., ROSENAU, W.: Lipoid Nephrosis in 31 Adult Patients: Renal Biopsy Study by Light, Electron and Fluorescence Microscopy with Experience in Treatment. Medicine (Baltimore) **49**, 321–341 (1970)

HYMAN, L. R., BURKHOLDER, P. M.: Focal Sclerosing Glomerulonephropathy with Segmental Hyalinosis. A Clinicopathologic Analysis. Lab. Invest. **28**, 533–544 (1973)

IVERSEN, P., BRUN, C.: Aspiration Biopsy of the Kidney. Amer. J. Med. **11**, 324–330 (1951)

JENNINGS, R. B., EARLE, F. P.: Post-streptococcal glomerulonephritis: histopathologic and clinical studies of the acute, subsiding acute and early chronic latent phases. J. Clin. Invest. **40**, 1525–1595 (1961)

JENSEN, M. K.: Chromosome Studies in Patients Treated with Azathioprine and Amethopterin. Acta med. scand. **182**, 445–455 (1967)

JONES, D. B.: Nephrotic glomerulonephritis. Amer. J. Path. **33**, 313–329 (1957)

Kimmelstiel, P., Osawa, G., Beres, J.: Some Glomerular Changes by Electron Microscopy with Predominant Mesangial Reaction. In: Proc. 3rd Int. Congr. Nephrol. Washington, 1966. Basel and New York: Karger, 1967

Kincaid-Smith, P.: The Clinical Value of Renal Biopsy. In: Proc. 3rd Int. Congr. Nephrol. Washington, 1966, Vol. II, pp. 17–32. Basel and New York: Karger, 1967

Kincaid-Smith, P.: The Treatment of Chronic Mesangiocapillary (Membranoproliferative) Glomerulonephritis with Impaired Renal Function. Med. J. Aust. (1972), 2, 583–587

Kincaid-Smith, P., Laver, M. C., Fairley, K. F.: Dipyridamole and anticoagulants in renal disease due to glomerular and vascular lesions. Med. J. Aust. (1970), 1, 145–151

Kincaid-Smith, P., Saker, B. M., Fairley, F. K.: Anticoagulants in "Irreversible" Acute Renal Failure. Lancet 1968 II, 1360–1363

Krumhaar, I., Reinschke, P., Peschel, H. G., Otto, F., Schwedtke, H.: Zur Problematik der klinischen und morphologischen Klassifizierung und Verlaufsbeobachtung von Glomerulonephritiden. Erste Ergebnisse in der Langzeittherapie. Dtsch. Gesundh.Wes. 26, 333–341 (1971)

Leonard, C. D., Nagle, R. B., Striker, G. E., Cutler, R. E., Scribner, B. H.: Acute glomerulonephritis with prolonged oliguria: an analysis of 29 cases. Ann. intern. Med. 73, 703–711 (1970)

Levy, M., Beaufils, H., Gubler, M. C., Habib, R.: Idiopathic recurrent macroscopic hematuria and mesangial IgA-IgG deposits in children (Berger's disease). Clin. Nephrol. 1, 63–69 (1973)

Masugi, M.: Über die experimentelle Glomerulonephritis durch das spezifische Antinierenserum. Ein Beitrag zur Pathogenese der diffusen Glomerulonephritis. Beitr. path. Anat. 92, 429–466 (1933–1934)

McGovern, V. J.: Persistent nephrotic syndrome; a biopsy study. Aust. Ann. Med. 13, 306–312 (1964)

McIntosh, R. M., Kaufman, D. B., Griswold, W., Urizar, R., Smith, F. G., Jr., Ver nier, R. L.: Azathioprine in Glomerulonephritis. A Longterm Study. Lancet 1972 I, 1085–1089

Meadow, S. R. Weller, O., Archibald, R. W. R.: Fatal systemic measles in a child receiving cyclophosphamide for nephrotic syndrome. Lancet 1969 II, 876–878

Meyer, D., Helmchen, U., Bohle, A.: Hypertensive glomeruläre Schäden. Verh. dtsch. Ges. Path. 57, 392 (1973)

Michael, A. F., Drummond, K. N., Good, R. A., Vernier, R. L.: Acute poststreptococcal glomerulonephritis—immune deposit disease. J. clin. Invest. 45, 237–248 (1966)

Michielsen, P., Lambert, P. P.: Effects du traitement par les corticostéroides et l'indomethacine sur la protéinurie. Soc. Méd. Hôp. Paris 118, 217–232 (1967)

Michielsen, P., Verberckmoes, R., Desmet, V., Hermerijcks, W.: Treatment for chronic glomerulonephritis with indomethacine. J. Urol. Néphrol. 75, 315–318 (1969)

Miller, D. G.: Alkylating agents and human spermatogenesis. J.A.M.A. 217, 1662–1665 (1971)

Miller, J. J., Cole, L. J.: Changes in mouse ovaries after prolonged treatment with cyclophosphamide. Proc. Soc. exp. Biol. Med. (N.Y.) 133, 190–193 (1970)

Morel-Maroger, L, L., Leatham, A., Richet, G.: Glomerular Abnormalities in Nonsystemic Disease. Relationship Between Findings by Light Microscopy and Immunofluorescence in 433 Renal Biopsy Specimens. Amer. J. Med. 53, 170–184 (1972)

Movat, H. Z.: Silver impregnation methods for electron microscopy. Amer. J. clin. Path. 35, 528–537 (1961)

Neustein, H. B., Davis, W.: Acute Glomerulonephritis. A Light and Electron Microscopic Study of Eight Serial Biopsy. Amer. J. clin. Path. 44, 613–626 (1965)

Okuda, R., Watanabe, Y., Yamamoto, Y., West, C. D.: The Origin of Membranoproliferative Nephritis. Amer. J. Dis. Child. 119, 281–295 (1970)

Olbing, H., Greifer, I., Bennett, B. P., Bernstein, J., Spitzer, A.: Idiopathic membranous nephropathy in children. Kidney Intern. 3, 381–390 (1973)

Quirin, H., Wehner, H., Weingard, D., Bohle, A., Kluthe, R.: Erfahrungen mit Indomethacin bei entzündlicher glomerulärer Erkrankung (Klinik und Morphologie). In: Medikamentöse Therapie bei Nierenerkrankungen (Hrsg. R. Kluthe, Stuttgart: Thieme 1971

REICHEL, W., FISCHBACH, H., QUELLHORST, E., SCHELER, F.: Spontanremission einer rapid progressiven Glomerulonephritis. Dtsch. med. Wschr. **99**, 523–526 (1974)

RENNER, R., EDEL, H. H., EIGLER, J., BUCHBORN, E.: Klinische und prognostische Bedeutung der histologischen Klassifizierung von Glomerulonephritiden. Klin. Wschr. **47**, 752–759 (1969)

Report by Medical Research Council Working Party: Controlled Trial of Azathioprine and Prednisone in Chronic Renal Disease. Brit. Med. J. **1971, 2**, 239–241

RICH, A. R.: A Hitherto Undescribed Vulnerability of the Juxtamedullary Glomeruli in Lipoid Nephrosis. Bull. Johns Hopkins Hosp. **100**, 173–186 (1957)

ROYER, P., HABIB, R., VERMEIL, G., MATHIEU, H., ALIZON, M.: Les Glomérulonéphritis prolongées de l'enfant. A propos de quatre aspects anatomiques révélés par la biopsie rénale. Ann. Pediat. **38**, 793–807 (1962)

SCHEINMAN, J. I., STAMLER, F. W.: Cyclophosphamide and fatal varicella. J. Pediat. **74**, 117 (1969)

SCHUBERT, G. E.: Die pathologische Anatomie des akuten Nierenversagens. Erg. allg. Path. path. Anat. **49**, 1–112 (1968)

SCHUBERT, G. E.: Pathologische Anatomie des akuten Nierenversagens. In: Pathogenese und Klinik des akuten Nierenversagens (Hrsg. U. GESSLER, K. SCHRÖDER, H. WEIDINGER). Stuttgart: Thieme 1971

SHIRES, D., HOLCOMB, A., CADE, J., LEVIN, D.: Treatment of chronic proliferative glomerulonephritis with heparin. Clin. Res. **14**, 378 (1966)

STRUNK, S. W., HAMMOND, W. S., BENDITT, E. P.: The resolution of acute glomerulonephritis. Lab. Invest. **13**, 401–429 (1964)

TRAVIS, L. B., DODGE, W. F., BEATHARD, G. A., SPARGO, B. H., LORENTZ, W. B., CARVAJAL, H. F., BERGER, M.: Acute glomerulonephritis in Children. Clin. Nephrol. **1**, 169–181 (1973)

VASSALLI, P., McCLUSKEY, R. T.: The pathogenic role of the coagulation process in rabbit Masugi nephritis. Amer. J. Path. **45**, 653–677 (1964)

VOLHARD, F., FAHR, TH.: Die Bright'sche Nierenkrankheit. Klinik — Pathologie — Atlas. Berlin: Springer 1914

WEGMANN, W., LEUMANN, E. P.: Glomerulonephritis associated with (infected) ventriculo-atrial shunt. Clinical and morphological findings. Virch. Arch. A **359**, 185–200 (1973)

WEHNER, H., FEURER, F., WEHNER, I.: Histometrical glomerular studies on the kidneys in multiple myeloma and in acute membranous glomerulonephritis (lipoid nephrosis)· Path. europ. **6**, 422–432 (1971)

WEHNER, H., MAJOREK, B., SCHÖLL, A., WÖRZ, U., SENTKER, H. J.: Histometrical glomerular studies in minimal proliferative intercapillary glomerulonephritis (minimal changes without nephrotic syndrome) with different clinical symptomatology. Klin. Wschr. **53**, 92–93, 1975

WEHNER, H., RENNER, E., EDEL, H. H., BUCHBORN, E., BOHLE, A.: Zur pathologischen Anatomie und Klinik der Glomerulonephritis. II. Die postakuten und chronischen Glomerulonephritiden. Klin. Wschr. **47**, 742–752 (1969)

WEST, C. D., McADAMS, A., McCONVILLE, J., DAVIS, N. C., HOLLAND, N. H.: Hypocomplementemic and normocomplementemic persistent (chronic) glomerulonephritis, clinical and pathological characteristics. J. Pediat. **67**, 1089–1112 (1965)

WHITE, R. H. R.: "Silent" Nephritis. A Study Based on Renal Biopsies. Guy's Hosp. Rep. **113**, 190–206 (1964)

WHITE, R. H. R., CAMERON, J. S., TROUNCE, J. R.: Immunosuppressive therapy in steroidresistant proliferative glomerulonephritis accompanied by the nephrotic syndrome. Brit. Med. J. **1966, 2**, 853–860 (1966)

Institute of Pathology, University of Tübingen, Federal Republic of Germany
(Director: Prof. Dr. A. Bohle)

Role of the Renin-Angiotensin System in Renal Hypertension. An Experimental Approach*

Udo Helmchen and Ursula Kneissler

With 20 Figures

Contents

I. Introduction 203

II. Methods 204
   1. Experimental Procedure 204
   2. Analytical Methods 205

III. Results 206
   1. Experiments in Normotensive Animals 206
   2. Two-Kidney Hypertension 208
   3. One-Kidney Hypertension 211

IV. Discussion 215
   1. Contribution of the RAS in Maintaining Normotension 215
   2. Contribution of the RAS in Initiating and Maintaining Renal Hypertension 221

V. Conclusion 230

References 231

I. Introduction

In 1898 Tigerstedt and Bergman first detected the existence of renal renin and discussed its possible role in the development of cardiac hypertrophy associated with various kidney diseases. Hartwich (1930) and Goldblatt et al. (1934) were able to produce persistent arterial hypertension in dogs by narrowing the renal arteries. Subsequently, a large number of findings accumulated in the field of renal hypertension. Most of the material has been covered in reviews edited by Braun-Menendez (1946), Page and McCubbin (1968), and Page and Bumpus (1974). There is general agreement that arterial hypertension, including renal hypertension, is a multifactorial disorder of regulation as anticipated by Page in 1949 when he proposed his concept known as the mosaic theory.

The following experimental study is mainly concerned with one aspect of this multifaceted complex: the renin-angiotensin system (RAS) and its role in renal hypertension.

Two facts have been repeatedly considered to argue against an important role of the RAS in renal hypertension:

1. The normal plasma renin activity (PRA) frequently observed in human beings and animals with renal hypertension.

* Supported by Deutsche Forschungsgemeinschaft.

2. The failure of active and passive immunization against angiotensin II to normalize arterial blood pressure in different forms of experimental renal hypertension.

A PRA, however, which is normal with respect to the average of normotensive controls does not necessarily indicate a normal regulation of renin release in hypertensive individuals. Furthermore, earlier conclusions based upon immunization studies may only be of limited value due to the possibility that macromolecular angiotensin II antibodies are unable to reach that vascular level where a competition with locally formed angiotensin II could occur. For this reason specific low molecular-weight angiotensin II antagonists might be more potent tools in approaching this problem.

The following experiments were designed to evaluate the regulation of renin release under normotensive and hypertensive conditions, and to reinvestigate the contribution of the RAS in maintaining normotension and renal hypertension by using a specific angiotensin II antagonist. Renal hypertension was induced in rats by constricting one renal artery with (one-kidney hypertension) or without (two-kidney hypertension) simultaneously removing the opposite kidney.

II. Methods

1. Experimental Procedure

Experimental Animals. All the experiments were carried out upon white male Wistar-type rats (Ivanovas, Kisslegg/Allg., Fed. Rep. of Germany), kept on a standard pellet diet (Altromin, R-10, Altrogge, Lage, Fed. Rep. of Germany). With the exception of one group of normotensive furosemide-treated rats and the anesthetized rats used in infusion experiments (see below), the animals had free access to tap water and food during the whole course of the experiment.

Renal Artery Constriction. Two-kidney hypertension was induced in animals (150–170 g) under ether anesthesia by placing a silver clip (0.2 mm I.D.) over the left renal artery, and leaving the contralateral kidney untouched (Pickering and Prinzmetal, 1938; Wilson and Byrom, 1939). One-kidney hypertension was similarly induced in animals (150–170 g) under ether anesthesia by removing the right kidney and constricting the left renal artery with a silver clip (0.2 mm I.D.).

Removal of the "clamped" kidneys in both the one- and the two-kidney models was performed after decapsulation under ether anesthesia. Removal of the renal artery clip (unclamping) was performed under ether anesthesia after the clamp was dissected free of surrounding connective tissue. In a sham-operated group the clamp was dissected free but not removed.

Furosemide Treatment in Normotensive and Hypertensive Rats. Normotensive animals (190–200 g) were given a single i.p. dose of 50 mg/kg of furosemide (Lasix, Hoechst, Fed. Rep. of Germany) after which the rats were divided in two groups. Group I had free access to tap water for the first 6 hours after injection. During the same period group II was given free access to 1 % NaCl instead of tap water.

Conscious rats with chronic (4–6 weeks) one-kidney hypertension were injected i.p. with 50 mg/kg furosemide. Six hours after administration of the diuretic a blood sample was assayed for PRA. The animals were then nephrectomized. Two hours later another blood sample was assayed for PRA. Blood pressure was measured before treatment, 6 hours after furosemide, and 2 hours after the subsequent nephrectomy.

Infusion of 1-Sar-8-Ile-Angiotensin II. Normotensive and hypertensive rats were anesthetized with Inactin (90 mg/kg i.p.) (Promonta, Hamburg, Fed. Rep. of Germany). The animals were placed on a temperature-regulated micropuncture table and a tracheostomy was performed. An indwelling polyethylene catheter was placed in the left femoral vein for infusion of saline or 1-Sar-8-Ile-angiotensin II (Beckman, Geneva, Switzerland). Another polyethylene catheter was inserted into the left femoral artery and connected to a pressure transducer (Statham P 23 Db) for continuous recording of blood pressure. Bolus injections of val-5-angiotensin-II-amide (Hypertensin, CIBA, Basle, Switzerland) were also given through the femoral vein catheter at doses of 2.5, 5.0 and 10.0 ng. Saline and the angiotensin II antagonist were infused by a micro-perfusion pump (Braun, Melsungen, Fed. Rep. of Germany) at the rate of 0.05 ml/min for 30 minutes. Pressor responses to exogenous angiotensin II were recorded before and after the infusion period.

One normotensive group and one one-kidney hypertensive group were given a single dose furosemide (50 mg/kg i.p.) 2 hours before starting the infusion of the angiotensin II analogue. In two two-kidney hypertensive rats the infusion of 1-Sar-8-Ile-angiotensin II was repeated after pretreatment with 50 mg/kg i.p. furosemide.

Systolic blood pressure was measured by tail plethysmography (BYROM and WILSON, 1938) under light ether anesthesia.

Blood samples were obtained by puncture of the retrooribtal venous plexus (NOELLER, 1955) under light ether anesthesia.

2. Analytical Methods

Measurement of PRA. PRA was determined by a micromethod as described by SCHAECHTELIN et al. (1967), and REGOLI et al. (1969). Briefly, peripheral blood was obtained (0.5 ml per sample) from retroorbital venous plexus. The samples were collected in polyethylene tubes and kept on ice until being centrifuged for 20 minutes at $800 \times g$ at $2°$ C, and the plasma separated immediately. 0.2 ml of plasma was acidified to pH 3.5 by adding 0.01 ml of 1.2 N HCl, and was maintained at this pH for 30 minutes at $0°$ C. Thereafter, the cooled plasma was brought to pH 5.2 by adding 0.005 ml of 1.2 N NaOH. The plasma was then transferred into a tube containing 0.8 ml of partially purified rat renin substrate, obtained from serum of nephrectomized rats (SCHAECHTELIN et al., 1966), to which 20 mM of EDTA had been added. This mixture was incubated for 4 hours at $40°$ C, and the enzymatic reaction was stopped by boiling for 5 minutes. In order to stabilize the angiotensin formed during incubation the pH was increased to 10.0 by adding 0.09 ml of 1.2 N KOH, and the mixture kept on ice. Before testing the angio-tensin concentration by its pressor effect in rats, the mixture was centrifuged for 20 min-utes at $800 \times g$ at $2°$ C. For the bioassay the supernatant was injected into rats which had been nephrectomized under ether anesthesia 24 hours before and anesthetized with a 20 % solution of urethane (1.4 g/kg s.c.). Pressor responses from the carotid artery (measured with a mercury manometer) were compared with the responses to solutions of val-5-angiotensin-II-amide (Hypertensin), dissolved in a glycine buffer solution at pH 10.0. The results were expressed as ng val-5-angiotensin-II-equivalents per ml of plasma. The variation coefficient calculated for this method was 8.7 % $(n=15)$. The recovery of val-5-angiotensin-II-amide added to the incubation mixture at doses of 50, 100 and 200 ng averaged 75 % $(n=21)$. There was a linear relationship between known doses of commercial, partially purified hog renin (Nutritional Biochemicals Corp., Cleve-land, Ohio, U.S.A.) incubated with the standard amount of partially purified rat renin substrate, and val-5-angiotensin-II-equivalents recovered by the bioassay.

Measurement of Renal Tissue Renin Activity (RRA). RRA was determined using a modification of the method described by SCHAECHTELIN et al. (1966): 100 mg of cortical tissue were peeled off the surface of the kidney and homogenized with 1.9 ml of 0.9 % solution of NaCl. This mixture was then acidified to pH 1.5 by adding 0.05 2N H_2SO_4 and kept at this pH at $0°$ C for 30 minutes. Reneutralization to pH 7.4 was achieved by adding 0.025 ml 2N NaOH. The mixture was then centrifuged for 15 minutes at $800 \times g$ at $2°$ C. The supernatant was diluted 25 times by adding 0.15 M phosphate buffer solution at pH 5.2. 0.2 ml of the diluted homogenate was then incubated for 30 minutes at $40°$ C with 0.8 ml of the partially purified renin substrate containing 20 mM EDTA. After incubation the same procedure was employed as described above for the plasma samples. Total renal renin activities were calculated by assuming that 20% of the total weight of each kidney was cortical tissue.

Extracellular volume was calculated by measuring the inulin space. Rats were bilaterally nephrectomized immediately before starting the experiment. Then 0.5 ml of 25% solution of inulin (Inutest, Laevosan Co., Linz, Austria) was injected into the left jugular vein. After 4 hours a sample was drawn from the retroorbital venous plexus. Inulin concentration was determined by using the method described by FUEHR et al. (1955).

Hematocrit values were determined in duplicate in blood obtained from the retroorbital venous plexus after spinning heparinized capillaries at 1000 ×g for 10 minutes.

Plasma sodium concentration was measured by flame photometry (Zeiss, PF 5).

Heart and kidney weights were measured in a precision balance (Mettler, HT 10).

Planimetric examinations of aortic and renal artery lumina were performed in perfusion-fixed vessels embedded in methacrylate, cut (0.5 μ thin sections) perpendicular to the longitudinal axis of the vessels and stained by a silver impregnation technique (MOVAT, 1961). Morphometry was performed by means of a Zeiss drawing tube in combination with a planimeter (Ott, Kempten, Fed. Rep. of Germany).

Granulation of the juxtaglomerular apparatus was assessed by the method of HARTROFT and HARTROFT (1953). Kidney slices were fixed in Bouin's fluid for 24 hours. 3–4 μ sections were prepared after paraffin embedding and stained for juxtaglomerular granules using Bowie's stain modified by SMITH (1966).

Statistical Analyses. Numerical data were given as means ± standard error (SE). Significance of differences was evaluated by Student's *t*-test after performing F- and Welch-tests. A *p*-value of less than 0.05 was considered significant.

III. Results

1. Experiments in Normotensive Animals

Furosemide Diuresis. The decrease in plasma volume occurring after the injection of 50 mg/kg furosemide was reflected in group I by the significant increase in the hematocrit. In these animals furosemide diuresis also caused a large increase of PRA but no significant change in systolic blood pressure. However, 6 hours after injecting furosemide none of these parameters (PRA, systolic blood pressure, and hematocrit) was significantly altered in group II (Table 1).

Table 1. Plasma renin activity (PRA), systolic blood pressure (BP), and hematocrit (HC) 6 hours after i.p. injection of 50 mg/kg furosemide into normotensive rats. The rats had free access to tap water (Group I) or to 1% NaCl solution (Group II) during the experiment. Numbers of experimental animals in brackets. The significance of differences (s. = significant; n.s. = not significant) refers to differences from untreated controls

	Untreated controls	Group I	Group II
PRA (ng A II eq/ml)	132.1 ± 11.6 (14)	504.2 ± 17.6 (6) s.	145.8 ± 17.6 (6) n.s.
BP (mm Hg)	106.3 ± 2.0 (12)	100.8 ± 1.6 (6) n.s.	105.0 ± 4.5 (6) n.s.
HC (%)	46.5 ± 0.5 (12)	55.7 ± 0.7 (6) s.	47.8 ± 0.7 (6) n.s.

Effect of 1-Sar-8-Ile-Angiotensin II in Normal and Furosemide-Treated Rats. The pressor response to bolus injections of 2.5, 5 and 10 ng angiotensin II was completely blocked in anesthetized rats after infusing 1-Sar-8-Ile-angiotensin II at 150 ng/kg/min for 30 minutes. During and after the perfusion

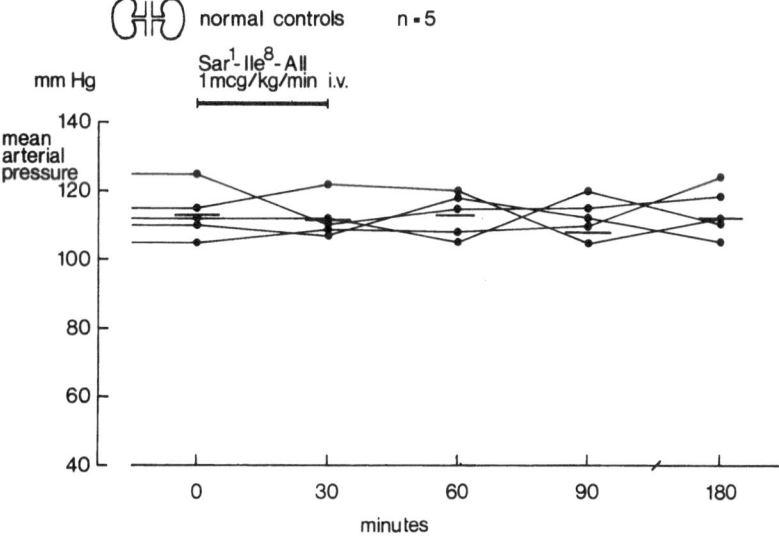

Fig. 1. Effect of 1-Sar-8-Ile-angiotensin II on mean arterial blood pressure of normotensive anesthetized rats

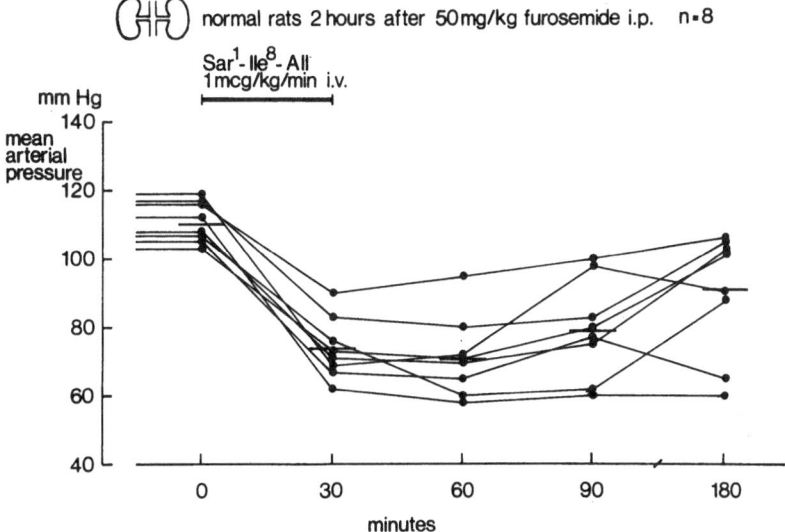

Fig. 2. Effect of 1-Sar-8-Ile-angiotensin II on mean arterial blood pressure in normotensive furosemide-treated rats

period mean arterial blood pressure remained unchanged in normal animals, even though the angiotensin II inhibitor was given at a higher dose (1 µg/ kg/min) in these experiments (Fig. 1). In contrast, the same dose of 1-Sar-8-Ile-angiotensin II lowered mean arterial blood pressure significantly in previously normotensive furosemide-treated rats (Fig. 2).

Table 2. Plasma renin activity (PRA), renal renin activity (RRA), systolic blood pressure (BP), hematocrit (HC), extracellular volume (ECV), plasma sodium concentration (P-Na), relative kidney weight (KW), and relative heart weight (HW) in two-kidney hypertensive rats. Period of hypertension: 4–6 weeks. Explanations as in Table 1

	Normotensive controls	Two-kidney hypertensive rats
PRA (ng A II eq/ml)	120.0 ± 8.0 (25)	172.7 ± 23.2 (11) (s.) clamped kidneys:
RRA (μg A II eq/kidney)	28.1 ± 1.5 (16)	53.0 ± 2.3 (10) (s.) untouched kidneys: 6.8 ± 2.4 (10) (s.)
BP (mm Hg)	112.8 ± 2.4 (25)	184.3 ± 5.8 (14) (s.)
HC (%)	48.3 ± 0.5 (20)	50.5 ± 0.7 (17) (s.)
ECV (ml/100 g b.w.)	22.9 ± 0.4 (18)	19.5 ± 0.4 (18) (s.)
P-Na (meq/l)	134.2 ± 0.4 (18)	132.0 ± 0.4 (18) (s.) clamped kidneys:
KW (mg/100 g b.w.)	342.5 ± 5.7 (18)	288.0 ± 9.3 (18) (s.) untouched kidneys: 385.3 ± 7.7 (18) (s.)
HW (mg/100 g b.w.)	302.4 ± 4.7 (18)	396.4 ± 8.2 (17) (s.)

2. Two-Kidney Hypertension

Table 2 shows that hypertension produced 6 weeks previously in rats by partially constricting one renal artery without touching the opposite kidney, was accompanied by a significant increase in renin activity in both the plasma and the clamped kidneys, whereas a significant renin depletion was found in the untouched kidneys. These differences in renal renin activities reflect neither hypertrophy of the untouched kidneys nor contraction of the clamped kidneys, because renin activities were always calculated for the whole renal cortex. The average hematocrit value was significantly increased in hypertensive rats. Extracellular volume and plasma sodium concentration were significantly decreased in the hypertensive group which also showed a significant gain in relative heart weight due to hypertrophied left ventricles.

Removal of the Clamped Kidney. Removing the clamped kidney in rats hypertensive for 4–6 weeks was followed by a significant fall in PRA and systolic blood pressure to low levels within 24 hours (Table 3). PRA was still significantly diminished after 5 days, but returned to control values 9 days after removal of the clamped kidney. Systolic blood pressure, being depressed 24 hours after operation, normalized within 2 days and remained normal during the following 3 weeks (Table 3). Average relative heart weight declined significantly within 1 day after nephrectomy and continued to fall until the end of the experiment (Table 3).

Effect of 1-Sar-8-Ile-Angiotensin II. The effect of infusion of 1-Sar-8-Ile-angiotensin II in 7 rats with two-kidney hypertension of 5 weeks duration is demonstrated in Fig. 3. When these anesthetized rats were infused with

Table 3. PRA, BP, and HW in normotensive controls and in two-kidney hypertensive rats before and after removing the clamped kidneys. Period of hypertension: 4–6 weeks. Explanations as in Table 2

	Normo-tensive controls	Hyper-tensive controls	Days after removing the clamped kidneys				
			1	2	5	12	21
BP (mm Hg)	112.8 ± 2.4 (25)	189.7 ± 3.8 (29) s.	91.4 ± 4.0 (7) s.	97.9 ± 3.8 (7) s.	103.6 ± 6.2 (7) n.s.	102.9 ± 6.7 (7) n.s.	121.4 ± 7.9 (7) n.s.
PRA (ng A II eq/ml)	120.0 ± 8.0 (25)	172.7 ± 23.3 (11) s.	29.2 ± 15.1 (7) s.	7.1 ± 5.8 (7) s.	39.3 ± 9.2 (7) s.	121.4 ± 10.1 (7) n.s.	114.3 ± 7.4 (7) n.s.
HW (mg/100 g b.w.)	302.4 ± 4.7 (18)	421.4 ± 3.4 (7) s.	394.7 ± 5.5 (6) s.	396.0 ± 12.2 (7) s.	382.6 ± 10.2 (7) s.	364.2 ± 7.8 (6) s.	316.6 ± 6.8 (7) n.s.

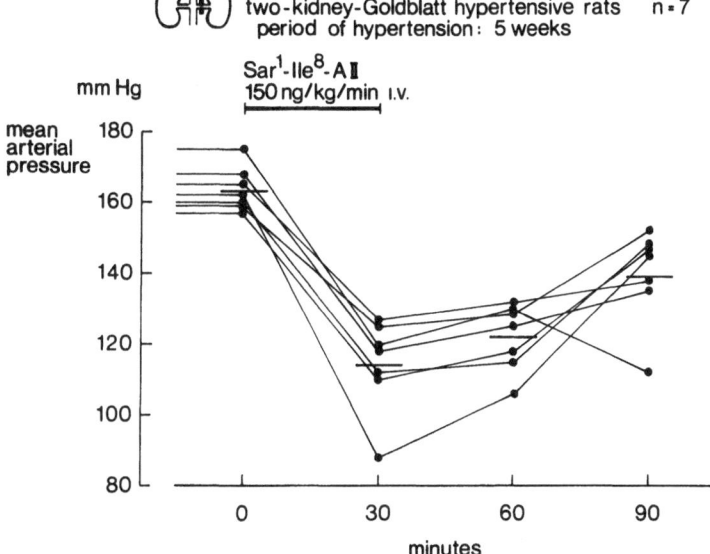

Fig. 3. Effect of 1-Sar-8-Ile-angiotensin II on mean arterial blood pressure of rats with two-kidney hypertension of 5 weeks duration

the angiotensin II analogue, mean arterial blood pressure fell significantly from an average of 163.9 ± 2.3 to 114.3 ± 5.0 mm Hg within 30 minutes of infusion and was still significantly decreased 30 and 60 minutes after termination of the infusion (122.3 ± 3.6 and 139.6 ± 5.1 mm Hg, respectively). Saline infusion at the same rate (0.05 ml/min) for 30 minutes into 3 two-kidney hypertensive rats did not significantly alter mean arterial blood pressure (Fig. 4). In rats hypertensive for 4 months mean arterial blood pressure fell significantly from 156.5 ± 4.8 to 137.0 ± 5.5 mm Hg during the 30 minutes infusion of 1-Sar-8-Ile-angiotensin II. Although the pressor response to the angiotensin II antagonist was significant, the effect was not as marked as

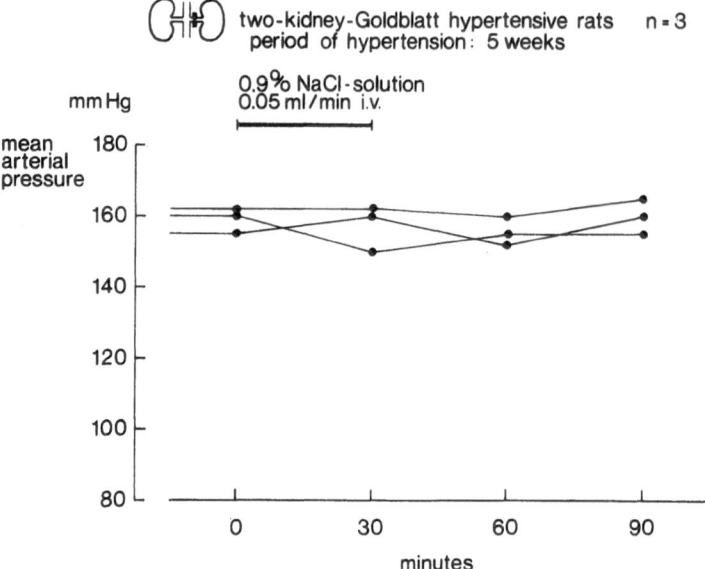

Fig. 4. Effect of infusion of 0.9% NaCl solution on mean arterial blood pressure of rats with two-kidney hypertension of 5 weeks duration

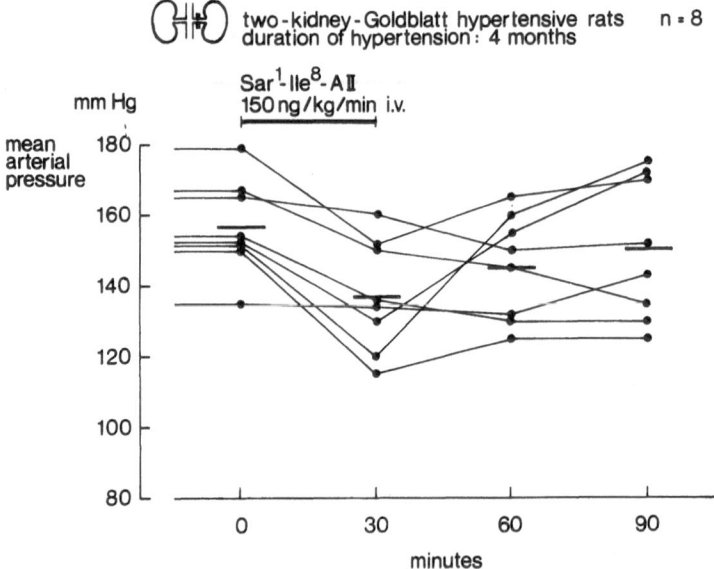

Fig. 5. Effect of 1-Sar-8-Ile-angiotensin II on mean arterial blood pressure of rats with two-kidney hypertension of 4 months duration

that observed in rats hypertensive for only 5 weeks and hypertension was already re-established 30 and 60 minutes after terminating the infusion (145.3 ± 5.3 and 150.3 ± 7.1 mm Hg, respectively) (Fig. 5). In two rats which

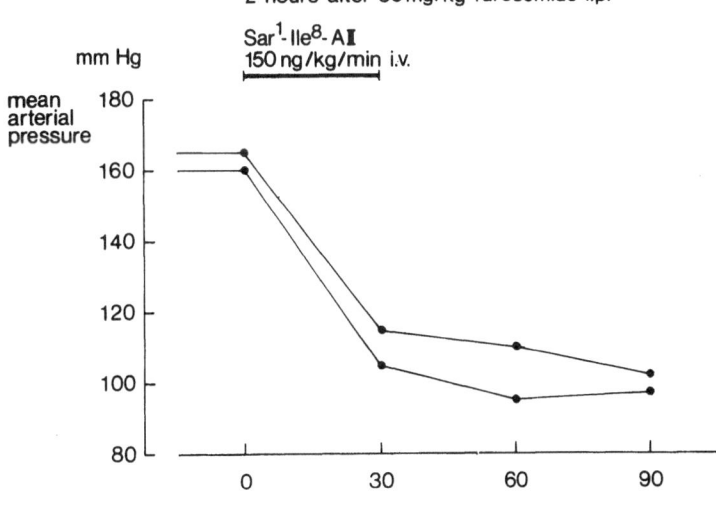

Fig. 6. Effect of 1-Sar-8-Ile-angiotensin II on mean arterial blood pressure 2 hours after furosemide injection into two-kidney hypertensive rats previously resistant to the angiotensin II inhibitor

did not respond initially to the inhibitor an infusion of 1-Sar-8-Ile-angiotensin II normalized mean arterial blood pressure after furosemide- induced sodium and volume depletion (Fig. 6).

3. One-Kidney-Hypertension

Table 4 shows various parameters obtained in hypertensive rats 6 weeks after partially constricting one renal artery and removing the opposite kidney. At that time mean PRA and RRA in hypertensive rats did not significantly differ from those in normotensive controls. Hematocrit, plasma sodium concentration and extracellular volume were not significantly changed when compared with normal controls. The mean relative weight of the sole remaining kidneys was significantly higher than that of normal kidneys, indicating a compensatory hypertrophy despite renal artery constriction. Considerable cardiac hypertrophy occurring in one-kidney hypertensive animals is indicated by a significant increase in relative heart weight.

Removal of the Sole Remaining Clamped Kidney. Nephrectomy performed 8 weeks after renal artery constriction did not normalize systolic blood pressure despite a significant fall of blood pressure which occurred 12 and 24 hours after nephrectomy (Table 5). No significant change in systolic blood pressure was observed in sham-operated one-kidney hypertensive rats (Table 5).

On the other hand, as demonstrated in Fig. 7, nephrectomy induced complete normalization of arterial blood pressure in chronic one-kidney hypertensive rats pretreated with furosemide. Furosemide diuresis per se, caused

Table 4. Data obtained from rats with one-kidney hypertension of 4–6 weeks duration.
Explanations as in Tables 1 and 2

	Normotensive controls	One-kidney hypertensive rats
PRA (ng A II eq/ml)	131.7 ± 6.7 (15)	123.1 ± 11.0 (13) n.s.
RRA (µg A II eq/kidney)	28.1 ± 1.5 (16)	31.5 ± 1.5 (10) n.s.
BP (mm Hg)	118.7 ± 1.8 (23)	194.6 ± 5.5 (13) s.
HC (%)	48.3 ± 0.6 (20)	48.1 ± 0.5 (17) n.s.
ECV (ml/100 g b.w.)	22.9 ± 0.4 (18)	21.8 ± 0.4 (17) n.s.
P-Na (meq/l)	134.2 ± 0.4 (19)	134.6 ± 0.2 (17) n.s.
KW (mg/100 g b.w.)	342.5 ± 5.7 (18)	437.6 ± 9.1 (17) s.
HW (mg/100 g b.w.)	302.4 ± 4.7 (18)	408.3 ± 9.6 (17) s.

Table 5. Systolic blood pressure before and after removing or sham-removing the sole
remaining clamped kidneys in rats with one-kidney hypertension of 8 weeks duration.
Explanations as in Table 1

	BP (mm Hg) before operation	BP (mm Hg) after operation		
		6 hours	12 hours	24 hours
Sham-nephrectomy	208.3 ± 5.2 (10)	210.2 ± 6.2 n.s.	212.8 ± 8.1 n.s.	206.5 ± 7.7 n.s.
Nephrectomy	215.3 ± 5.3 (14)	191.6 ± 9.3 n.s.	165.6 ± 6.9 s.	162.9 ± 8.5 s.

by a single i.p. injection of 50 mg/kg furosemide, resulted in a significant increase of PRA within 6 hours, at a time when no normalization of blood pressure had occurred. However, PRA virtually disappeared and systolic blood pressure fell to normal levels within 2 hours after subsequent removal of the sole remaining clamped kidney (Fig. 7).

Effect of Unclamping on Systolic Blood Pressure and PRA. Fig. 8 shows that removal of the renal artery clip in chronic one-kidney hypertensive rats was followed by a significant fall in systolic blood pressure within 90 minutes to levels which were, nevertheless, still elevated. Systolic blood pressure had returned to normal 6 hours after unclamping and was significantly below that of normal controls 24 hours later. Systolic blood pressure was not significantly influenced by sham-unclamping (Fig. 8). Fig. 9 demonstrates changes in PRA in these animals: PRA in rats with chronic one-kidney hypertension did not

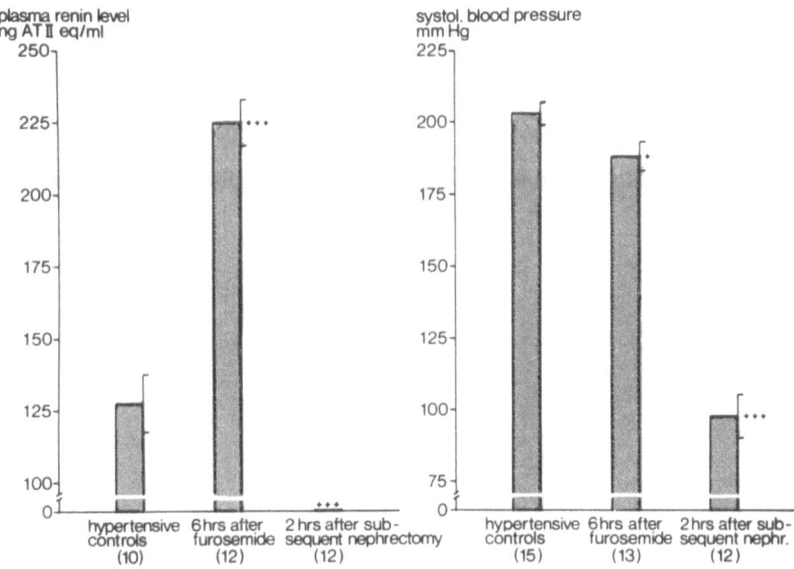

Fig. 7. The effect of furosemide (50 mg/kg i.p.) and subsequent nephrectomy on plasma renin levels and systolic blood pressure in chronic, one-kidney hypertension. The term plasma renin level refers to plasma renin activity. Columns are means ± SE. Numbers of experimental animals in brackets. The significance of differences, shown by *$p<0.05$, **$p<0.01$, ***$p<0.001$; n.s. = not significant refers to differences from normal controls. (HELMCHEN et al., 1974)

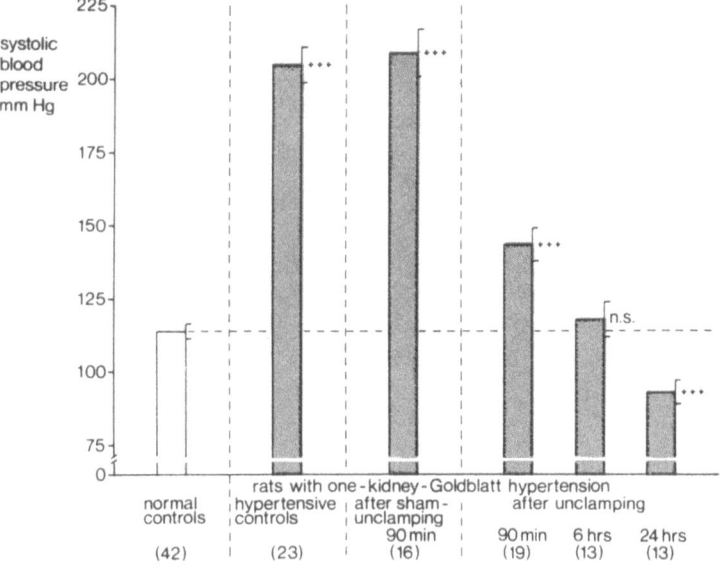

Fig. 8. Systolic blood pressure in normal controls and in rats with chronic, one-kidney hypertension before and after unclamping or sham-unclamping. Explanations as in Fig. 7. (HELMCHEN et al., 1974)

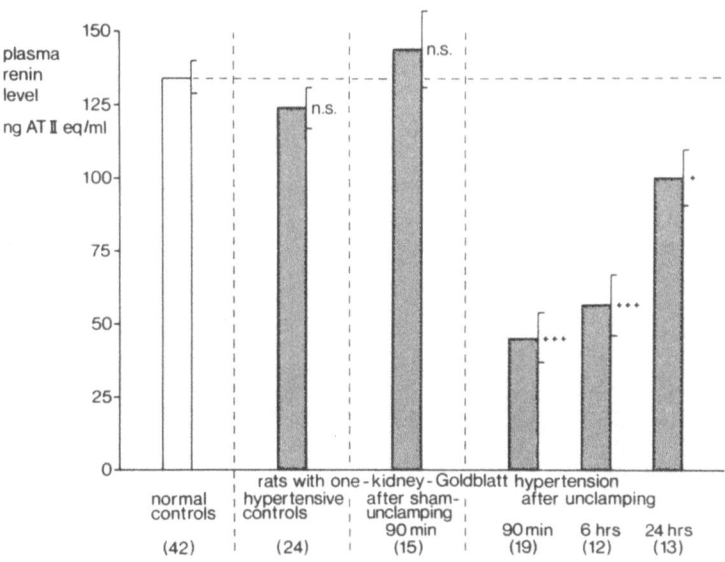

Fig. 9. Plasma renin levels in normal controls and in rats with chronic, one-kidney hypertension before and after unclamping or sham-unclamping. Explanations as in Fig. 7. (Helmchen *et al.*, 1974)

significantly differ from that in normotensive controls. Sham-unclamping did not induce a significant change in PRA within 90 minutes. Unclamping, however, did result in a significant decrease of PRA to less than half its normal value during the first 90 minutes, after which PRA began to rise during the subsequent 6 hours and, by the end of the experiment, had attained a value inter-mediate between normal and that observed 90 minutes after unclamping.

Morphologic Changes Occurring After Removing the Renal Artery Clip. As shown in Fig. 10 unclamping was followed by reopening of the previously constricted part of the renal arterial lumen, which became significantly en-larged during the first 24 hours even when compared with corresponding mean values of uninephrectomized normotensive rats of the same age (Fig. 11). As a consequence of the sudden exposure to a high filling pressure after un-clamping, focal hypertensive lesions developed in renal arterial and glomerular vessels hitherto "protected" against hypertension by the renal artery clip (Fig. 12). Hypertensive lesions consisted mainly of plasma insudation into the walls of interlobular arteries and afferent arterioles (Fig. 13) and of aneurysms in the glomerular capillaries (Fig. 14). Although renal perfusion pressure probably increased immediately after unclamping, afferent arterioles at the level of the juxtaglomerular apparatus were rarely affected (Fig. 15), and the juxtaglomerular index, as determined 90 minutes after unclamping, was significantly higher than that prevailing during the chronic stage of one-kidney hypertension (Fig. 16).

Effect of 1-Sar-8-Ile-Angiotensin II. Although 1-Sar-8-Ile-angiotensin II, infused at a rate of 150 ng/kg/min, significantly lowered mean arterial blood

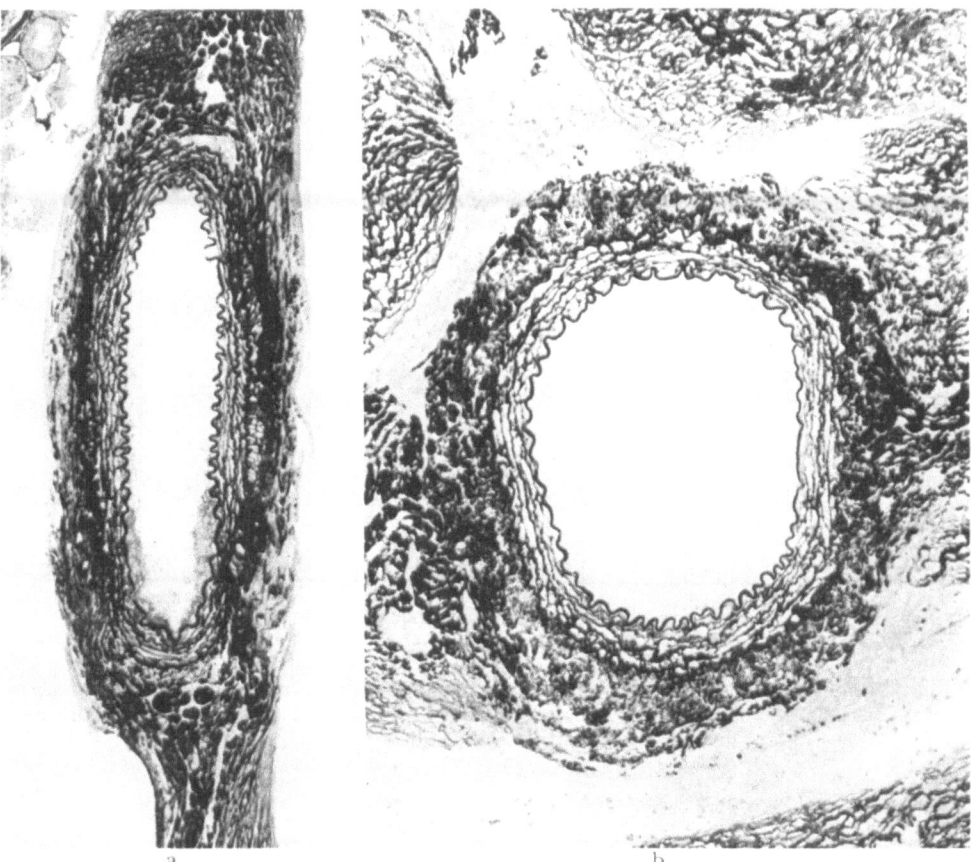

Fig. 10. a Clamped (intrastenotic) part of the renal artery in chronic one-kidney hypertension. b Previously clamped part of the renal artery 24 hours after unclamping. Methacrylate embedding, silver impregnation (MOVAT), ×130

pressure from an average of 169.1 ± 2.0 to 159.4 ± 3.3 mm Hg within an infusion period of 30 minutes, arterial blood pressure was not normalized. Animals were still hypertensive at the end of the experiment (159.1 ± 2.1 mm Hg) (Fig. 17). Furosemide diuresis resulting from an i.p. injection of 50 mg/kg furosemide failed to normalize mean arterial blood pressure in 5 rats also hypertensive for 5 months. However, subsequent administration of 1-Sar-8-Ile-angiotensin II resulted in normalization of mean arterial blood pressure during or after the infusion period (Fig. 18).

IV. Discussion

1. Contribution of the RAS in Maintaining Normotension

Renin (TIGERSTEDT and BERGMAN, 1898), an enzyme (BRAUN-MENENDEZ et al., 1940; PAGE and HELMER, 1940) produced, stored, and secreted by the epitheloid cells of the juxtaglomerular apparatus (GOORMAGHTIGH, 1939; MARSHALL and WAKERLIN, 1949; COOK, 1958; EDELMAN and HARTROFT, 1961;

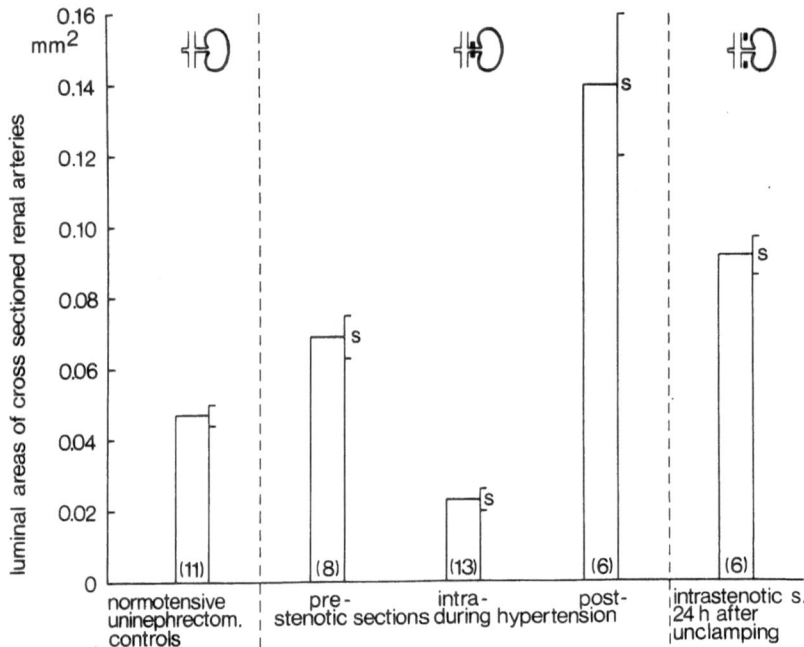

Fig. 11. Lumina of cross-sections of the renal artery in normotensive uninephrectomized rats and in chronic, one-kidney hypertensive rats. Compare the luminal size of the "intrastenotic" parts before and after unclamping

ROBERTSON et al., 1966; SUTHERLAND, 1970), acts on the plasma globulin angiotensinogen to release the decapeptide angiotensin I which is converted by pulmonary and plasma enzymes to the octapeptide angiotensin II (see PAGE and McCUBBIN, 1968; PAGE and BUMPUS, 1974). Although renin activity was also found in various organs, including brain (FISHER-FERRARO et al., 1971; GANTEN et al., 1971, 1972; MINNICH et al., 1972), salivatory glands (WERLE et al., 1962, 1968; OLIVER and GROSS, 1966; BING et al., 1967), uterus (BING et al., 1967; FERRIS et al., 1967), placenta (STAKEMAN, 1960; GROSS et al., 1964a; ZIEGLER et al., 1967), and arterial vessel walls (DENGLER, 1956; GOULD et al., 1964; GENEST et al., 1969; ROSENTHAL et al., 1969; HAYDUK et al., 1970, 1972; GANTEN et al., 1972), tissue renin reaches its highest value in the renal cortex (HAYDUK et al., 1970; GANTEN et al., 1972). After bilateral nephrectomy, PRA fell to either undetectable or extremely low values within a few hours (SCHAECHTELIN et al., 1964; GANTEN et al., 1972). Thus, the level of PRA depends mainly on renal renin release.

The effector component of the RAS, angiotensin II, may influence the level of arterial blood pressure directly or indirectly. In addition to its vascular action, it stimulates aldosterone and catecholamine secretion, alters renal hemodynamics, thereby changing sodium and water excretion, and activates the central and peripheral sympathetic nervous system (PAGE and McCUBBIN, 1968; PAGE and BUMPUS, 1974).

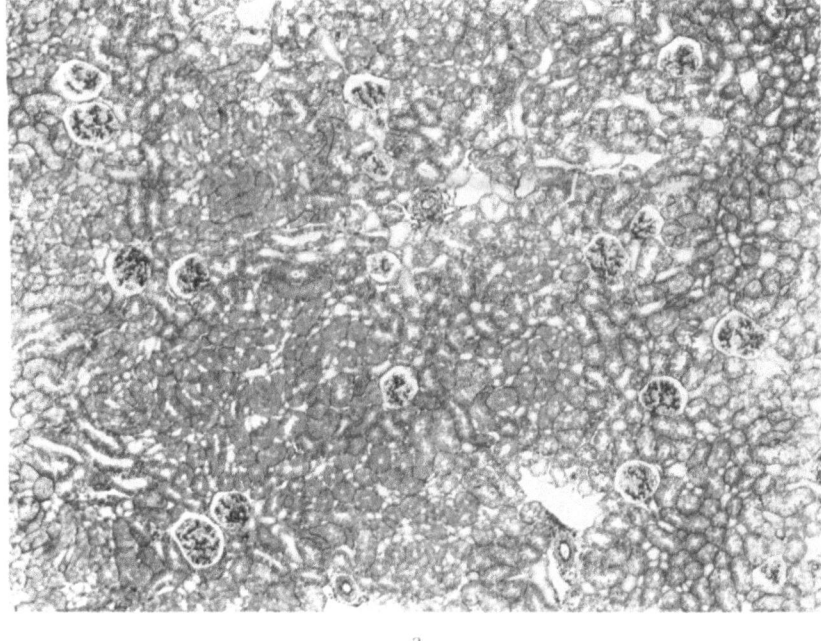

a

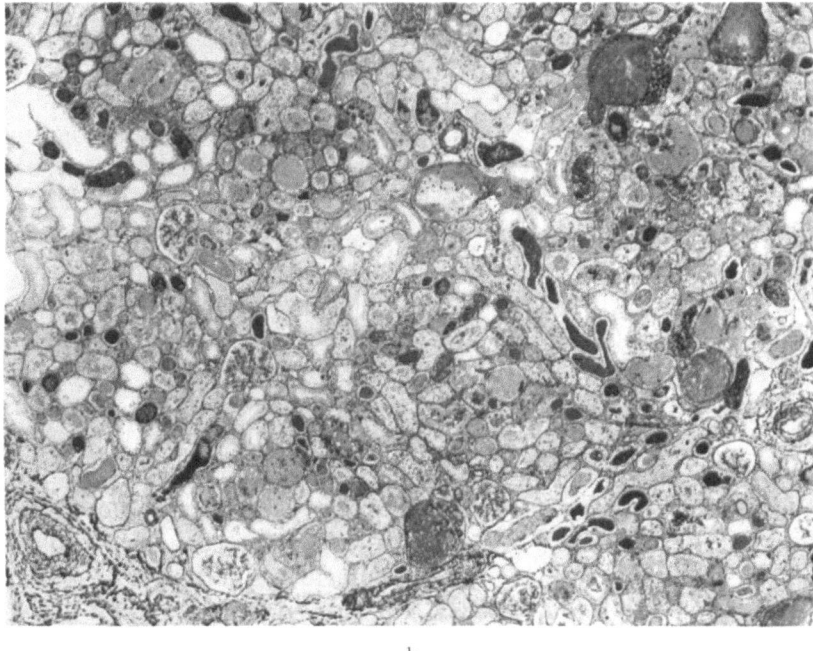

b

Fig. 12a and b. Renal cortex of sole remaining kidneys in chronic, one-kidney hypertension before (a) and after (b) unclamping. Normal cortical structure in (a), and widespread acute hypertensive lesions in (b) with prominent glomerular aneurysms and tubular casts. Methacrylate embedding, silver impregnation (MOVAT), ×120

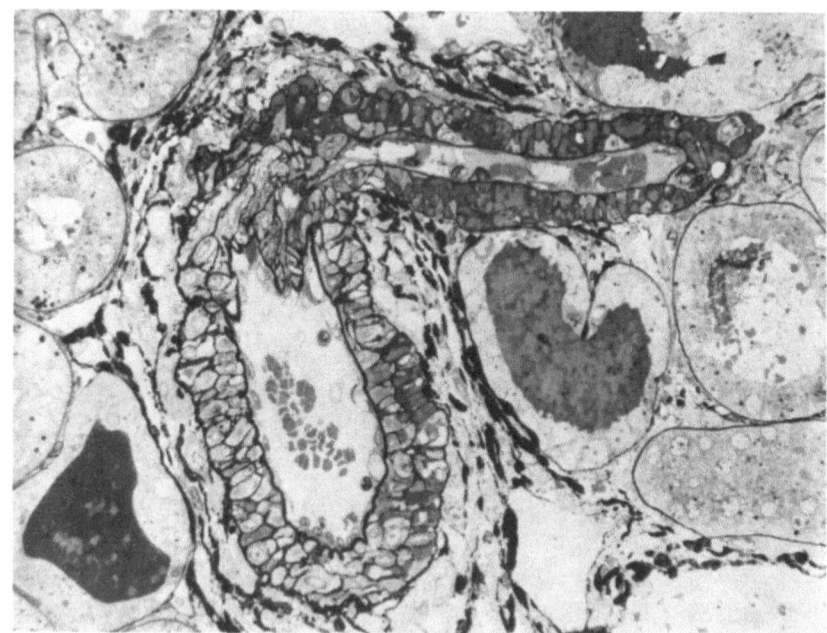

Fig. 13. 24 hours after unclamping a chronic, one-kidney hypertensive rat: interlobular artery branching into an afferent arteriole with plasma insudations in the focally necrotic media. Two tubuli surrounding the interlobular artery are filled with hyalin material and red cells. Methacrylate embedding, silver impregnation (Movat), ×360

During the past six years several specific inhibitors of angiotensin II have been developed, and seem to provide a powerful tool for investigating the physiology and pathophysiology of the RAS (Khairallah et al., 1970; Marshall et al., 1970; Pals et al., 1971; Türker et al., 1971; Khosla et al., 1972, 1975; Regoli and Park, 1972; Yamamoto et al., 1972; for more literature see Khosla et al., 1974). The essential prerequisites for developing angiotensin II analogues were the identification of the amino acid sequence of angiotensin II by Skeggs et al. (1956), and the synthesis of angiotensin II by Bumpus et al. (1957) and by Schwyzer et al. (1957). The blocking agents, now available, are angiotensin II analogues apparently acting as specific competitive antagonists at the receptor sites for angiotensin II. In order to be considered as potent angiotensin II antagonists these compounds must be shown to fulfill a number of criteria, including specificity (for instance no blockade of norepinephrine-induced blood pressor responses), a capacity to block the musculotropic and adrenotropic effects of angiotensin II, a lack or near-lack of agonistic properties and, finally, a prolonged biological half-life (Davis et al., 1974).

One of the analogues, 1-Sar-8-Ile-angiotensin II, which was used in the present study, has been shown to be an antagonist of angiotensin II in vitro (Türker et al., 1972; Yamamoto et al., 1972) and in vivo (Bumpus et al., 1973; Sweet et al., 1973, 1974). In 1-Sar-8-Ile-angiotensin II the positions 1and 8 in

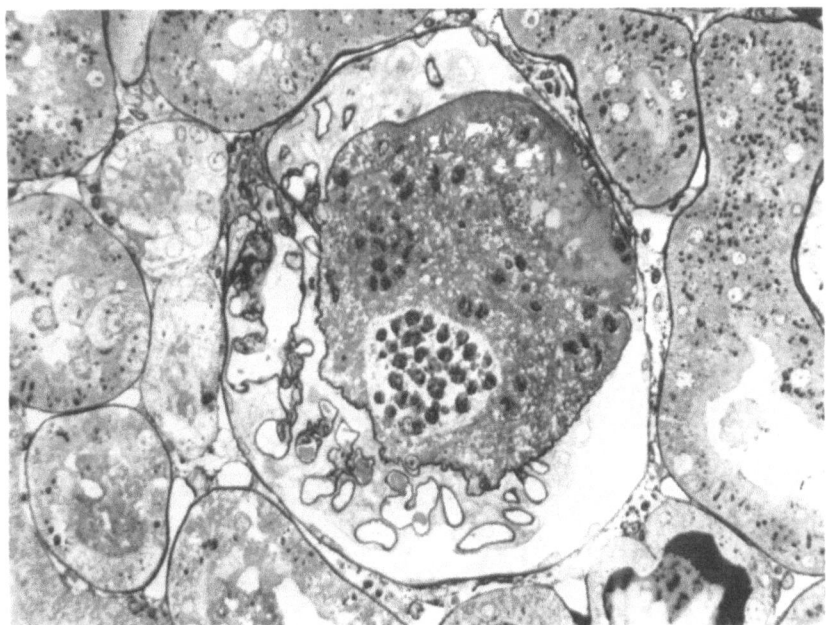

Fig. 14. 24 hours after unclamping a chronic, one-kidney hypertensive rat: glomerular aneurysm surrounded by the basement membrane and filled with red cells, leucocytes, and plasmic material. Methacrylate embedding, silver impregnation (Movat), ×440

the amino acid sequence of the parent peptide were substituted by sarcosine and isoleucine, respectively. Substitution of isoleucine in position 8 was shown to be responsible for the antagonistic potency, whereas insertion of sarcosine in position 1 prolongs the duration of action either by protecting 1-Sar-8-Ile-angiotensin II from enzymatic degradation or by increasing the binding affinity of the analogue for the receptor site (Hall et al., 1974).

Considering that angiotensin II, on a weight basis, is the most potent vasopressor substance known, and that normal plasma renin and angiotensin II levels probably reach the pressor-effective range (Imbs et al., 1967; Bianchi et al., 1968; Worcel et al., 1969; Chinn and Düsterdieck, 1972), a fall of arterial blood pressure a priori might be expected in normal animals following administration of the specific angiotensin II antagonist. However, infusion of 1-Sar-8-Ile-angiotensin II at a dose higher than needed for blocking the response to exogenous angiotensin II failed to lower mean arterial blood pressure in normotensive anesthetized rats (Fig. 1). Similar results were observed by Bumpus et al. (1973) in normotensive anesthetized rats after infusion of 8-Ile-angiotensin II, as well as by Gavras et al. (1973) using the angiotensin II antagonist 1-Sar-8-Ala-angiotensin II in normotensive rats. These findings parallel the fact that disappearance of PRA after bilateral nephrectomy does not cause hypotension.

In contrast, infusion of 1-Sar-8-Ile-angiotensin II lowered mean arterial blood pressure within 30 minutes in furosemide-treated (i.e. sodium- and

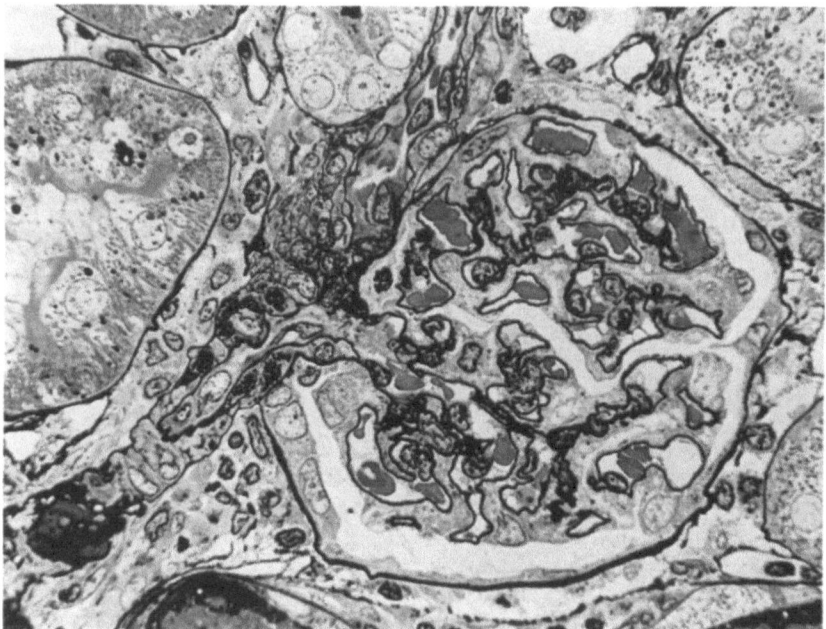

Fig. 15. 24 hours after unclamping a chronic, one-kidney hypertensive rat: glomerulus with adjacent afferent and efferent arterioles. Vas afferens with a focal plasma insudation proximal to intact granulated juxtaglomerular cells. Methacrylate embedding, silver impregnation (Movat), ×720

volume-depleted) normotensive rats (Fig. 2). In agreement with earlier studies in man and animals (Fraser et al., 1965; Klaus et al., 1968; Meyer et al., 1968; Oelkers et al., 1970) furosemide diuresis induced a large and significant increase of PRA which could be prevented by drinking 1% NaCl solution during the course of the experiment (Table 1). The significant fall of mean arterial blood pressure induced by 1-Sar-8-Ile-angiotensin II in furosemide-treated rats clearly indicates that normotension, persisting despite a considerable volume depletion, as reflected by the significant rise of the average hematocrit value (Table 1), was maintained by the RAS. It appears that, under these acute experimental conditions, other humoral and neural mechanisms also involved in blood pressure control (Guyton et al., 1972) were not adequate to counterbalance the blocked function of the RAS. This compensatory role of the RAS acting to maintain arterial blood pressure within normal limits against blood pressure lowering influences is not limited to furosemide-induced acute sodium and water losses. The RAS was also found to counteract a potential fall of normal arterial blood pressure under several conditions known to be accompanied by enhanced renin release. 1-Sar-8-Ala-angiotensin was shown to lower arterial blood pressure significantly in dogs after dietary sodium depletion, bilateral adrenalectomy and thoracic caval constriction (Johnson and Davis, 1973a, b; Davis et al., 1974; Spielman and Davis, 1974). The same blood-pressure-lowering effect obtained in dietary

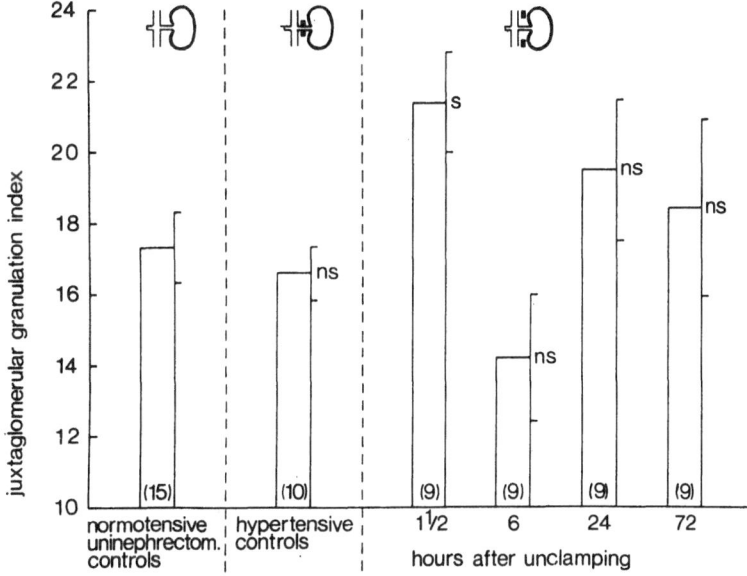

Fig. 16. Juxtaglomerular index in normotensive, uninephrectomized rats and in chronic, one-kidney hypertensive rats before and after unclamping

sodium-depleted rats has been described by GAVRAS et al. (1973). Moreover, HABER et al. (1975) reported severe hypotension in sodium-depleted and upright-tilted volunteers when the conversion of angiotensin I to angiotensin II was blocked by administration of a converting enzyme inhibitor.

Thus, as suggested by DAVIS et al. (1974), the RAS may provide a powerful and previously underestimated counteracting mechanism which is capable of maintaining arterial blood pressure at normal or near normal levels in potential hypotensive situations.

2. Contribution of the RAS in Initiating and Maintaining Renal Hypertension

Although the ultimate intrarenal mechanism responsible for renin release has not yet been identified, a number of factors, including arterial blood pressure, effective blood volume, sodium balance, autonomic nervous system, catecholamines, and angiotensin II are known to participate in the control of renin secretion (DAVIS, 1974). If a disturbance in the control of renin secretion is to be definitely shown to play a role in the pathogenesis of renal hypertension, an altered relationship between one or more of these factors and renin release must be postulated. In this respect, the physiologic role of arterial blood pressure in controlling renin secretion warrants particular attention.

Under acute experimental conditions there is evidence that an inverse correlation exists between the level of renal perfusion pressure and renal

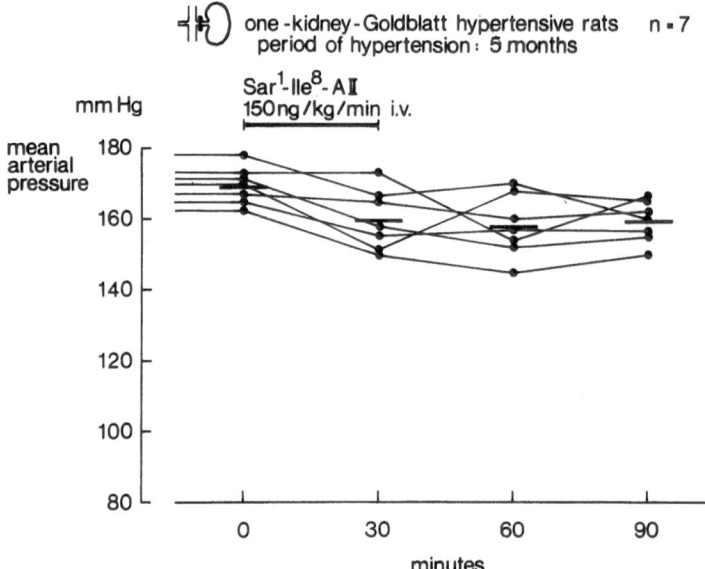

Fig. 17. Effect of 1-Sar-8-Ile-angiotensin II on mean arterial blood pressure of rats with one-kidney hypertension of 5 months duration

renin release (Skinner et al., 1964; Imbs et al., 1970; Krahé et al., 1972; Hofbauer et al., 1974; Kaloyanides et al., 1974). Moreover, the decrease of renin activity occurring in the untouched kidneys of two-kidney hypertensive rats, despite a significant fall in extracellular volume and plasma sodium concentration (Table 2), as well as the secretory insufficiency of the untouched kidneys observed after removing the clamped kidneys (Table 3), suggest that renin release is also suppressed by increased renal perfusion pressure under chronic conditions.

Thus, in the hypertensive state, an intact regulatory influence of arterial blood pressure on the RAS should be reflected by a fall in PRA to low levels. Consequently, not only the increased PRA of the two-kidney hypertensive rats (Table 2), but also the "normal" PRA of the one-kidney hypertensive rats (Table 4), might indicate an irregular control of the RAS with respect to the prevailing high systemic blood pressure.

It is assumed that the clamp on the renal artery, narrowing the arterial lumen approximately to half of the control value (Fig. 11), might falsify the afferent information necessary for an appropriate feedback mechanism at the level of the juxtaglomerular apparatus, thereby preventing the expected depression of renin secretion. This hypothesis (Lee, 1969) was confirmed by the "unclamping" experiments performed in chronic one-kidney hypertensive rats (Helmchen et al., 1974). Removing the clamp from the renal artery and thereby exposing the kidney to the elevated systemic arterial blood pressure, resulted in a significant fall of PRA within 90 minutes (Fig. 9). This occurred at a time when the blood pressure of these animals, despite a significant

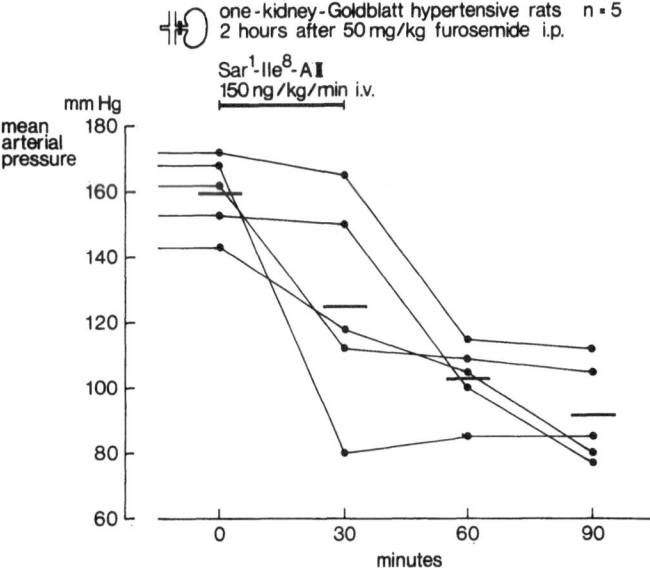

Fig. 18. Effect of furosemide diuresis and subsequent administration of 1-Sar-8-Ile-angiotensin II on mean arterial blood pressure of rats with one-kidney hypertension of 5 months duration

fall, was still elevated (Fig. 8). Between 6 and 24 hours after unclamping PRA rose, but did not reach normal levels (Fig. 9), while systolic blood pressure continued to fall (Fig. 8).

Thus, removal of the renal artery clip and subsequent perfusion of the kidney at high arterial pressure obviously depressed renin secretion. However, even the lowest PRA measured 90 minutes after unclamping probably does not represent the PRA appropriate to the systemic hemodynamic conditions of the chronic one-kidney hypertensive animals for the following reasons:

1. The influence of surgery per se, reflected by the slight increase of PRA in sham-unclamped hypertensive rats (Fig. 9).

2. The blood pressure fall, already significant 90 minutes after unclamping (Fig. 8).

3. A loss of sodium and water occurring immediately after unclamping (LIARD and PETERS, 1970).

4. The biological half-life of PRA of approximately 30 minutes (SCHAECHTELIN et al., 1964).

Therefore, the appropriate level of PRA during the chronic stage of one-kidney hypertension would be expected to be even lower than that determined 90 minutes after unclamping.

Though the blood pressure effect appears to dominate in depressing renin release after unclamping, it is impossible to decide whether a *baroreceptor* mechanism (TOBIAN, 1960), a *macula densa* mechanism (THURAU and SCHNER-

Mann, 1965; Vander, 1967; Schnermann et al., 1970; Thurau et al., 1972; Thurau, 1974), or both were involved. As shown by Liard and Peters (1970, 1973), unclamping the renal artery in rats with chronic one-kidney hypertension consistently caused a large increase of sodium and water excretion in agreement with earlier findings of Selkurt (1951), Thurau and Deetjen (1962), and Lowitz et al. (1968) that an increase in renal perfusion pressure induced diuresis and natriuresis. Recently, Liard et al. (1974) also reported a fall of PRA accompanied by an increase of urinary volume following cessation of the renal artery constriction in sinoaortic baroreceptor-denervated dogs with one-kidney hypertension. Thus, an additional influence reaching the juxtaglomerular apparatus from the tubular site cannot be excluded under these experimental conditions.

It is very likely that the increased peripheral PRA in two-kidney hypertension also reflects an irregular feedback control of renin release in the clamped kidneys with increased renin activity (Table 2). Compared with the decreased renin activity in the untouched "hypertensive" kidneys, which might be considered as nearly appropriate with respect to the systemic hemodynamics, the renin content of the clamped kidneys appears to be eight times too high (Table 2). After removing the clamped kidney, PRA, which is then only dependent upon renin derived from the previously renin-depleted, untouched kidney, fell to very low levels within 24 hours despite subnormal systolic blood pressure (Table 3). This probably reflects the appropriate secretory insufficiency of the renin-producing juxtaglomerular cells prevailing during the hypertensive stage in the untouched kidney. The increased ability to enhance peripheral PRA in response to various hypotensive stimuli observed in two-kidney hypertensive rats (Helmchen et al., 1972a) may thereby be explained in terms of the inappropriately stimulated juxtaglomerular apparatus of the clamped kidney.

In fact, the low PRA measured 24 hours after removing the clamped kidneys (Table 3) cannot be related to the PRA, which would be actually appropriate to the hypertensive stage, since arterial blood pressure had already fallen at this time (Table 3). In addition, a fall of angiotensin II concentration in plasma, secondary to the diminished PRA observed after removing the clamped kidney (Table 3), might have affected renin secretion in the remaining kidney as well (Fourcade et al., 1971; Guyton et al., 1974).

The data presented here indicate a disturbed regulation of renin release in both one- and two-kidney hypertension due to a falsification of regulatory influences resulting from the presence of the clamp on the renal artery. Obviously, neither humoral nor neural factors, otherwise known to be involved in the control of renin secretion, were capable of compensating for the falsified information transmitted hemodynamically to the juxtaglomerular apparatus of the clamped kidneys.

Before discussing the possible role of the RAS in renal hypertension, it is necessary to consider changes in renal sodium and water excretion consistently accompanying renal artery constriction. According to the experiments of

SELKURT (1951) and THURAU and DEETJEN (1962) and to the results of a systems analysis (GUYTON et al., 1972, 1974), any elevation of arterial blood pressure is expected to be accompanied physiologically by an increased excretion of sodium and water. These increases observed after elevation of renal perfusion pressure are probably due to an enhanced filtration rate in non-autoregulated juxtamedullary glomeruli as well as to a decreased fluid reabsorption in the loop of Henle (STUMPE et al., 1969, 1970, 1971). In contrast, the excretory function of the clamped kidney in two-kidney hypertension was depressed in both the acute (GUIGNARD et al., 1970) and the chronic stages (LOWITZ et al., 1968; KRAMER and OCHWADT, 1972). In one-kidney hypertension, urinary volume normalized in the chronic stage following a period of decreased urinary output during the first few days after renal artery constriction (GROSS et al., 1964b, 1965). However, even the normalized urinary output observed in chronic one-kidney hypertensive rats may indicate an excretory kidney function inappropriately depressed with respect to systemic arterial hypertension. This hypothesis is supported by the unclamping experiments performed in rats (LIARD and PETERS, 1970) and in dogs (LIARD et al., 1974), resulting in a large increase of renal sodium and water excretion occurring immediately after releasing renal artery constriction. Despite the sodium and water retention observed in chronic one-kidney hypertension (TOBIAN et al., 1969; BRUNNER, 1970), it appears that no other mechanism was able to override the hemodynamical signal falsified by the renal artery clamp. Thus, constricting the renal artery does not only lead to an inappropriately elevated renin release, but also results in sodium and water excretion being inappropriately depressed in relation to the hypertensive stage (GUYTON et al., 1974; HELMCHEN and LIARD, 1974).

The question now arises whether or not the demonstrated disturbance in the control of renin release may possess significance in the genesis of both forms of experimental renal hypertension.

In the past a variety of experimental procedures has been applied in an attempt to elucidate this crucial point: unilateral and bilateral nephrectomy (see PAGE and McCUBBIN, 1968), immunization with preparations of renin (WAKERLIN and JOHNSON, 1941; DEODHAR et al., 1964; WEISER et al., 1969; HILL et al., 1970), immunization with angiotensin II (HEDWALL, 1968; CHRISTLIEB et al., 1969; EIDE and AARS, 1969, 1970; JOHNSTON et al., 1970; BRUNNER et al., 1972; EIDE, 1972; MACDONALD et al., 1972), the application of a phospholipid renin preinhibitor (SEN et al., 1968, 1969), and the administration of a converting enzyme-inhibiting pentapeptide (KRIEGER et al., 1971) or nonapeptide (MILLER et al., 1972; AYERS et al., 1974).

First reports concerning the antihypertensive effect of specific angiotensin II antagonists (BRUNNER et al., 1971; PALS et al., 1971; BUMPUS et al., 1973; BING and NIELSEN, 1973; GAVRAS et al., 1973; AYERS et al., 1974; SWEET et al., 1973, 1974) appear to confirm expectations that these angiotensin II analogues would provide an effective tool in analyzing the contribution of the RAS in different forms of renal hypertension.

In the present experiments, the specific antagonist 1-Sar-8-Ile-angio-
tensin II was used to reinvestigate the role of angiotensin II in one- and two-
kidney hypertension

In rats with two-kidney hypertension of 5 weeks duration, the angiotensin II inhibitor produced an immediate normalization of mean arterial
blood pressure which remained normal for 30 minutes after terminating infusion of 1-Sar-8-Ile-angiotensin II (Fig. 3). An unspecific blood pressure
lowering effect under these conditions was excluded by infusing 0.9% NaCl
solution at the same rate as used in the previous experiment (Fig. 4).

These results suggest that two-kidney hypertension in these experimental
rats was mediated entirely by endogenously formed angiotensin II. Similar observations obtained in two-kidney hypertensive rats after infusion of 1-Sar-8-
Ala-angiotensin II or 8-Ile-angiotensin II were described by Brunner el at.
(1971) and Bumpus et al. (1973), respectively.

On the basis of these findings, normalization of blood pressure, frequently
reported to occur following the removal of the clamped kidneys in two-kidney
hypertensive animals (Pickering and Prinzmetal, 1938; Wilson and Byrom,
1941; Floyer, 1951; Regoli et al., 1962; Schaechtelin et al., 1963; Masson
et al., 1965), actually does seem to be a result of the fall of PRA occurring
under these circumstances (Table 3). In contrast, some investigators (Hedwall, 1968; Eide, 1972; Macdonald et al., 1972) using active immunization
against angiotensin II suggested that angiotensin II is not involved in pathogenesis of two-kidney hypertension. However, several reasons could account
for the failure to lower blood pressure by immunological procedures:

(a) Active immunization against angiotensin II stimulates the endogenous
renin production and secretion (Christlieb et al., 1969; Oster et al., 1974).
This is of particular importance in view of the finding that (b) angiotensin II
is also formed locally in the vascular wall (Swales and Thurston, 1973)
as postulated by Daum et al. (1966). These latter sites are inaccessible to
large angiotensin II antibody molecules but easily accessible to the low-
molecular-weight angiotensin II analogues (Thurston and Swales, 1974)
which also stimulate endogenous renin secretion (Bumpus et al., 1973; Johnson
and Davis, 1973; Ayers et al., 1974). (c) Active immunization to angiotensin II
does not exclude the possibility that amounts of free plasma angiotensin II,
adequate to influence arterial blood pressure, could contribute to hypertension
(Walker et al., 1972).

1-Sar-8-Ile-angiotensin II significantly lowered the average mean arterial
blood pressure in chronic one-kidney hypertension of 5 months duration but
failed to abolish hypertension (Fig. 17) even though the pressor response to
exogenous angiotensin II immediately after terminating the infusion of the
angiotensin II inhibitor was blocked. Similar results were reported after
infusion of 8-Ile-angiotensin II into rats with one-kidney hypertension of
more than 30 weeks duration (Bumpus et al., 1973). Moreover, Brunner et al.
(1971) and Gavras et al. (1973) noted the failure of 1-Sar-8-Ala-angiotensin II
to normalize arterial blood pressure in one-kidney hypertension of 4–6 weeks

duration. BING and NIELSEN (1973), using very high doses of 1-Sar-8-Ala-angiotensin II, observed a blood-pressure-lowering effect of this compound in chronic one-kidney hypertension. Even in this latter case, most of the rats still remained hypertensive. Similarly, hypertension also persisted in the chronic stages of this kind of experimental renal hypertension after administration of a converting enzyme-blocking pentapeptide (KRIEGER et al., 1971).

These data seem to exclude an important role for angiotensin II in the maintenance of chronic one-kidney hypertension, thereby possibly also explaining the failure of nephrectomy in normalizing blood pressure observed under these conditions (PICKERING, 1945; FLOYER, 1951; LIARD, 1969; ROMERO et al., 1972) (Table 5).

However, removal of the sole remaining clamped kidney (LIARD, 1971, 1973) (Fig. 7) or administration of angiotensin II analogues in chronic one-kidney hypertensive rats, previously sodium- and volume-depleted, normalized arterial blood pressure regardless of whether sodium and volume depletion was caused by furosemide diuresis (Fig. 7, 18) or by a prolonged dietary sodium deprivation (GAVRAS et al., 1973). Furosemide diuresis per se did not normalize blood pressure (Figs. 7, 18) even though the acute sodium and water excretion exceeded that observed during the first 6 hours after unclamping (LIARD, 1973; HELMCHEN and LIARD, 1974).

The blood pressor response to angiotensin II antagonists observed in chronic one-kidney hypertensive rats after sodium and volume depletion resembles that obtained in acute one-kidney hypertension when nephrectomy (PICKERING, 1945; LIARD, 1969; ROMERO et al., 1972) or administration of the converting enzyme-blocking nonapeptide (MILLER et al., 1972, 1975; AYERS et al., 1974) or angiotensin II antagonists (AYERS et al., 1974; SWEET et al., 1974) were shown to prevent or to abolish hypertension in different species.

These results suggest that the RAS, stimulated in both acute one-kidney hypertensive rats (KOLETSKY et al., 1971; HELMCHEN et al., 1972b) and in sodium- and volume-depleted chronic one-kidney hypertensive rats (Fig. 7), is responsible for initiating and maintaining hypertension under these conditions.

How can the pathogenic mechanisms inducing and maintaining both forms of experimental renal hypertension be characterized?

The following concept is based upon the assumption that the physiological capability of the kidney to counterbalance hypotensive stimuli is the key for understanding renal hypertension. Any lowering of renal perfusion pressure, normally signaling systemic arterial hypotension, is accompanied by an increased renin release and by a decreased urinary output. It has been demonstrated that both renal mechanisms, the RAS (DAVIS et al., 1974) (Fig. 2) and the renal-body fluid system (GUYTON et al., 1972, 1974), are important factors in stabilizing normal blood pressure against various potential hypotensive stimuli. A comparable situation is assumed to be caused by any partial constriction of the renal artery resulting in a persisting dissociation between systemic and renal arterial blood pressure (Braun-Menendez, 1946; Skinner *et al.*, 1964; Ziegler and Janzik, 1968; Lowitz *et al.*, 1969; Koletsky *et al.*, 1971; Kramer *et al.*, 1971; Ferrario and McCubbin, 1973), thereby simulating hypotension to the kidney in the presence of systemic normotension, or simulating normotension after systemic hypertension has been established. This may lead to a functional state of the RAS and of the renal excretory mechanism that, though appropriate to poststenotic hemodynamics, are, respectively, inappropriately activated or depressed in relation to the circulatory system, thereby inducing or maintaining arterial hypertension instead of normotension.

Consequently, renal hypertension may be considered to depend principally upon two different mechanisms:

The first consists of an inappropriately stimulated RAS acting directly through its vasoconstrictor effects and indirectly by activating both aldosterone biosynthesis and secretion and the central and peripheral sympathetic nervous system (for literature, see Page and Bumpus, 1974). The second concerns the inappropriately controlled renal-body fluid mechanism. Renal output of water and salt, inappropriately reduced by clamping the renal artery, causes retention of water and salt if a normal intake is continued. Subsequently, expansion of body fluid leads to a sequence of events finally culminating in an increase in both total peripheral resistance and arterial blood pressure due to a phenomenon known as total circulatory autoregulation (Bayliss, 1902; Borst and Borst de Geus, 1963; Guyton *et al.*, 1970, 1972; Coleman *et al.*, 1971; Wilson *et al.*, 1971).

Accordingly, it may be assumed that renal hypertension will be only abolished by manipulations which provide for the correction of both renal mechanisms.

This is the case in chronic one-kidney hypertension. Neither furosemide or dietary-induced sodium- and water-depletion nor suppression of the renin-angiotensin effects by nephrectomy or angiotensin II antagonists, lowered arterial blood pressure when applied separately. Under these conditions abolishing one of these mechanisms unmasked the effectiveness of the other which then predominated. Normotension could only be achieved by successively or simultaneously influencing both pathogenic mechanisms as provided by unclamping the renal artery or by administration of angiotensin II analogues in previously sodium- and volume-depleted animals (Fig. 18).

It is conceivable that the contribution of the RAS in maintaining chronic one-kidney hypertension becomes minimal after attaining steady-state conditions. However, any reduction of hypertension may lead to a tendency for the poststenotic renal perfusion pressure to fall from normal to subnormal levels, at least temporarily. This in effect may simulate systemic arterial hypotension and inappropriately reactivate the counterregulatory role of both the incretory and excretory renal mechanisms as observed in the acute hypertensive stage. If the hypotensive stimulus is provided by sodium and volume depletion, the RAS may then become the only pressor-effective renal mechanism.

It remains to explain that acute one-kidney hypertension and acute and chronic two-kidney hypertension have been shown to depend only upon an inappropriately stimulated renin-angiotensin mechanism. The different significance of the RAS and the renal-body fluid mechanism during the acute and chronic stage of one-kidney hypertension is assumed to reflect the situation occurring after lowering systemic arterial blood pressure in normal animals. As demonstrated by GUYTON et al. (1972), the RAS and the renal-body fluid system, each considered to be a pressor-control system, differ markedly with respect to their response times. While the vasoconstrictor effect of the RAS operates within minutes, the renal body fluid pressor control mechanism reaches its highest degree of effectiveness within one week (GUYTON et al., 1972). Reducing the renal perfusion pressure by clamping the sole remaining kidney seems to provoke the same sequence of events, leading to a normalization of renal perfusion pressure at the price of systemic arterial hypertension. Thus, the predominant role of the RAS during the acute stage of one-kidney hypertension may be explained by the physiological delay in pressor effectiveness of the renal-body fluid mechanism.

In two-kidney hypertension, diminished salt and water output of the clamped kidney was demonstrated to be compensated for, or even over-compensated for, by an increased sodium and water excretion by the untouched kidney (LOWITZ et al., 1968; GUIGNARD et al., 1970; KRAMER et al., 1972), frequently leading to a sodium and volume depletion (GOTZEN et al., 1969, 1971) (Table 2). Under these conditions the predominance of the RAS in maintaining hypertension becomes apparent. In this context it is also worth mentioning that during the first three weeks of two-kidney hypertension a mild sodium retention may occur (MOEHRING et al., 1971). Nevertheless, the RAS is assumed to be the dominant pathogenic factor, since it probably acts by affecting the excretory function of the untouched kidney, diminishing its sodium and water excretion either by an increase of intrarenal vascular resistance or by a renal aldosterone effect (FOURCADE et al., 1971; GUYTON et al., 1974). If such a secondary inappropriate aldosterone secretion really plays an important role, it is conceivable that, during this early stage, the angiotensin II antagonists 1-Sar-8-Ile-angiotensin II and 1-Sar-8-Ala-angiotensin II might be less effective in lowering arterial blood pressure than removing the clamped kidney. Both analogues, though potent and specific blockers of the pressor response to angiotensin II, are much less effective inhibitors of aldosterone biosynthesis (STEELE and LOWENSTEIN, 1974; BRAVO et al., 1975). This might explain the failure of 1-Sar-8-Ala-angiotensin II to normalize blood pressure in two-kidney hypertensive rabbits (JOHNSON et al., 1975).

On the other hand, the period of dominance of the RAS in maintaining two-kidney hypertension may be limited by the occurrence of widespread hypertensive vascular lesions in the untouched kidney (Fig. 19). The vas-

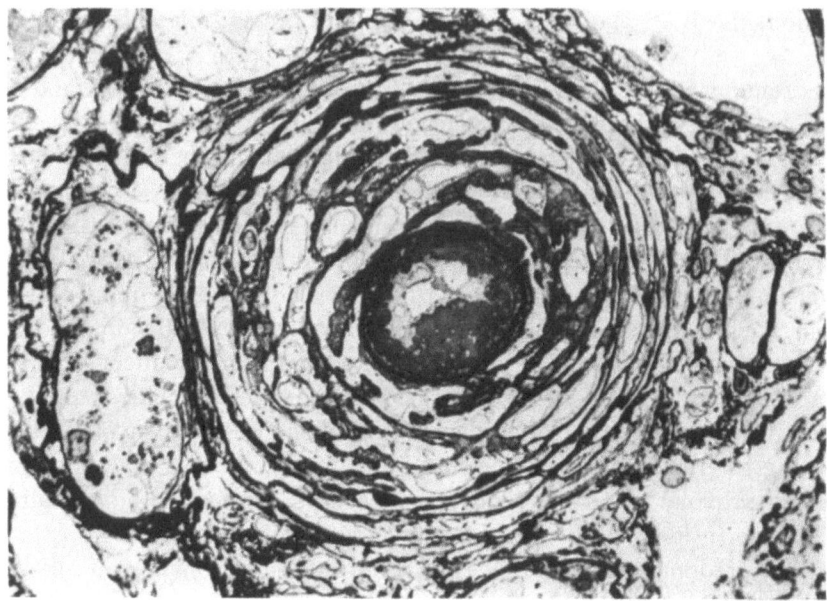

Fig. 19. Interlobular artery with a lumen narrowed by subendothelial plasma insudation and "onion-like" cell proliferation in the intima and media. Untouched kidney of a rat with two-kidney hypertension of 12 months duration. Methacrylate embedding, silver impregnation (Movat), ×880

cular changes do not only seem to reactivate the previously inactivated renin producing juxtaglomerular cells (Fig. 20), but also to depress the excretory function of the affected kidney (Helmchen, 1974). Similar morphological changes may be responsible for the lesser degree of blood pressure reduction in response to the administration of 1-Sar-8-Ile-angiotensin II in long-standing two-kidney hypertension (Fig. 5). In a preliminary experiment 1-Sar-8-Ile-angiotensin II became pressor-effective in two of those previously inhibitor-resistant rats after furosemide diuresis (Fig. 6). Thus, under these circumstances, the two-kidney hypertension is considered to become similar to chronic one-kidney hypertension with respect to the underlying pathogenic mechanism.

V. Conclusion

Renal hypertension experimentally elicited by partially constricting one renal artery may depend principally on an inappropriately stimulated RAS as well as on an inappropriately depressed renal sodium and water excretion. Both mechanisms were demonstrated to be operating in chronic one-kidney hypertension, and it is likely that they are also responsible for sustaining two-kidney hypertension after widespread hypertensive vascular lesions had developed in the untouched kidney. Acute one-kidney hypertension may depend only on the direct and/or indirect pressor effects of the RAS due to the delayed pressor response of sodium and water retention. In two-kidney hypertension, the sodium and volume factor may be abolished by an excessive

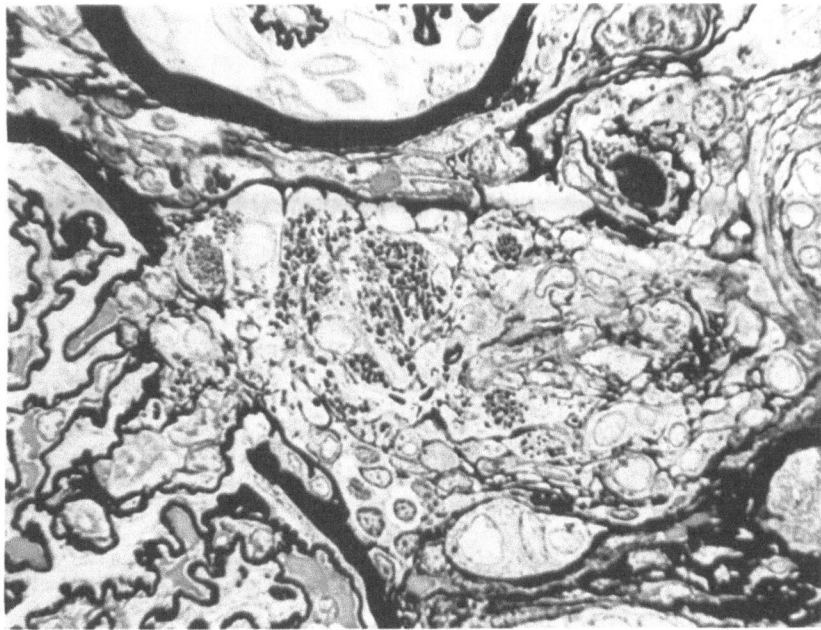

Fig. 20. Hyperplastic juxtaglomerular apparatus with granules in numerous epitheloid cells in an untouched kidney of a rat with two-kidney hypertension of 12 months duration. Methacrylate embedding, silver impregnation (Movat), ×1100

urinary output through the untouched kidney, and the RAS will be the only pathogenic factor as long as no obstructive intrarenal vascular lesions affect the excretory renal function.

On the basis of the findings presented here, renal hypertension seems to reflect the misdirected potency of the kidney to counterbalance hypotensive stimuli by incretory and excretory mechanisms.

References

Ayers, C. R., Vaughan, E. D., Yancey, M. R., Bing, K. T., Johnson, C. C., Morton, A. C.: Effect of 1-Sarcosine-8-Ala angiotensin II and converting enzyme inhibitor on renin release in dog acute renovascular hypertension. Circulat. Res. **34/35**, Suppl. I, 27–33 (1974)

Bayliss, W. M.: On the local reactions of the arterial wall to changes of internal pressure. J. Physiol. (Lond.) **28**, 220–231 (1902)

Bianchi, G., Brown, J. J., Lever, A. F., Robertson, J. I. S., Roth, N.: Changes of plasma renin concentration during pressor infusions of renin in the conscious dog: The influence of dietary sodium intake. Clin. Sci. **34**, 303–314 (1968)

Bing, J., Eskildsen, P. C., Faarup, P., Frederiksen, O.: Location of renin in kidneys and extrarenal tissues. Circulat. Res. **20/21**, Suppl. II, 3–11 (1967)

Bing, J., Nielsen, K.: Role of the renin-system in normo- and hypertension. Acta path. microbiol. scand. Section A **81**, 254–262 (1973)

Borst, J. G. G., Borst de Geus, A.: Hypertension explained by Starling's theory of circulatory homeostasis. Lancet **I**, 677–682 (1963)

Braun-Menendez, E., Fasciolo, J. C., Leloir, L. F., Munoz, J. M.: The substance causing renal hypertension. J. Physiol. (Lond.) **98**, 283–298 (1940)

Braun-Menendez, E., Fasciolo, J. C., Leloir, L. F., Munoz, J., Taquini, A. C.:
Renal Hypertension. Springfield, Ill.: Thomas, 1946

Bravo, E. L., Khosla, M. C., Bumpus, F. M.: Vascular and adrenocortical responses
to a specific antagonist of angiotensin II. Amer. J. Physiol. 228, 110–114 (1975)

Brunner, H.: Gesteigerter Na-Umsatz bei renal hypertonischen Ratten. Naunyn-
Schmiedebergs Arch. exp. Pharmak. 267, 278–292 (1970)

Brunner, H. R., Chang, P., Wallach, R., Sealey, J. E., Laragh, J. H.: Angiotensin II
vascular receptors: Their avidity in relationship to sodium balance, the autonomic
nervous system and hypertension. J. Clin. Invest. 51, 58–67 (1972)

Brunner, H. R., Kirshman, J. D., Sealey, J. E., Laragh, J. H.: Hypertension of
renal origin: evidence for two different mechanisms. Science 174, 1344–1346 (1971)

Bumpus, F. M., Schwarz, H., Page, I. H.: Synthesis and pharmacology of the octapeptide angiotonin. Science 125, 886–887 (1957)

Bumpus, F. M., Sen, S., Smeby, R. R., Sweet, C., Ferrario, C. M., Khosla, M. C.: Use
of angiotensin II antagonists in experimental hypertension. Circulat. Res. 32/33,
Suppl. I, 150–158 (1973)

Byrom, F. B., Wilson, C.: A plethysmographic method for measuring systolic blood
pressure in the intact rat. J. Physiol. (Lond.) 93, 301–304 (1938)

Chinn, R. H., Düsterdieck, G.: The response of blood pressure to infusion of angiotensin II: Relation to plasma concentrations of renin and angiotensin. Clin. Sci. 42,
489–504 (1972)

Christlieb, A. R., Biber, T. U. L., Hickler, R. B.: Studies on the role of angiotensin
in experimental hypertension: an immunologic approach. J. clin. Invest. 48, 1506–
1518 (1969)

Coleman, T. G., Granger, H. J., Guyton, A. C.: Whole-body circulatory autoregulation
and hypertension. Circulat. Res. 28/29, Suppl. II, 76–87 (1971)

Cook, W. F., Pickering, G. W.: The location of renin in the rabbit kidney. J. Physiol.
(Lond.) 149, 526–536 (1959)

Daum, A., Uehlecke, H., Klaus, D.: Unterschiedliche Beeinflussung der Blutdruck-
wirkung von Renin und Angiotensin durch Aminopeptidase. Naunyn-Schmiedeberg's
Arch. exp. Path. Pharmak. 254, 327–333 (1966)

Davis, J. O.: The control of renin release. In: Hypertension Manual (ed. J. H. Laragh),
p. 142–196. New York: Yorke Medical Books, Dun-Donnelley, 1974

Davis, J. O., Freeman, R. H., Johnson, J. A., Spielman, W. S.: Agents which block
the action of the renin-angiotensin system. Circulat. Res. 34, 279–285 (1974)

Dengler, H.: Über einen reninartigen Wirkstoff in Arterienextrakten. Naunyn-Schmiedeberg's Arch. exp. Path. Pharmak. 227, 481–487 (1956)

Deodhar, S. D., Haas, E., Goldblatt, H.: Induced changes in the antigenicity of
renin and the production of antirenin to homologous renin and to human renin.
Canad. Med. Ass. 90, 236–238 (1964)

Edelman, R., Hartroft, P. M.: Localization of renin in juxtaglomerular cells of rabbit
and dog through the use of the fluorescent-antibody technique. Circulat. Res. 9,
1069–1077 (1961)

Eide, I.: Renovascular hypertension in rats immunized with angiotensin II. Circulat.
Res. 30, 149–157 (1972)

Eide, I., Aars, H.: Renal hypertension in rabbits immunized with angiotensin. Nature
222, 571 (1969)

Eide, I., Aars, H.: Renal hypertension in rabbits immunized with angiotensin II.
Scand. J. Clin. Lab. Invest. 25, 119–128 (1970)

Ferrario, C. M., McCubbin, J. W.: Renal blood flow and perfusion pressure before
and after development of renal hypertension. Amer. J. Physiol. 224, 102–109 (1973)

Ferris, T. F., Gorden, P., Mulrow, P. J.: Rabbit uterus as a source of renin. Amer.
J. Physiol. 212, 698–702 (1967)

Fisher-Ferraro, C., Nahmod, V. E., Goldstein, J. J., Finkielman, S.: Angiotensin
and renin in rat and dog brain. J. Exp. Med. 133, 353–361 (1971)

Floyer, M. A.: The effect of nephrectomy and adrenalectomy upon the blood pressure
in hypertensive and normotensive rats. Clin. Sci. 10, 405–421 (1951)

Fourcade, J. C., Navar, L. G., Guyton, A. C.: Possibility that angiotensin resulting
from unilateral kidney disease affects contralateral renal function. Nephron 8, 1–16
(1971)

FRASER, R., JAMES, V. H. I., BROWN, J. J., ISAAC, P., LEVER, A. F., ROBERTSON, J. I. S.: Effect of angiotensin and of furosemide on plasma aldosterone, corticosterone, cortisol and renin in man. Lancet **289**, 989–991 (1965)

FÜHR, J., KACZMARCZYK, J., KRUTTGEN, C. D.: Eine einfache colorimetrische Methode zur Inulinbestimmung für Nieren-Clearance-Untersuchungen bei Stoffwechselgesunden und Diabetikern. Klin. Wschr. **33**, 729–730 (1955)

GANTEN, D., GRANGER, P., GANTEN, U., BOUCHER, R., GENEST, J.: An intrinsic renin-angiotensin system in the brain. In: Hypertension '72 (eds. J. GENEST and E. KOIW), pp. 423–432. Berlin-Heidelberg-New York: Springer 1972

GANTEN, D., MARQUEZ-JULIO, A., GRANGER, P., HAYDUK, K., KARSUNKY, K. P., BOUCHER, R., GENEST, J.: Renin in dog brain. Amer. J. Physiol. **221**, 1733–1737 (1971)

GAVRAS, H., BRUNNER, H. R., VAUGHAN, E. D., LARAGH, J. H.: Angiotensin-sodium interaction in blood pressure maintenance of renal hypertensive and normotensive rats. Science **180**, 1369–1371 (1973)

GENEST, J., SIMARD, S., ROSENTHAL, J., BOUCHER, R.: Norepinephrine and renin content in arterial tissue from different vascular beds. Canad. J. Physiol. Pharmacol. **47**, 87–91 (1969)

GOLDBLATT, H., LYNCH, J., HANZAL, R. F., SUMMERVILLE, W. W.: Studies on experimental hypertension. I. The production of persistent elevation of systolic blood pressure by means of renal ischemia. J. Exp. Med. **59**, 347–379 (1934)

GOORMAGHTIGH, N.: Existence of an endocrine gland in the media of the renal arterioles. Proc. Soc. Exp. Biol. (N.Y.) **42**, 688–689 (1939)

GOTZEN, R., HERBERG, C., SCHULTZE, G., LOHMANN, F. W.: Statischer Druck, Blutvolumen und zentralvenöser Druck bei renovasculärer Hypertonie. Arch. Kreisl.-Forsch. **66**, 66–79 (1971)

GOTZEN, R., SCHULTZE, G.: Das Blutvolumen in den verschiedenen Stadien der tierexperimentellen renovasculären Hypertonie. Verh. Dtsch. Ges. Inn. Med. **75**, 194–197 (1969)

GOULD, A. B., SKEGGS, L. T., KAHN, J. R.: The presence of renin activity in blood vessel walls. J. Exp. Med. **119**, 389–399 (1964)

GROSS, F., BRUNNER, H., ZIEGLER, M.: Renin-angiotensin system, aldosterone, and sodium balance. Rec. Progr. Hormone Res. **21**, 119–167 (1965)

GROSS, F., SCHAECHTELIN, G., BRUNNER, H., PETERS, G.: The role of the renin-angiotensin system in blood pressure regulation and kidney function. Canad. Med. Ass. J. **90**, 258–262 (1964b)

GROSS, F., SCHAECHTELIN, G., ZIEGLER, M., BERGER, M.: A renin-like substance in the placenta and uterus of the rabbit. Lancet **1964a I**, 914–916

GUIGNARD, J. P., FILLOUX, B., PETERS, G.: Urinary acidification and electrolyte excretion in renal hypertensive rats. Nephron **7**, 430–446 (1970)

GUYTON, A. C., COLEMAN, T. G., BOWER, J. D., GRANGER, A. J.: Circulatory control in hypertension. Circulat. Res. **26/27**, Suppl. II, 135–147 (1970)

GUYTON, A. C., COLEMAN, T. G., COWLEY, A. W., MANNING, R. D., NORMAN, R. A., FERGUSON, J. D.: A systems analysis approach to understanding longe-range arterial blood pressure control and hypertension. Circulat. Res. **35**, 159–175 (1974)

GUYTON, A. C., COLEMAN, T. G., COWLEY, A. W., SCHEEL, K. W., MANNING, R. D., NORMAN, R. A.: Arterial pressure regulation. Overriding dominance of the kidneys in long-term regulation and in hypertension. Amer. J. Med. **52**, 584–594 (1972b)

GUYTON, A. C., COLEMAN, T. G., GRANGER, H. J.: Circulation: Overall regulation. Ann. Rev. Physiol. **34**, 13–46 (1972a)

HABER, E., SANCHO, J., RE, R., BURTON, J., BARGER, A. C.: The role of the renin-angiotensin-aldosterone system in cardiovascular homeostasis in normal man. Clin. Sci. **48**, Suppl. II, 49–52 (1975)

HALL, M. M., KHOSLA, M. C., KHAIRALLAH, P. A., BUMPUS, F. M.: Angiotensin analogs: The influence of sarcosine substituted in position 1. J. Pharmacol. Exp. Ther. **188**, 222–228 (1974)

HARTROFT, P. M., HARTROFT, W. S.: Studies on renal juxtaglomerular cells. I. Variations produced by sodium chloride and desoxycorticosterone acetate. J. Exp. Med. **97**, 415–428 (1953)

HARTWICH, A.: Der Blutdruck bei experimenteller Urämie und partieller Nierenausscheidung. Z. ges. exp. Med. **69**, 462–481 (1930)

Hayduk, K., Boucher, R., Genest, J.: Renin activity content in various tissues of dogs under different physiopathological states. Proc. Soc. Exp. Biol. (N.Y.) **134**, 252–255 (1970)

Hayduk, K., Ganten, D., Boucher, R., Genest, J.: Arterial and urinary renin activity. In: Hypertension '72 (eds. J. Genest and E. Koiw), pp. 435–443. Berlin-Heidelberg-New York: Springer 1972

Hedwall, P. R.: Effect of rabbit antibodies against angiotensin II on the pressor response to angiotensin II and renal hypertension in the rat. Brit. J. Pharmacol. **34**, 623–629 (1968)

Helmchen, U.: Renin and the juxtaglomerular apparatus in experimental post-Goldblatt hypertension. Kidney Internat. **5**, 308, 1974 (abstr.)

Helmchen, U., Kneissler, U., Churchill, P., Peters-Haefeli, L., Schaechtelin, G., Peters, G.: Plasma renin activity in renal hypertensive rats. Pflügers Arch. **332**, 232–238 (1972a)

Helmchen, U., Kneissler, U., Liard, J. F., Peters, G.: Renin secretion in the earliest stage of Goldblatt-type hypertension in rats. Klin. Wschr. **50**, 841–844 (1972b)

Helmchen, U., Kneissler, U., Peters, G.: Disturbances of the control of renin secretion in chronic one-kidney-Goldblatt hypertension in the rat. Pflügers Arch. **348**, 197–204 (1974)

Helmchen, U., Liard, J. F.: Die Regulation der Reninfreisetzung und der Natrium- und Wasserausscheidung bei experimenteller renaler Hypertonie (one-kidney-Gold-blatt hypertension). In: Hypertension (eds. A. Distler and H. P. Wolff) pp. 52–56. Stuttgart: G. Thieme 1974

Hill, R. W., Chester, J. E., Wisenbaugh, P. E.: The effect of intravenous antirenin injection on chronic experimental and acute renin-induced hypertension. Lab. Invest. **22**, 404–410 (1970)

Hofbauer, K. G., Zschiedrich, H., Hackenthal, E., Gross, F.: Function of the renin-angiotensin system in the isolated perfused rat kidney. Circulat. Res. **34/35**, 193–201 (1974)

Imbs, J. L., Brown, J. J., Davies, D. L., Lever, A. F., Robertson, J. I. S.: Plasma renin concentration in conscious rabbits during pressor infusions of renin. Clin. Sci. **32**, 83–88 (1967)

Imbs, J. L., Velly, J., Fontaine, J. L., Schwartz, J.: Contrôle de la sécrétion de rénine. Nephron **7**, 499–511 (1970)

Johnson, J. A., Davis, J. O.: Angiotensin II: Important role in the maintenance of arterial blood pressure. Science **179**, 906–907 (1973a)

Johnson, J. A., Davis, J. O.: Effects of a specific competitive antagonist of angiotensin II on arterial pressure and adrenal steroid secretion in dogs. Circulat. Res. **32**, Suppl. I, 159–168 (1973b)

Johnson, J. A., Davis, J. O., Braverman, B.: Role of angiotensin II in experimental renal hypertension in the rabbit. Amer. J. Physiol. **228**, 11–16 (1975)

Johnston, C. I., Hutchinson, J. S., Mendelsohn, F. A.: Biological significance of renin angiotensin immunization. Circulat. Res. **26/27**, Suppl. II, 215–222 (1970)

Kaloyanides, G. J., Bastron, R. D., Dibona, G. F.: Impaired autoregulation of blood flow and glomerular filtration rate in the isolated dog kidney depleted of renin. Circulat. Res. **35**, 400–412 (1974)

Khairallah, P. A., Toth, A., Bumpus, F. M.: Analogs of angiotensin II. Mechanism of receptor interaction. J. Med. Chem. **13**, 181–184 (1970)

Khosla, M. C., Hall, M. M., Smeby, R. R., Bumpus, F. M.: Agonist and antagonist relationships in 1 and 8 substituted analogs of angiotensin II. J. Med. Chem., 1975, in press

Khosla, M. C., Leese, R. A., Maloy, W. L., Ferreria, A. T., Smeby, R. R., Bumpus, F. M.: Synthesis of some analogs of angiotensin II as specific antagonists of the parent hormone. J. Med. Chem. **15**, 792–795 (1972)

Khosla, M. C., Smeby, R. R., Bumpus, F. M.: Structure-activity relationship in angiotensin II analogs. In: Angiotensin (eds. I. H. Page and F. M. Bumpus), pp. 126–161. Berlin-Heidelberg-New York: Springer 1974

Klaus, D., Bocskor, A., Seif, F.: Regulation der Reninsekretion bei Aldosteronmangel und bei Aldosteronismus. Ergebnisse mit einem Renin-Stimulations- und Suppressionstest. Klin. Wschr. **46**, 1195–1200 (1968)

KOLETSKY, S., PAVLICKO, K. M., RIVERA-VELEZ, J. M.: Renin-angiotensin activity in hypertensive rats with a single ischemic kidney. Lab. Invest. 24, 41–44 (1971)

KRAHÉ, P., ORTH, H., MIKSCHE, U., GROSS, F.: Renin release and reninsubstrate reaction in the isolated perfused rabbit kidney. Kidney Internat. 2, 6–10 (1972)

KRAMER, P., OCHWADT, B.: Sodium excretion in Goldblatt-hypertension. Pflügers Arch. 332, 332–346 (1972)

KRAMER, P., RUMPF, K. W., OCHWADT, B.: Hämodynamische Charakteristika einer experimentellen Nierenarterienstenose bei der Ratte. In: Renale Elimination von Pharmaka (eds. R. HEINTZ and H. HOLZHÜTER), pp. 655–661. Aachen 1972

KRIEGER, G. M., SALGADO, H. C., ASSAN, C. J., GREENE, C. L. J., FERREIRA, S. H.: Potential screening test for detection of overactivity of renin angiotensin system. Lancet 1972 I, 269–271

LEE, M. R.: Renin and Hypertension. A Modern Synthesis. London: Lloyd-Luke 1969

LIARD, J. F.: Effect de l'ablation partielle ou totale du tissu rénal sur l'hypertension rénovasculaire du rat. Experientia (Basel) 25, 934–935 (1969)

LIARD, J. F.: Sodium retention versus renin angiotensin system in experimental renal hypertension. Canad. J. Physiol. Pharmacol. 51, 238–241 (1973)

LIARD, J. F., COWLEY, A. W., McCAA, R. E., GUYTON, A. C.: Renin, aldosterone, body fluid volumes, and the baroreceptor reflex in the development and reversal of Goldblatt hypertension in conscious dogs. Circulat. Res. 34, 549–560 (1974)

LIARD, J. F., PETERS, G.: Mechanism of the fall in blood pressure after "unclamping" in rats with Goldblatt-type hypertension. Experientia (Basel) 26, 743–745 (1970)

LOWITZ, H. D., STUMPE, K. O., OCHWADT, B.: Natrium- und Wasserresorption in den verschiedenen Abschnitten des Nephrons beim experimentellen Hochdruck der Ratte. Pflügers Arch. 304, 322–335 (1968)

LOWITZ, H. D., STUMPE, K. O., OCHWADT, B.: Mikropunktionsuntersuchung der geklammerten Niere bei einseitig nephrektomierten Ratten mit experimentellem renalen Hochdruck. Pflügers Arch. 309, 212–223 (1969)

MACDONALD, G. J., BOYD, G. W., PEART, W. S.: Renal hypertension and angiotensin antibodies. Amer. Heart J. 83, 137–139 (1972)

MARSHALL, G. R., VINE, W., NEEDLEMAN, P.: A specific competitive inhibitor of angiotensin II. Proc. Natl. Acad. Sci. 67, 1624–1626 (1970)

MASSON, G. M. C., KASHII, C., MATSUNAGA, M., PAGE, I. H.: Effect of removal of a clipped kidney or cessation of renin administration on hypertension. Proc. Soc. Exp. Biol. 120, 640–644 (1965)

MEYER, P., MENARD, J., PAPANICOLAOU, N., ALEXANDRE, J. M., DEVAUX, C., MILLIEZ, P. Mechanism of renin release following furosemide diuresis in rabbit. Amer. J. Physiol. 215, 908–915 (1968)

MILLER, E. D., SAMUELS, A. I., HABER, E., BARGER, A. C.: Inhibition of angiotensin conversion in experimental renovascular hypertension. Science 177, 1108–1109 (1972)

MILLER, E. D., SAMUELS, A. I., HABER, E., BARGER, A. C.: Inhibition of angiotensin conversion and prevention of renal hypertension. Amer. J. Physiol. 228, 448–453 (1975)

MINNICH, J. L., GANTEN, D., BARBEAU, A., GENEST, J.: Subcellular localization of cerebral renin-like activity. In: Hypertension '72 (eds. J. GENEST and E. KOIW), pp. 432–435. Berlin-Heidelberg-New York: Springer 1972

MÖHRING, J., NÄUMANN, H. J., MÖHRING, B., PHILIPPI, A., GROSS, F.: Sodium balance and plasma renin activity in renal hypertensive rats. Europ. J. Clin. Invest. 1, 384 (1971) (abstr.)

MOVAT, H. Z.: Silver impregnation methods for electron microscopy. Amer. J. Clin. Path. 35, 528–537 (1961)

NÖLLER, H. G.: Die Blutentnahme aus dem retroorbitalen Venenplexus. Klin. Wschr. 33, 770–771 (1955)

ÖLKERS, W., MAGNUS, R., SAMWER, K. F.: Das Verhalten der Plasmareninkonzentration nach akuter Natriurese und nach Orthostase bei Gesunden und Hypertonikern. Klin. Wschr. 48, 598–607 (1970)

OLIVER, W. J., GROSS, F.: Verhalten des Renin-ähnlichen Prinzips in der Speicheldrüse der weißen Maus unter verschiedenen Bedingungen. Naunyn-Schmiedeberg's Arch. Exp. Path. Pharmak. 255, 55–56 (1966)

Oster, P., Hackenthal, E., Vecsei, P., Gless, K. H., Möhring, J., Gross, F.: Effect of active immunization against angiotensin II on the renin-angiotensin-aldosterone system of rabbits. In: Hypertension (eds. A. Distler and H. P. Wolff), pp. 62–69. Stuttgart: G. Thieme 1974

Page, I. H.: Pathogenesis of arterial hypertension. JAMA 140, 451–457 (1949)

Page, I. H., Bumpus, F. M.: Angiotensin. Berlin-Heidelberg-New York: Springer 1974

Page, I. H., Helmer, O.: A cristalline pressor substance (angiotonin) resulting from the reaction between renin and renin-activator. J. Exp. Med. 71, 29–42 (1940)

Page, I. H., McCubbin, J. W.: Renal Hypertension. Chicago: Year Book Med. Publ. 1968

Pals, D. T., Masucci, F. D., Denning, G. S., Sipos, F., Fessler, D. C.: Role of the pressor action of angiotensin II in experimental hypertension. Circulat. Res. 29, 673–681 (1971)

Pickering, G. W.: The role of the kidney in acute and chronic hypertension following renal artery constriction in the rabbit. Clin. Sci. 5, 229–247 (1945)

Pickering, G. W., Prinzmetal, M.: Experimental hypertension of renal origin in the rabbit. Clin. Sci. 3, 357–368 (1938)

Regoli, D., Brunner, H., Peters, G., Gross, F.: Changes in renin content in kidneys of renal hypertensive rats. Proc. Soc. Exp. Biol. (N.Y.) 109, 142–145 (1962)

Regoli, D., Park, W. K.: Pressor and myotropic effect and antagonistic properties of several analogs of angiotensin II. Canad. J. Physiol. Pharmacol. 50, 99–112 (1972)

Regoli, D., Schaechtelin, G., Peters, G.: The renin activity of rat plasma. In: Progress in Nephrology (eds. G. Peters and F. Roch-Ramel), pp. 335–336. Berlin-Heidelberg-New York: Springer 1969

Robertson, A. L., Smeby, R. R., Bumpus, F. M., Page, I. H.: Production of renin by human juxtaglomerular cells in vitro. Circulat. Res. 18/19, Suppl. I, 131–142 (1966)

Romero, J. C., Kozak, T. J., Hoobler, S. W.: The effect of nephrectomy and of renomedullary extracts on the blood pressure of experimentally hypertensive rabbits. Proc. Soc. Exp. Biol. (N.Y.) 140, 651–656 (1972)

Rosenthal, J., Boucher, R., Rojo-Ortega, J. M., Genest, J.: Renin activity in aortic tissue of rats. Canad. J. Physiol. Pharmacol. 47, 53–56 (1969)

Schaechtelin, G., Chomety, F., Regoli, D., Peters, G.: Dosage de l'activité réninique d'extraits tissulaires par incubation avec un substrat naturel purifié. Helv. Physiol. Acta 24, 89–105 (1966)

Schaechtelin, G., Regoli, D., Gross, F.: Bio-assay of circulating renin-like pressor material by isovolemic cross circulation. Amer. J. Physiol. 205, 303–306 (1963)

Schaechtelin, G., Regoli, D., Gross, F.: Quantitative assay and disappearance rate of circulating renin. Amer. J. Physiol. 205, 1361–1364 (1964)

Schaechtelin, G., Regoli, D., Peters, G.: Microméthode pour le dosage de l'activité réninique dans 0.2 ml de plasma de rat. Helv. Physiol. Acta 25, CR 222–CR 223 (1967)

Schnermann, J., Wright, F. S., Davis, J. M., v. Stackelberg, W., Grill, G.: Regulation of superficial nephron filtration rate by tubulo-glomerular feedback. Pflügers Arch. 318, 147–175 (1970)

Schwyzer, R., Iselin, B., Kappeler, H., Riniker, B., Rittel, W., Zuber, H.: Synthese von Hypertensin-peptiden. Chimia (Aarau) 11, 335–336 (1957)

Selkurt, E. E.: Effect of pulse pressure and mean arterial pressure modification on renal hemodynamics and electrolyte and water excretion. Circulation 4, 541–551 (1951)

Sen, S., Smeby, R. R., Bumpus, F. M.: Antihypertensive effect of an isolated phospholipid. Amer. J. Physiol. 214, 337–341 (1968)

Sen, S., Smeby, R. R., Bumpus, F. M.: Plasma renin activity in hypertensive rats after treatment with renin preinhibitor. Amer. J. Physiol. 216, 499–503 (1969)

Skeggs, L. T., Kahn, J. R., Shumway, N. P.: Purification of hypertensin II. J. Exp. Med. 103, 301–307 (1956)

Skinner, S. L., McCubbin, J. W., Page, I. H.: Control of renin secretion. Circulat. Res. 15, 64–76 (1964)

Smith, C. L.: Rapid demonstration of juxtaglomerular granules in mammalians and birds. Stain Technol. 41, 291–294 (1966)

SPIELMAN, W. S., DAVIS, J. O.: The renin-angiotensin system and aldosterone secretion during sodium depletion in the rat. Circulat. Res. **35**, 615–624 (1974)

STAKEMAN, G.: A renin-like pressor substance found in the placenta of the rat. Acta path. microbiol. Scand. **60**, 350–354 (1960)

STEELE, J. M., JR., LOWENSTEIN, J.: Differential effects of an angiotensin II analogue on pressor and adrenal receptors in the rabbit. Circulat. Res. **35**, 592–600 (1974)

STUMPE, K. O., LOWITZ, H. D., OCHWADT, B.: Function of juxtamedullary nephrons in normotensive and chronically hypertensive rats. Pflügers Arch. **313**, 43–52 (1969)

STUMPE, K. O., LOWITZ, H. D., OCHWADT, B.: Fluid reabsorption in Henle's loop and urinary excretion of sodium and water in normal rats and rats with chronic hypertension. J. Clin. Invest. **49**, 1200–1212 (1970)

STUMPE, K. O., LOWITZ, H. D., OCHWADT, B.: Beschleunigte Natriurese und Diurese beim Hochdruck: Folge einer Resorptionshemmung in der Henleschen Schleife. Pflügers Arch. **330**, 290–301 (1971)

SUTHERLAND, L. E.: A fluorescent antibody study of juxtaglomerular cells using the freeze-substitution technique. Nephron **7**, 512–523 (1970)

SWALES, J. D., THURSTONE, H.: Generation of angiotensin II at peripheral vascular level: studies using angiotensin II antisera. Clin. Sci. **45**, 691–700 (1973)

SWEET, C. S., FERRARIO, C. M., KHOSLA, M. C., BUMPUS, F. M.: Antagonism of peripheral and central effects of angiotensin II by (1-sarcosine, 8-isoleucine) angiotensin II. J. Pharmacol. Exp. Ther. **185**, 35–41 (1973)

SWEET, C. S., FERRARIO, C. M., KOSOGLOV, A., BUMPUS, F. M.: Cardiovascular evaluation of (1-sarcosine-8-isoleucine) angiotensin II and its effects on blood pressure of conscious renal hypertensive dogs. Rec. Adv. Physiol. Pharmacol. (1974) 257–267

THURAU, K.: Intrarenal actions of angiotensin. In: Angiotensin (eds. I. H. PAGE and F. M. BUMPUS), pp. 475–489. Berlin-Heidelberg-New York: Springer 1974

THURAU, K., DAHLHEIM, H., GRÜNER, A., MASON, J.: Activation of renin in the single juxtaglomerular apparatus by sodium chloride in the tubular fluid at the macula densa. Circulat. Res. **30/31**, Suppl. II, 182–186 (1972)

THURAU, K., DEETJEN, P.: Die Diurese bei arteriellen Drucksteigerungen. Bedeutung der Hämodynamik des Nierenmarkes für die Harnkonzentrierung. Pflügers Arch. **274**, 567–580 (1962)

THURAU, K., SCHNERMANN, J.: Die Natriumkonzentration an den Macula-densa-Zellen als regulierender Faktor für das Glomerulumfiltrat (Mikropunktionsuntersuchungen). Klin. Wschr. **43**, 410–413 (1965)

THURSTON, H., SWALES, J. D.: Action of angiotensin antagonists and antiserum upon the pressor response to renin: Further evidence for the local generation of angiotensin II. Clin. Sci. **46**, 273–276 (1974)

TIGERSTEDT, R., BERGMAN, P. G.: Niere und Kreislauf. Scand. Arch. Physiol. **8**, 223–271 (1898)

TOBIAN, L.: Interrelationship of electrolytes, juxtaglomerular cells, and hypertension. Physiol. Rev. **40**, 280–312 (1960)

TOBIAN, L., COFFEE, K., McCREA, P.: Contrasting exchangeable sodium in rats with different types of Goldblatt hypertension. Amer. J. Physiol. **217**, 458–460 (1969)

TÜRKER, R. K., HALL, M. M., YAMAMOTO, M., SWEET, C. S., BUMPUS, F. M.: A new, long-lasting competitive inhibitor of angiotensin. Science **177**, 1203–1205 (1972)

VANDER, A. J.: Control of renin release. Physiol. Rev. **47**, 359–382 (1967)

WAKERLIN, G. E., JOHNSON, C. A.: Reductions in blood pressure of renal hypertensive dogs by hog renin. Proc. Soc. Exp. Biol. (N.Y.) **46**, 104–108 (1941)

WALKER, W. G., RUIZ-MAZA, F., HORVAT, J. S.: Demonstration of free (unbound) angiotensin II in immunized rabbits (abstr.). Proc. 5th Int. Congr. Nephrol., p. 115

WEISER, R. A., JOHNSON, A. G., HOOBLER, S. W.: The effect of antirenin on the blood pressure of the rat with experimental renal hypertension. Lab. Invest. **20**, 326–331 (1969)

WERLE, E., BAUMEISTER, K., SCHMAL, A.: On the renin-like enzyme in the submaxillary gland of the white mouse. Naunyn-Schmiedeberg's Arch. Exp. Path. Pharmak. **244**, 21–30 (1962)

WERLE, E., TRAUTSCHOLD, I., KRAMMER, K., SCHMAL, A.: Anreicherung und Immunspezifität des Isorenins der Glandula submaxillaris der Maus. Hoppe-Seylers Z. Physiol. Chem. **349**, 1441–1448 (1968)

Wilson, C., Byrom, F. B.: Renal changes in malignant hypertension. Experimental evidence. Lancet 1939 I, 136–139

Wilson, C., Byrom, F. B.: The vicious circle in chronic Bright's disease. Experimental evidence from the hypertensive rat. Quart. J. Med. 10, 65–93 (1941)

Wilson, C., Ledingham, J. M., Floyer, M. A.: Experimental renal and renoprival hypertension. In: The Kidney (eds. Ch. Rouiller and A. F. Muller), pp. 155–247. New York-London: Acad. Press 1971

Worcel, M., Meyer, P., d'Auriac, G. A., Milliez, P.: Role of angiotensin in normal blood pressure regulation. Pflügers Arch. 310, 251–263 (1969)

Yamamoto, M., Türker, R. K., Khairallah, P. A., Bumpus, F. M.: A potent competitive antagonist of angiotensin II. Europ. J. Pharmacol. 18, 316–322 (1972)

Ziegler, M., Janzik, W.: Renin-Angiotensin-System und intrarenaler Gefäßwiderstand. Urologe 7, 115–118 (1968)

Ziegler, M., Riniker, B., Gross, F.: Nature of the pressor substance in rabbit placenta. Biochem. J. 102, 28–32 (1967)

Medizinische Universitäts-Poliklinik Münster

New Clinical Syndromes
under Regular Intermittent Hemodialysis

H. Loew, A. Samizadeh and E. Heilmann

With 12 Figures

Contents

1.   Introduction (H. Loew) 239
2.   Cardiovascular System (H. Loew) 240
3.   Carbohydrate and Fat Metabolism (H. Loew) 243
4.   Polyneuropathy (H. Loew) 245
5.   Gonadal Dysfunction (H. Loew) 246
6.   Bone Disease (A. Samizadeh) 246
6.1.   Pathogenesis 247
6.1.1. Renal Acidosis 247
6.1.2. Hyperphosphatemia 247
6.1.3. Vitamin D$_3$ Metabolism 248
6.1.4. Parathyroid Hormone 250
6.2.   Bone Disease Under Chronic Hemodialysis Treatment 252
6.3.   The Influence of Dialysis Treatment Itself on Renal Bone Disease 252
6.4.   The Clinical Syndrome of Renal Bone Disease 253
6.5.   Roentgenological Appearance of Renal Bone Disease 253
6.6.   Other Diagnostic Procedures 253
6.7.   Therapy of Renal Bone Disease 254
7.   Anemia (E. Heilmann) 256
7.1.   Introduction 256
7.2.   Pathogenesis 256
7.3.   Treatment 262
7.4.   Summary 264
References 265

1. Introduction

H. Loew

Until about 1960, patients with progressive renal failure inevitably died from uremia. Therapy was symptomatic only and prolongation of life to any significant degree was not possible. Within the past 15 years many thousands of patients have survived end-stage renal failure by intermittent hemodialysis treatment.

This form of treatment consists of the transfer of solutes of the blood up to a molecular weight of about 2000 through a cellophane membrane into a rinsing fluid composed of water to which sodium, calcium, potassium, and a bicarbonate buffer have been added. The patient undergoes this treatment 3 times a week for 5 to 10 hours each time. His blood is pumped at a rate of 150 to 250 ml/min through the dialyser. A subcutaneous fistula between the radial artery and a superficial vein of the forearm is usually used as a permanent blood access to allow these flow rates. The arterialised vein becomes distended and can be punctured with needles of adequate size three times a week for many years. During the treatment the patient receives heparin to prevent his blood from clotting in the dialyser. In this way the accummulation of water and certain metabolic waste products can be kept at a tolerable level, permitting a life free of uremic complaints.

In Europe, about 40 patients per million enter the state of terminal renal insufficiency each year and need regular hemodialysis treatment or renal transplantation. In Europe today, about 60 patients per million are already under chronic hemodialysis treatment; and until 1978, there will be more than 120 patients per million surviving under regular hemodialysis or after having had renal transplantation. The 6-year survival under regular dialysis treatment in Europe so far is 70% [17]. Many patients will survive more than 10 years [25]. The main causes of death in this patient group are vascular problems (52%) and infections (15%) [17]. At the present time, severe atherosclerosis after prolonged maintenance hemodialysis seems to be the most important limiting factor of this treatment [25].

Since patients with severe renal failure or without kidneys can survive for many years with the artificial kidney, the pathophysiology of the syndrome of chronic uremia has become of much more practical interest than formerly, when all patients with progressive renal failure died. Since the artificial kidney is a relatively poor prothesis for the real organ, not all symptoms of chronic uremia can be alleviated. Anemia, secondary hyperparathyroidism, cardiovascular alterations, polyneuropathy, and hyperlipemia are the main problems of patients undergoing regular hemodialysis treatment. Beside these, patients may show a pathologic blood coagulability, disturbances of certain endocrine functions—most importantly a lowered secretion of sexual hormone, pathologic glucose utilization, and changes of the skin. Probably no organ system is without alteration during long-term hemodialysis treatment. As renal anemia and the altered calcium and phosphorous metabolism, including bone disease of chronic uremia, have been studied extensively in the past, these conditions will be discussed in two separate chapters. In the following, some aspects of the alteration of the cardiovascular system, of polyneuropathy, the impaired sexual function, and the hyperlipemia of patients under chronic hemodialysis treatment will be summarized.

2. Cardiovascular System

H. Loew

Hypertension is a main cause of complications during chronic renal failure and regular hemodialysis. As a rule, hemodialysis treatment allows normalization of the blood pressure either by itself or with tolerable amounts of anti-hypertensive drugs [12]. According to current thought, the diseased kidney causes hypertension by activation of the renin angiotensin system and retention of sodium and water primarily in the late stages of renal insufficiency [16].

The role of plasma renin in hypertension of patients receiving maintenance hemodialysis is not well-understood .While patients with normal blood pressure under dialysis treatment tend to have normal plasma renin levels, those who remain hypertensive in spite of intensive dialysis treatment often have elevated renin levels. On the other hand, plasma renin activities do not correlate with the blood pressure. Good correlations were found between plasma renin activity and plasma sodium concentration and dietary sodium intake [13]. Bilateral nephrectomy usually leads to better control of severe hypertension under dialysis treatment [31]. Patients with resistent hypertension and high plasma renin activity seem to respond better to nephrectomy than those hypertensives with normal or low renin levels [37]. However, high levels of plasma renin concentration do not exclude a good response of hypertension to hemodialysis treatment alone [13]. The blood pressure of anephric patients is usually very sensitive to hydration. Overhydration causes a rise in blood pressure, increase of the cardiac output and an elevation of the peripheral resistance [11].

Bilateral nephrectomy for arterial hypertension should only be performed in cases of malignant hypertension when all other measures, such as intensive dialysis treatment with adequate water and salt restriction, have failed to control the blood pressure. The patient definitely benefits even from poorly functioning kidneys. Nephrectomy always leads to a decrease of the hematocrit, and the solute excretion by the kidney even at a glomerular filtration rate of as little as 1 ml/min seems to be beneficial for the patient. Polyneuropathy, for instance, is seen more frequently in anephric patients than in those with some residual renal excretory function.

Before chronic hemodialysis offered a life prolonging treatment to patients with endstage renal failure, little attention was paid to the hypertension during chronic renal insufficiency. It was even thought that elevation of the blood pressure might be an important compensatory mechanism raising the perfusion of the diseased kidney. Today long-standing untreated hypertension during the period of chronic renal failure has become an important factor worsening the prognosis during maintenance hemodialysis. As can be expected, the cardiac size of hemodialysis patients correlates with the degree and duration of hypertension [8]. We correspondingly found a correlation between the degree of change in the EKG and the level of blood pressure elevation, as in cases of hypertensives without kidney disease (Fig. 1).

In addition to hypertension, anemia, the increased volume load carried by the arteriovenous fistula, intermittent overhydration, and occasionally pericarditis and cardiomyopathy affect the heart during regular hemodialysis. The shunt flow of the subcutaneous arteriovenous fistula, which is usually used today as a regular blood access for maintenance hemodialysis treatment

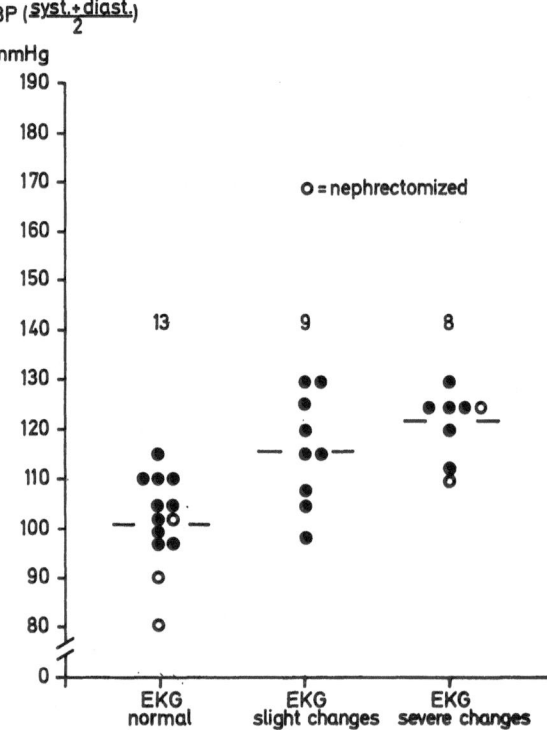

Fig. 1 Blood pressure and EKG findings of 30 patients under regular hemodialysis
treatment

can be considerable. Various authors have measured flow rates from as little
as 150 ml/min up to more than 2 liters/min depending on the type and site
of the fistula, on the examination techniques applied, and on the group of
patients studied [1, 24, 34]. The flow rate of the fistula also depends on the
cardiac output and amounts up to more than 20% thereof [24, 34]. The flow
rate also depends on the blood pressure [2].

Generally the uremic patient without cardiac failure seems to have an
elevated cardiac output even before an arteriovenous fistula for hemodialysis
treatment has been created [29]. Dialysis patients were found to have a
significantly elevated resting cardiac output. SILL found in a group of 7 patients
on chronic hemodialysis with hematocrits between 20 and 24 a resting cardiac
output of 14.9 l/min as compared to only 6.3 l/min in a normal control
group. After closure of the fistula for 15 minutes, the cardiac output decreased
to 12.2 l/min. The high cardiac output in this group of patients was caused
by elevated stroke volume at normal pulse rates.

These figures, however, cannot be considered representative for the average
dialysis patient. Other researchers have found lower figures for the cardiac
output of hemodialysis patients [24].

The cardiac reserve of patients under chronic hemodialysis is reduced.
Patients with normal resting pulmonary artery pressure tend to develop patho-

logic pressure increase during low exercise [33]. In single cases the heart of the dialysis patient can also be affected by uremic pericarditis and cardio-myopathy [7]. Pericardial effusion, which is seen fairly frequently in patients under long term hemodialysis, does not, in our experience, seem to alter the patient's condition greatly although it is found mostly in patients not doing well under the dialysis treatment in other respects. Pericardiac effusion, how-ever, might become a sudden problem when, in rare instances during hemo-dialysis, the patient's blood is heparinised and he develops a hemorrhagic effusion which can cause a cardiac tamponade [28].

3. Carbohydrate and Fat Metabolism

H. LOEW

Chronic uremia accompanies carbohydrate intolerance, as has been known for many years. However, diabetes mellitus does not occur as a result of chronic uremia. Different from juvenile diabetics, patients with uremia always have high basal serum insulin levels and respond on a subnormal level to parenterally administered insulin. This indicates a resistence of the peripheral tissue to insulin under uremia, which delays glucose assimilation [5, 6, 18, 20, 27]. Intensive hemodialysis reduces carbohydrate intolerance, which led to the assumption that some uremic toxin causes insulin resistence in uremia [20].

From the clinical point of view, a more serious problem is hyperlipemia in chronic uremic patients, since this seems to be the main factor contributing to accelerated atherosclerosis seen in patients after several years of regular hemodialysis.

We observed that 31 of 46 patients under chronic hemodialysis had hyper-triglyceridemia ranging from upper normal limit of 175 mg% to more than 500 mg%. Cholesterol levels were normal in two-thirds of the patients and only slightly elevated in the others (Fig. 2).

We also found that the frequency of hypertriglyceridemia increases as renal function deteriorates and is highest in the terminal stage of chronic uremia when regular hemodialysis is indicated. In our patient group there was no correlation of triglyceride blood levels to age and body weight. The most significant observation was that the blood pressure of our patients correlated well with the triglyceride levels (Fig. 3).

A six-month course of regular hemodialysis did not seem to affect tri-glyceride blood levels. Patients who had hypertriglyceridemia before dialysis treatment had a constant hyperlipemia under chronic dialysis treatment but none who had normal blood levels at the beginning developed hypertri-glyceridemia during a 6-month period of dialysis treatment.

Chronically uremic patients with hypertriglyceridemia resemble patients with Type IV hyperlipemia in many respects. In both frequently occur glucose intolerance, hyperuricemia, elevated basal insulin levels, and a tendency toward accelerated atherogenesis. But other than those in Type IV hyperlipemia,

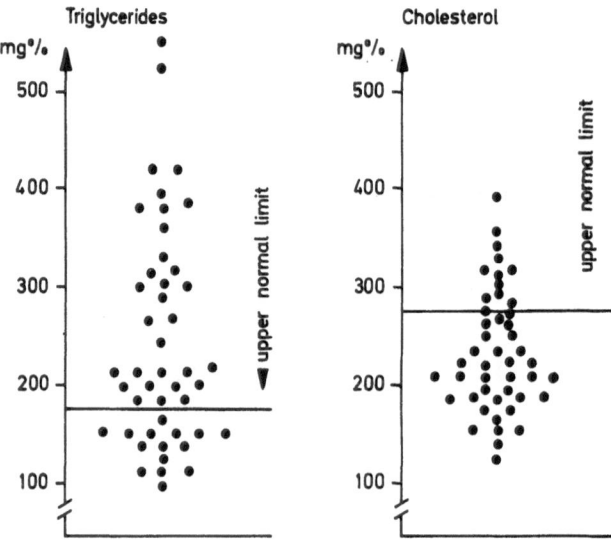

Fig. 2. Triglyceride and cholesterol blood levels of 46 patients under regular hemodialysis treatment

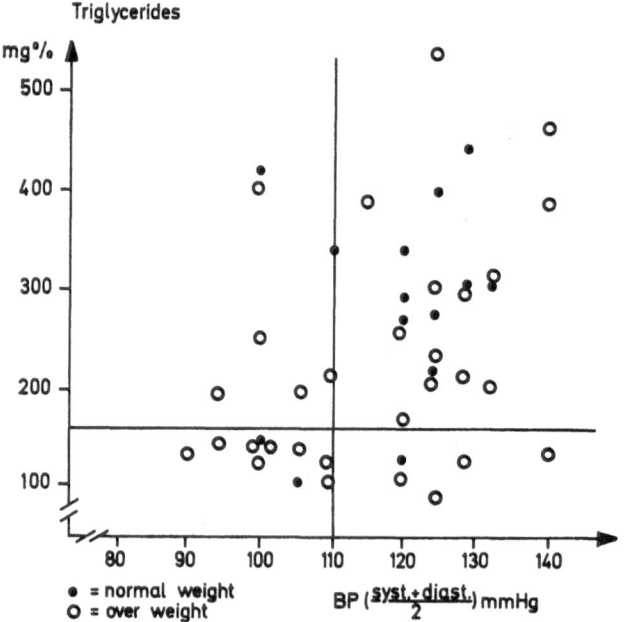

Fig. 3. Triglyceride blood levels and blood pressure of 44 patients under regular hemodialysis treatment

chronically uremic patients are not obese and do not show elevation of plasma triglyceride levels in response to a fat-free, high-carbohydrate diet.

The pathomechanisms of hyperlipemia in uremia are unknown. The main abnormality in uremic patients is an elevation of the very-low-density lipoprotein. This is obviously synthetized in the liver in excess, which could be the result of the accumulation of certain aminoacids in uremia. Also, the elevated serum insulin levels may have some influence on the production of lipoproteins in the liver, as insulin promotes aminoacids entry into cells. A third mechanism resulting in elevated serum triglyceride levels could be the reduced clearance of triglycerides from the serum by the peripheral tissue. The fact that the post-heparin lipolytic activity in patients under chronic dialysis is reduced favors this view. Triglyceride clearance from the serum is induced by the enzyme lipoprotein lipase which can normally be stimulated by the administration of heparin. In contrast to patients with Type I hyperlipemia, which is induced by a hereditary lack of lipoprotein lipase, chylomicronemia is absent in uremic patients. This in turn could mean that there is not a general lack of lipoprotein lipase in uremics but mainly a resistence of tissue to heparin. An excellent survey of the present knowledge of the disorders of carbohydrate and lipid metabolism in uremia is given by BAG-DADE [4].

At the present it is not clear how to manage hyperlipemia during chronic intermittent hemodialysis.

4. Polyneuropathy

H. LOEW

Peripheral neuropathy is a typical complication of chronic uremia; it may lead to severe paralysis and muscle wasting of the extremities in those patients who survive endstage renal failure on intermittent dialysis treatment [3, 21, 23, 24, 32]. Primarily affected are the sensory and motor neurons of the peripheral nerves of the lower extremities.

The patient exhibits the "restless leg" syndrome, burning of the skin, paraesthesias, and muscle weakness. The histopathology of the nerve shows segmental demyelinisation and, in severe cases, axon degeneration [2, 21]. Also, the cochleo-vestibular nerve can be involved, and the patient may develop vertigo or loss of hearing [39]. There is no doubt that neuropathy is caused by some uremic toxin not yet identified. Since most patients today are dialysed 3 times a week for a total of 24 to 30 hours, neuropathy has become a relatively rare event when compared to the early period of regular hemodialysis, when dialysis treatment was given only twice weekly. DOBBEL-STEIN [14] found that the frequency of neuropathy among 900 German dialysis patients correlated inversely with the dialysis time per week.

Uremic polyneuropathy can be detected before the patient has any complaints by determination of the motor nerve conduction time or the vibratory sensitivity [19, 21]. If uremic polyneuropathy does not respond to intensive dialysis treatment, renal transplantation will usually reverse this condition. Beside the peripheral neuropathy, there seems to exist a specific uremic myopathy [15, 26]. Cerebral dysfunctions with loss of consciousness or seizures are a rare complication during regular dialysis, and are primarily caused by rapid changes of extracellular water and electrolyte composition. Slight changes of the EEG during dialysis treatment, however, can be observed frequently [22, 40, 41].

5. Gonadal Dysfunction

H. Loew

Patients under chronic hemodialysis treatment are infertile as a rule. Only in rare instances have male dialysis patients fathered children and female patients given birth to children [10].

An andrologic examination of 10 of our hemodialysis patients revealed in all of them an azoospermia or oligospermia. Basal plasma testosterone levels in 24 of our male dialysis patients were significantly lowered (Fig. 4). The testosterone production of the dialysis patients did not respond to human chorionic gonadotropin, and basal luteotropic hormone levels were slightly elevated [38].

Hypogonadism in chronic uremia therefore seems to be a primary testicular insufficiency. Biopsies of the testicle of chronic uremic patients have been done only rarely. Bundschu [9] found interstitial calcium phosphate deposits in a few cases of testicular biopsies. The patients rarely complain of being infertile. Their major problem is impotence, which depends on other factors beside hypogonadism.

6. Bone Disease

A. Samizadeh

Uremic bone disease had not been a problem of great clinical significance until patients with terminal renal failure received a chance to survive for many years by means of intermittent chronic dialysis treatment. Patients under long-term chronic hemodialysis treatment may develop advanced renal osteodystrophy and suffer from pathological bone fractures, especially of the vertebrae.

Today, renal bone disease has become one of the most intensively studied complications of chronic uremia and has stimulated the investigation of the action of vitamin D and parathyroid hormone on calcium metabolism. Multiple factors have been found to be causes of bone disease as a consequence of chronic uremia. The most important ones under discussion at present are secondary hyperparathyroidism [59, 120] and abnormalities in vitamin D metabolism [3, 120].

Stanbury [123] proposed already in 1962 a classification of renal bone disease in azotemic osteomalacia and azotemic hyperparathyroidism. Garner and Ball [43] again in 1966 and Binswanger *et al.* in 1971 [12] reported on osteomalacia as a consequence of chronic renal failure. A combination of disturbed bone mineralization and hyperparathyroidism was found in patients with chronic renal failure by Jowsey *et al.* [68], Hitt *et al.* [62], Krempien

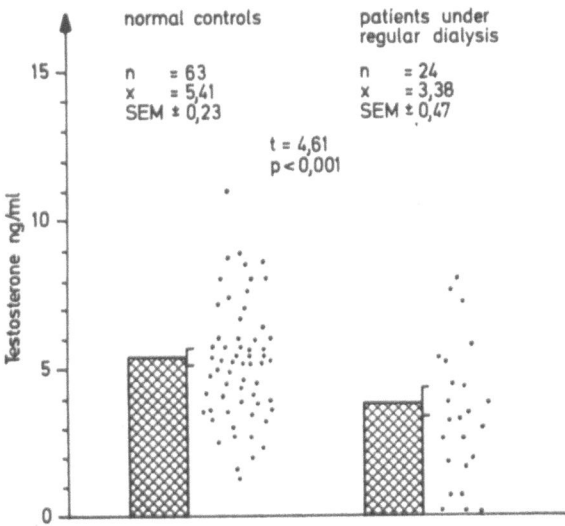

Fig. 4. Basal plasma testosterone levels of healthy males (age: 20–60 years) and male patients under regular hemodialysis treatment

et al. [76] and DUURSMA *et al.* [35]. Osteoporosis and osteosclerosis have also been observed [25].

6.1. Pathogenesis
6.1.1. Renal Acidosis

The early concept of ALBRIGHT that the metabolic acidosis of patients with chronic renal failure was the main cause of renal bone disease [1] could not be confirmed by many other investigators [7, 21, 83, 108, 111].

6.1.2. Hyperphosphatemia

Phosphate in vivo as well as in vitro stimulates bone formation, diminishes bone resorption and reduces the sensitivity of bone for parathyroid hormone [103]. The phosphate retention in renal failure was thought by some investigators to be the key disturbance leading to uremic bone disease. BRICKER [16, 125] postulates that very early in chronic renal failure when the first nephrons are destroyed and glomerular filtration rate diminishes, phosphate secretion is also reduced. Consequently, the serum phosphate concentration tends to rise which in turn causes a fall in ionised serum calcium concentration leading to an increase in parathyroid hormone secretion. The increased parathyroid hormone activity reduces tubular phosphate resorption and compensates for the reduction in glomerular phosphate filtration keeping the serum phosphate level constant until renal function deteriorates further. On the contrary, hypocalcemia sometimes can be observed in early renal failure before hyperphosphatemia develops [38, 39]. The thesis of BRICKER cannot explain many observations in renal failure; for instance, disturbance of bone mineralization and the reduction of intestinal calcium absorption which can be observed in experimental renal failure a few hours after reduction of renal function.

6.1.3. Vitamin D_3 Metabolism

These observations made it likely that vitamin D plays a role in renal bone disease. Renal osteomalacia cannot be morphologically separated from classical osteomalacia, due to lack of vitamin D, and can be detected early in the course of chronic renal failure before the development of azotemia. It seems to be unrelated to the level of the serum calcium concentration and the calcium-phosphate product in the blood. It is caused by a blocked mineralization of the osteoid which is resistant to physiologic doses of vitamin D [72, 84, 85, 100, 116]. The vitamin D serum level is normal in uremic individuals [13, 98]. The degree of osteomalacia correlates with the duration of chronic renal failure. LIU and CHU [84] were the first to show that the abnormalities of calcium metabolism in uremia can be corrected by high doses of vitamin D. This was confirmed later on by several other investigators [19, 115, 117]. HESCH et al. found the intestinal calcium absorption to be diminished at an early stage of renal failure when serum phosphate levels were still normal [59, 60]. There was no correlation seen between serum creatinine concentration and the degree of decrease in calcium absorption. An understanding of the complex role of vitamin D in renal bone disease began when radioactive vitamin D was synthesised. DE LUCA, AVIOLI et al. [4, 5, 6, 28, 30] could demonstrate for the first time multiple metabolites of vitamin D in men by the use of $1,2\text{-}{}^3H$ vitamin D_3. BLUNT and his group were able to isolate the first biologically potent metabolite of vitamin D_3 and identified it as 25-hydroxycholecalciferol [13]. This metabolite is the circulating form of vitamin D_3 and stimulates intestinal calcium resorption and the mobilization of calcium from bone [8, 23, 24, 53, 63, 101, 116]. The 25-hydroxycholecalciferol seems to be formed mainly in the liver [98, 99] although the kidney is able to form this metabolite of vitamin D_3 [52, 53] as well.

During the following period of intensive investigation of vitamin D metabolism, other metabolites were found which were even more potent than 25-hydroxycholecalciferol. FASER and KODICEK [36, 73] in 1970 and, at the same time, LAWSON et al. [81] found 1,25-dihydroxycholecalciferol to be a very potent metabolite of vitamin D_3. It was found in the kidneys of chicken and derives mainly from mitochondria of the renal cortex [73]. The kidney therefore can be considered an endocrine organ which forms and secretes 1,25-hydroxycholecalciferol [29, 45, 46, 73, 90]—the biologically active form of vitamin D, especially for the mucosa of the gut [14, 15, 40, 41, 64, 65, 91, 129]. This metabolite also plays a role in the calcium mobilization from the bone, as it is highly concentrated in the nucleus of bone cells [54, 104, 114].

The formation of 1,25-dihydroxycholecalciferol correlates with the serum level of parathyroid hormone. A decrease of serum calcium concentration is

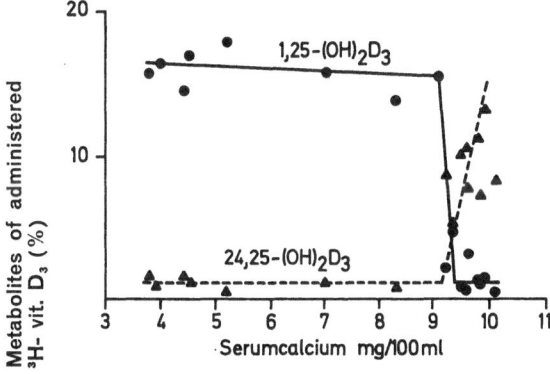

Fig. 5. Relationship between serum calcium level and vitamin D₃-metabolites 1,25-dihydr-oxycholecalciferol and 24,25-dihydroxycholecalciferol (DE LUCA *et al.* [13])

followed by an increased secretion of parathyroid hormone, which in turn causes an increased gastrointestinal calcium resorption induced by an increased rate of 1,25-dihydroxycholecalciferol formation. The rate of formation of 1,25-dihydroxycholecalciferol is reduced at elevated serum calcium levels [31].

The amount of calcium in the diet also seems to play a role in the regulation of 1,25-dihydroxycholecalciferol formation. DE LUCA *et al.* [31] found that a low-calcium diet increases the rate of intestinal calcium resorption, and that diet rich in calcium causes a reduction of enteral calcium resorption.

At the same time the formation of 1,25-dihydroxycholecalciferol is increased or decreased. During reduction of 1,25-dihydroxycholecalciferol formation, 24,25-dihydroxycholecalciferol is produced at an increased rate. The biological activity of the latter metabolite has not yet been clarified [15, 31, 92] (Fig. 5).

The regulation of 1,25-dihydroxycholecalciferol formation is closely related to the parathyroid gland [42, 106]. In the experimental animal, the 1,25-dihydroxycholecalciferol formation ceases within 48 hours after parathyroidectomy even when the animal is fed a low-calcium diet [42] (Fig. 6). At the same time the production of 24,25-dihydroxycholecalciferol increases. The application of parathyroid hormone promptly stimulates 1,25-dihydroxycholecalciferol in these animals. Thus, the parathyroid hormone can be considered a tropic hormone for the 1,25-dihydroxycholecalciferol formation [26, 29].

The serum phosphate level also plays an important role in the regulation of 1,25-dihydroxycholecalciferol formation. Hypophosphatemia in some way independently of parathyroid hormone stimulates the formation of this metabolite. The ability to form 1,25-dihydroxycholecalciferol correlates with the concentration of anorganic phosphate in the renal cortex. A low concentration of anorganic phosphates in the kidneys stimulates 1,25-dihydroxycholecalciferol formation, whereas high phosphate concentration seems to stimulate the formation of 24,25-dihydroxycholecalciferol [31] (Fig. 7).

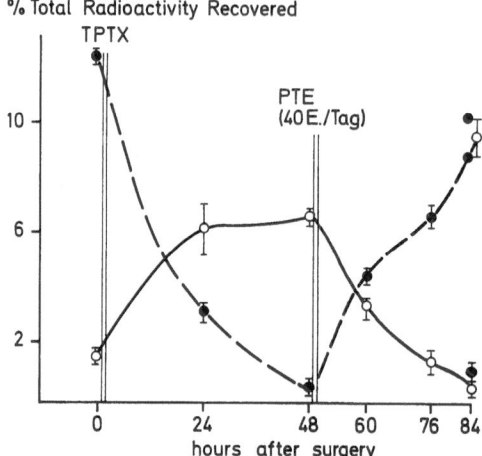

Fig. 6. Effect of thyroparathyroidectomy (TPTX) and therapy with parathyroid extract (PTE) on the rate of production of 1,25-dihydroxycholecalciferol (---) and 24,25-dihydroxycholecalciferol (—) in rats. TPTX results in a rapid fall of the serum concentration of 1,25-dihydroxycholecalciferol while the concentration of 24,25-dihydroxycholecalciferol rises. This effect can be reversed by the administration of PTE

Whether or not the mineral content of bone itself has some influence on the regulation of intestinal calcium absorption and 1,25-dihydroxycholecalciferol formation is still an open question [114].

The intestinal calcium resorption depends on a carrier, the calcium binding protein, which is built by the mucosa of the ileum under the influence of 1,25-dihydroxycholecalciferol and a calcium dependent ATP-ase [22, 33, 75, 87, 93, 97, 127, 128, 130, 134, 135, 136]. All these findings show that vitamin D metabolism is regulated by a complex mechanism in which the amount of ionized calcium in the extracellular fluid, the phosphate concentration in the renal cortex, and the parathyroid hormone play important roles. Due to the key position of the kidneys in vitamin D_3 metabolism no 1,25-dihydroxycholecalciferol can be detected in the serum after bilateral nephrectomy [88, 89]. Also, individuals with far-advanced renal failure show a significantly reduced transformation of 25-hydroxycholecalciferol into 1,25-dihydroxycholecalciferol [51]. Some formation of 1,25-dihydroxycholecalciferol has been found down to a glomerular filtration rate of about 3 ml/min [58, 114, 116]. There also exists a resistance of the tissues against 1,25-dihydroxycholecalciferol in chronic uremic patients [61]. Uremia by itself seems to cause a disturbance of intestinal calcium absorption [108, 114, 115].

6.1.4. Parathyroid Hormone

The serum parathyroid hormone level is already elevated when renal function is impaired only slightly. The parathyroid hormone level in chronic renal disease is higher on the average than in primary hyperparathyroidism

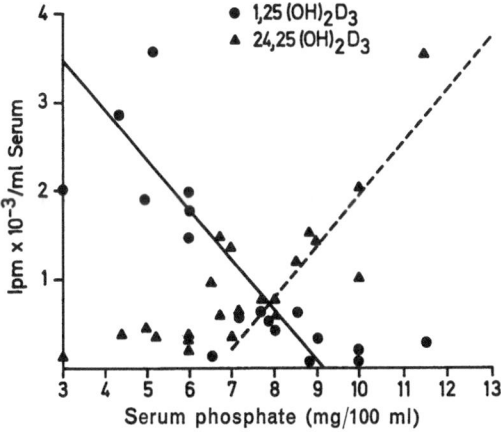

Fig. 7. Relationship between serum phosphorus level and the serum concentration of vitamin D_3-metabolites 1,25 - and 24,25-dihydroxycholecalciferol (DeLuca *et al.* [31])

[11, 26, 100, 107]. In the earlier stages of chronic renal failure there is a correlation between serum parathyroid hormone concentration and the serum creatinine concentration [37, 107]. No close correlation could be found between serum parathyroid hormone level and the degree of bone disease in patients with chronic renal disease [54].

The increased parathyroid hormone production accompanies hyperplasia of the parathyroid gland [112]. Parathyroid hormone synthesis and secretion is controlled by the level of the ionized serum calcium [120]. This is true also of uremic patients. To a small degree parathyroid hormone synthesis and secretion also depend on magnesium concentration in the serum. Raisz *et al.* [104] were able to show that hyperphosphatemia does not, as has been postulated, stimulate the secretion of parathyroid hormone since hyperphosphatemia lowers the serum calcium level [111]. Many patients with chronic renal insufficiency seem to be resistant to parathyroid hormone [123]. This resistance to parathyroid hormone in uremia probably is due to the lack of biological active metabolites of vitamin D_3, as has been described before [105]. Parathyroid hormone can affect the bone only in the presence of normal vitamin D activity. This probably explains why in uremic patients, in spite of the very high parathyroid hormone levels, the serum calcium level remains low and cannot be elevated by mobilization of calcium from the bone, the so-called "hypocalcemic hyperparathyroidism" [124].

From all these details the fact emerges that reduced formation of 1,25-dihydroxycholecalciferol is the basic disturbance in the pathogenesis of renal bone disease. The reduction of formation of this vitamin D metabolite is not only due to a loss of renal parenchyma but is also caused by an inhibited synthesis due to hyperphosphatemia early in renal failure. Because of the lack of 1,25-dihydroxycholecalciferol, intestinal calcium resorption and calcium mobilization from the bone are reduced, and the ability of parathyroid hormone to elevate the serum calcium level is impaired.

6.2. Bone Disease Under Chronic Hemodialysis Treatment

The frequency of bone disease among patients under chronic hemodialysis seems to depend mainly upon the skill of the physician in checking patients for symptoms of this complication. As a rule uremic bone disease is not completely corrected by regular hemodialysis treatment. Ritz et al. [111] studied 300 hemodialysis patients and found in 47% symptoms of a pathologic calcium metabolism. The degree of bone disease correlated to the duration of dialysis treatment. In an early observation by Drukker [34], 30% of chronic uremic patients show a decrease of bone disease under chronic dialysis treatment, in 33% symptoms remained unchanged and in 37% bone disease was progressive. Experimental data make it unlikely that hemodialysis treatment can change the disturbance of the vitamin D function on the tissues [121]. But it could be expected that along with the reduction of the serum phosphate level the resistence of bone against parathyroid hormone is reduced and that the elevation of the serum calcium level reduces parathyroid hormone secretion [111].

6.3. The Influence of Dialysis Treatment Itself on Renal Bone Disease

If the water used for the dialysis fluid is softened only and not completely demineralized, the possibility for fluorine intoxication exists [109]. Some investigators found high fluorine concentrations in the bone of dialysis patients. It has also been discussed whether the chronic use of aluminium hydroxide, which is taken by all patients under chronic dialysis to minimize phosphate resorption from the intestine, leads to an accummulation of this metal in the bone [109].

Heparin, which is used during each hemodialysis treatment, causes a mobilization of calcium and phosphate, and increases the calcium-phosphate product in the serum [74].

The role of magnesium in the pathogenesis of renal bone disease is not precisely known. If magnesium, as postulated by some authors, suppresses parathyroid hormone secretion, the magnesium level in the dialysis fluid used at the present should be raised [18].

The level of calcium concentration in the dialysis fluid is an important factor. It should be high enough to allow the serum calcium level of the patient to become normal. It should also be high enough to stop negative calcium balance in chronic uremic patients. If too high, on the other hand, it causes hypercalcemia and tissue calcification [9, 10, 17, 44, 56, 79, 102]. The highest serum dialysate concentration of 4 mval/l is proposed by a group of the Mayo Clinic who observed a normalization of the parathyroid hormone level and a reduction of the serum phosphate level in patients under regulaɪ dialysis with high dialysate calcium concentration [111].

The remarkably elevated serum phosphate level in dialysis patients is not only due to reduced renal elimination but also to the reduced formation of energy-rich phosphate compositions resulting from toxic disturbance of the metabolism [55]. Phosphate elimination through hemodialysis and reduced resorption resulting from the use of oral aluminium hydroxide lead to a negative phosphate balance, which decreases the resistence of bone to parathyroid hormone and reduces the chance of tissue calcification.

6.4. The Clinical Syndrome of Renal Bone Disease

The patient suffers from bone pain, especially in the pelvic area and the heels, if he has any complaints related to renal bone disease at all. Periarticular deposits of hydroxylapatite can cause sudden joint pain, especially in the hands, the elbows, and the shoulders (Fig. 8). This occurs when the calcium phosphate product is significantly elevated. Calcium hydroxylapatite can be deposited in the human tissues only when the calcium phosphate product in the serum supercedes an upper normal limit of 40. Uremic patients tolerate a calcium phosphate product up to 75 [122]. This is probably due to renal acidosis. This arthritis—resembling clinically acute gouty arthritis—is caused by the deposition of calcium phosphate microcrystals in the synovial fluid and the periarticular tissue. Calcium phosphate deposition in the conjunctivae causes the so-called "red-eye" syndrome. Beside these massive calcium phosphate depositions, metastatic calcifications are also found in other tissues, extracellular (especially along the basement membrane) and intracellular, extra- and intramitochondrial [109]. A well-known phenomenon in dialysis patients is a homogenous calcification of the vessels. Different from artherosclerosis, the calcification of the vessels seen in dialysis patients begins in the peripheral vessels of the fingers and toes independent of blood pressure and calcium phosphate product in the serum. Histologically, these calcifications are found primarily in the media of the vessel wall [79, 82, 95, 96].

6.5. Roentgenological Appearence of Renal Bone Disease

In the early stage of renal insufficiency, x-ray examination of the hands shows a longitudinal separation of the cortical bone of the phalanges, the skull shows multiple small holes of osteolysis which, on the roentgenogram, gives the appearance of the so-called "pepper and salt" skull. A typical finding is the acroosteolysis of the lateral end of the clavicle. The finger bones characteristically show resorption of the subperiosteal bone, mainly along the radial side of the middle phalanx of the second finger (Fig. 8). Relatively rarely, the spine shows osteosclerosis of the upper and lower layer of the vertebrae, known by the roentgenologist as "rugger jersey" spine. LOOSER's zones as a specific finding related to osteomalacia are seen only rarely. The roentgenograms of the extremities characteristically show vessel calcification.

6.6. Other Diagnostic Procedures

Beside the roentgenological examination, the histologic examination of the bone is the most specific method to diagnose renal bone disease. JOWSEY

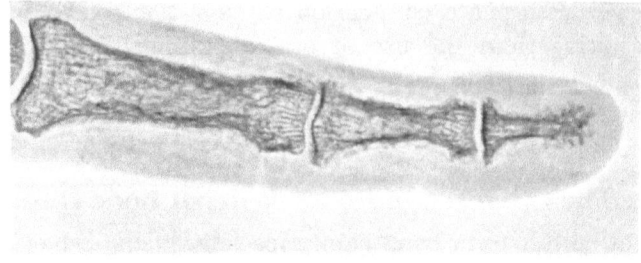

A

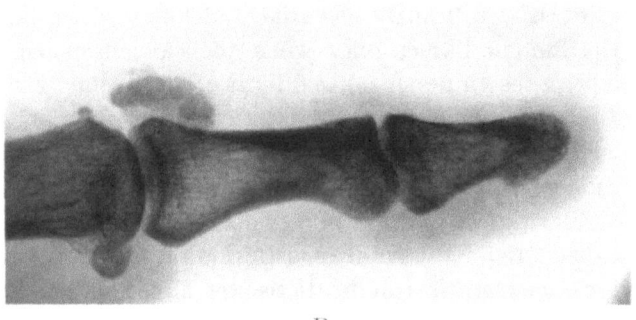

B

Fig. 8. A. Xeroradiogram of the index finger of a patient with renal bone disease showing severe osteoclasia, especially subperiosteal bone resorption, the typical appearance of the skeletal changes of hyperparathyroidism with kind permission of Dr. Peters, Radiologische Klinik, University of Münster. B. Radiogram of the thumb of a patient under regular hemodialysis treatment with metastatic periarticular calcification due to a high serum phosphate level

et al., Ingham *et al.*, Kuhlencordt *et al.*, Delling, Schultz *et al.* [27, 66, 67, 68, 76, 77, 118] have investigated the histologic appearance of renal bone disease and have proposed a histologic classification of renal bone disease.

Biochemical methods and the diagnosis of renal bone disease include the estimation of the parathyroid hormone with a radioimmuno assay and the estimation of intestinal calcium absorption [59, 60]. Routine procedures are the estimation of serum calcium phosphate and alkaline phosphatase levels. The alkaline phosphatase is elevated in renal bone disease as a result of increased osteoblastic activity.

6.7. Therapy of Renal Bone Disease

According to what is now known about the pathogenesis of renal bone disease, successful therapy must eliminate the vitamin D resistence and the stimulation of the parathyroid hormone. The effect of such therapy is best when started early in the course of renal disease [59, 115, 116).

All patients under chronic hemodialysis and with chronic renal failure before regular dialysis treatment should be given aluminium hydroxide orally which binds phosphate of the food resulting in a decreased serum phosphate level. This in turn causes a decrease of the parathyroid hormone level. An overdose of aluminium hydroxide can cause hypophosphatemia resulting in an undermineralisation of the bone similar to osteomalacia, and should therefore be avoided.

High doses of oral calcium gluconate (1.5 to 2 g per day) can compensate for the reduced calcium resorption rate of the intestine [20].

Fluorine has a positive effect on bone formation. This effect diminishes after several months [78]. Whether fluorine is also useful in renal bone disease has not yet been studied. Side effects of fluorine therapy are nausea, abdominal pain, joint pain—especially in the feet and knees—and transient osteomalacia.

It has been shown that in order to prevent calcium loss through dialysis a calcium concentration in the dialysis bath of 3 or more mval/l is necessary. The dialysate calcium concentration primarily used in Germany today is 3.5 mval/l. It has not yet been established whether this calcium concentration has a positive effect on renal bone disease.

Treatment of renal osteodystrophy with vitamin D_3 and vitamin D_3 metabolites (or analogues thereof) has not yet been established. High doses of vitamin D_3 can raise the intestinal calcium absorption in hemodialysis patients [57, 114]. The administration of vitamin D_3, however, can only be useful as long as sufficient amounts of 1,25-dihydroxycholecalciferol can be synthesized by the diseased kidneys. It has been shown that 25-hydroxycholecalciferol in high doses can be effective in the intestines and in bone without being transformed into 1,25-dihydroxycholecalciferol [31, 32, 132]. But uncertainty exists whether or not it also heals bone disease. As 25-hydroxycholecalciferol is less toxic than vitamin D_3, it seems to be advantageous to vitamin D_3 itself. The best results were obtained with 1,25-dihydroxycholecalciferol after it had been synthesized. In very small doses, it normalizes calcium absorption of the intestine. Vitamin D_3 analogues like 5,6-trans-cholecalciferol and 5,6-trans-25-hydroxycholecalciferol are under investigation, But their therapeutic value has not been established yet. The disadvantage of vitamin D_3 is the small range between therapeutic doses and toxic doses [80, 86, 94, 114]. Clinically, vitamin D intoxication is identical with the hypercalcemia syndrome. This consisty of renal, intestinal, cardial, neurological, and psychic symptoms [138]. In the future, it is likely that the less toxic vitamin D metabolites will be used exclusively in the treatment of renal osteodystrophy [2, 113].

A new possibility to treat renal bone disease has been introduced by Kaye et al. [69, 70, 71], Suda et al. [126], Harrison et al. [48, 49, 50], and Hallik et al. [47], who have used dihydrotachysterol and observed an improvement of the intestinal calcium resorption and a regression of uremic bone disease in their dialysis patients. Dihydrotachysterol is hydroxylated in the liver to form 25-hydroxydihydrotachysterol, which is active without being metabolized in the kidney. Dihydrotachysterol has the advantage over vitamin D in being less toxic because it cummulates less. Older patients seem to be more sensitive to dihydrotachysterol [138] during long-time therapy with this drug. As with any other vitamin D-like substance, patients must be watched closely [119, 137].

Severe secondary hyperparathyroidism can probably only be treated by parathyroidectomy. DELLING et al. [118] have seen a significant effect on the bone after successful subtotal parathyroidectomy. Parathyroidectomy seems to be indicated only if there is severe progressive osteoclasia with hyper-calcemia or hyperphosphatemia causing recurrent calcium-phosphate deposits in the tissues.

7. Anemia

E. HEILMANN

7.1. Introduction

Since BRIGHT's report of 1835 [12], anemia is known as one of the earliest and most characteristic manifestations of chronic renal disease. Prior to the widespread therapeutic use of hemodialysis, anemia was a minor problem for patients suffering from renal failure and azotemia. Intermittent hemo-dialysis was introduced some 15 years ago as a new therapeutic method in chronic renal failure [90], but anemia is still an important problem menacing the patient's life expectancy. Recovery of physical ability will always depend on the improvement of anemia [95]. Long-term effects of anemia on the myocardium—such as fatty degeneration [14] and increased cardiac output [82]—have a substantial influence on the prognosis of dialysis patients.

Anemia occurs eventually in every patient with chronic renal failure. Although many studies [61, 62, 67, 71, 72] point to a correlation between the degree of uremia and the severity of anemia, there is a wide variation in time of onset and progression of anemia in patients on intermittent hemo-dialysis. But no relationship seems to exist between intensity of anemia and the etiology of renal disease [6]. In a state of chronic renal failure the hemato-crit will not fall below a certain minimum. Patients on intermittent hemo-dialysis show a hematocrit between 14 and 38%, with an average of 23%, which is quite independent of the creatinine level [48].

This review intends to cover the present knowledge about pathogenesis of anemia in patients on regular hemodialysis and to discuss the currently available and the prospective methods of therapy.

7.2. Pathogenesis

Anemia in patients on intermittent hemodialysis has a complex patho-genesis influenced by various factors. The most important causes seem to be a toxic influence on erythropoiesis, an accelerated red cell loss due to hemolysis and bleeding, deficiency of iron, folic acid, vitamin B_{12}, pyridoxine, aminoacids, and erythropoietin. The main cause of renal anemia lies in the relative failure of the bone marrow to respond to anemia in the manner of an organism with normal kidney functions. Prior to the discovery of erythropoietin, BRIGHT [12] and VOLHARD [97] had believed that urea and certain other substances, normally excreted in the urine but now retained, were responsible for toxic damage of the bone marrow, and for the resulting impairment of erythropoiesis. But is was proved by BECKER [5], BOCK [9], and KELLER [63] that neither urea nor creatinine are causing toxic bone marrow depression. RENNER [87] found various substances in the dialysis fluid after extracorporeal hemodialysis, among them phenole derivatives, guanidine, and aromatic amines, and he was able to demonstrate their toxic effect.

ADAMSON [1] and ESCHBACH [32] proved that uremic toxines could damage the bone marrow, but that their role in the pathogenesis of anemia was quantitatively negligible.

Various investigators [6, 19, 34, 49, 76, 94, 96] have demonstrated increased *hemolysis* in patients with renal insufficiency; there seems to be, however, no relation between the degree of azotemia and the amount of hemolysis. When azotemia is controlled by intermittent hemodialysis, some hemolytic component will still remain.

Several characteristic signs of hemolysis—such as increased indirect bilirubin, increased lactate-dehydrogenase in the serum, and reticulocytosis—were not demonstrated in this context, a slight hemolysis can be detected by chrom-51-tagging of erythrocytes [46, 60]. Some investigators have reported a shorter erythrocyte life-span in patients on regular hemodialysis. KELLER [63], ESCHBACH *et al.* [32], GIOVANETTI [42], SHAW [94], ESSERS [34], and DESFORGES [19] found the survival time of erythrocytes reduced to one-half or two-thirds of the normal values. According to BLUMBERG [7], the average life-span, as measured by chrom-51-tagging, would be 19 days. Our studies showed a medium span of 20 days [49].

Different results were obtained in studies of the role attributed to red cell enzymes in correlation to hemolysis in patients with renal failure [10, 41, 55, 81]. Erythrocytic enzymes in patients on intermittent hemodialysis were evaluated in the hematology laboratories of Freiburg University [49]*. The calculations yielded normal or slightly elevated values (Fig. 9). Higher values are characteristic of a young erythrocyte population associated with increased hemolysis [54, 84, 89]; they show, however, no features typical for renal anemia. Impairment of glycolysis seems improbable, according to studies of BLUMBERG [6], since concentration of organic phosphates is not increased in general.

---

* Hexokinase; phosphoglucomutase; aldolase; 2,3-diphosphoglyceratmutase; 6-P-gluconatdehydrogenase; P-fructokinase; glutathionreductase; glucose-6-p-dehydrogenase; pyruvatkinase; enolase; mono-p-glyceratmutase; glucose-P-isomerase; glycerinaldehyd-3-P-dehydrogenase; lactat-dehydrogenase; 3-P-glycerat-1-kinase; reduced glutathion; triose-P-isomerase; adenylatkinase.

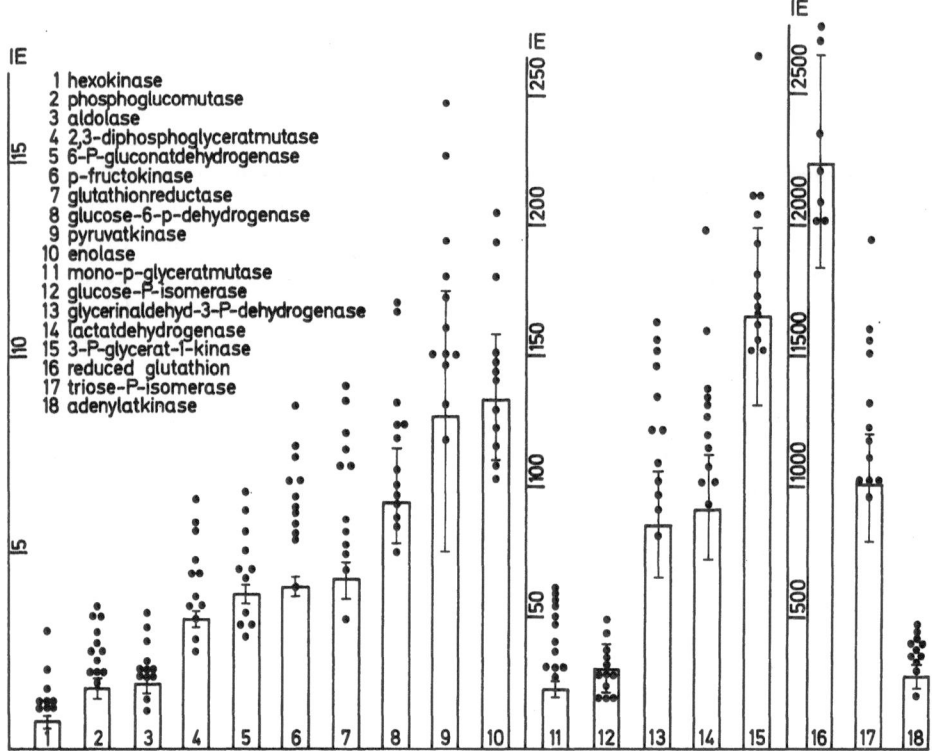

Fig. 9. Erythrocytic enzymes in patients on intermittent hemodialysis

To evaluate the red blood cell trauma caused by the hemodialyser, the free hemoglobin was determined in the plasma before and after dialysis. HYDE and SATTLER [56] have found by means of plasma-hemoglobin evaluation, a slight hemolysis in the closed system of artificial kidneys of various types *(Kiil, Klung, Miniklung, Twin Coil)*. The extent of hemolysis was not correlated to the membrane surface area. Our observations [52] starting from normal values, showed a rising amount of free hemoglobin in the plasma after treatment with different methods of hemodialysis (Fig. 10). The hemolytic component of renal anemia must be due to the uremic environment, but not to a primary cellular defect or mechanical destruction. Of all uremic toxines recently investigated for their potential hemolytic activity, guanidine derivates are most likely to act as hemolytic agents [87].

Until now, *iron deficiency* has been regarded as a minor cause of renal anemia [6, 10, 63]. But in regular hemodialysis, iron deficiency seems in fact to play an important role in the development of anemia. Frequent blood sampling, dialysis itself and gastrointestinal bleeding, reduced iron resorption, and low intake of iron are suspected as the responsible factors. BLUMBERG [6] calculated a loss of 2 to 5 liters of blood per annum caused by dialysis and blood sampling for routine laboratory investigations. We must add blood loss by puncture of the A-V-fistulas, and by occult bleeding from the gastro-

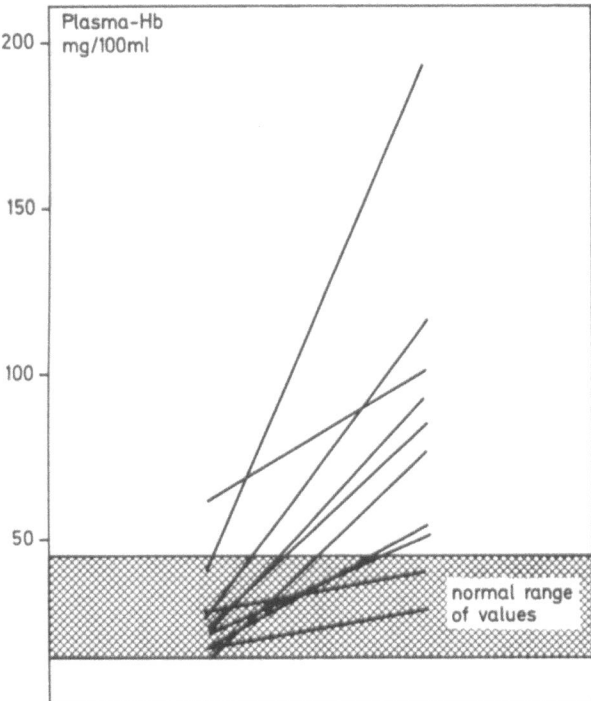

Fig. 10. Plasma hemoglobin in patients with renal insufficiency before and after an 8 hour hemodialysis

intestinal tract. KOCH and other authors [30, 98] found a mean annual iron loss of 2.13 ± 0.92 g by exploring data from [59] Fe whole-body measurements. EDWARDS et al. [22] estimated a daily iron loss between 5 and 6 mg. A reduced iron resorption by dialysis patients was proven by BLUMBERG [8] and BODDY et al. [11]. ESCHBACH et al. [28] demonstrated that iron re-absorption in the dialysis patient is subject to the influence of iron balance depending on iron stores in the bone marrow.

Our central European diet has a normal iron content of 5.5 mg/1000 cal [75]; compared with this, many dialysis patients living on a low meat diet without iron supplementation, will certainly suffer from severe iron deficiency. For diagnosis of this defect, no reliable criteria can be found in the determination of serum iron.

The resulting values oscillate between higher and lower rates and do not reflect the iron stores in the bone marrow [52]. A reliable parameter of the actual iron level of the organism, can be found in the amount of iron deposits within the reticulum cells of the bone marrow. Histologic or cytologic evaluation of iliac creast biopsies after staining with prussian blue allows exact definition of these values. The increase in total iron binding capacity of the serum provides a chemical evidence of iron deficiency in the blood (Fig. 11) [51].

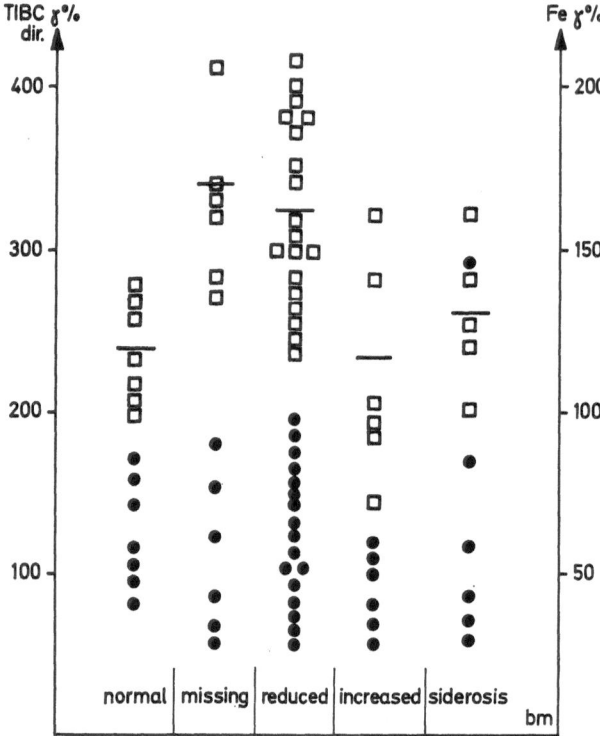

Fig. 11. Correlation between serum iron (Fe), total iron bindung capacity (TIBC) and iron contents (hemosiderin in bone marrow (bm) in patients on permanent hemodialysis

Pyridoxine, which is necessary for hemosynthesis, may be lost in the dialysis fluid [26].

GIORDANO [41] had found a certain deficit in *aminoacids*, especially histidine, in his dialysis patients; but substitution of these substances failed to promote a convincing improvement in hematopoiesis.

Folic acid is a dialysable co-enzyme needed for normal red cell production. In 1963 LASKER *et al.* [68] were first to report lower levels of folic acid in the plasma of dialysis patients. HAMPERS *et al.* [47] reported about 10 patients, of whom five showed megaloblastic changes in the bone marrow, while nine of them had lowered levels of folic acid in the plasma. He recommended that patients on long-term hemodialysis should receive folic acid supplementation. WHITEHEAD [99], JOIST [59] and MACKENZIE *et al.* [70] conclude from their studies that in adequately dialysed patients lowered folic acid will normally have no decisive influence on the pathogenesis of renal anemia.

No symptoms are found in patients on intermittent dialysis of deficiency of *vitamin B$_{12}$*, which is tightly bound to plasma proteins, and which is fortunately not dialysable. Vitamin B$_{12}$ values in the serum were reported as normal by MACKENZIE [70] and HAMPERS [47] in their patients on intermittent hemodialysis. We performed a radioimmunoassay for vitamin B$_{12}$, before and after an 8 hours dialysis. The levels were within the normal range, without lowering during dialysis.

Whereas the excretory function of the kidney and its role in regulating fluid volume and blood pressure is clearly defined and explained, recent investigations have shown the importance of endocrinous renal influence on erythropoiesis. In 1906, CARNOT and DEFLANDRE [15] were the first to assume a humoral factor regulating the amount of red cells, which they called hemato-poietin.

Some fifty years later REISSMANN [85] and ERSLEV [23, 24] investigated the humoral mechanism destined to regulate erythropoiesis. JACOBSON *et al.* [57] associated this *erythropoietin* production with the kidney. GORDON *et al.* [16, 17, 43, 44] described a small mitochondrial fraction of the kidney con-taining a factor REF—the renal erythropoietic factor which is inactive in itself, but distinctively capable of promoting erythropoiesis after incubation with a globuline in the plasma. REF is clearly distinguished from renin [101]. Several investigators [80, 86] presumed that REF acts like an enzyme upon a liver-derived globulin fraction of the plasma, thereby producing an erythropoiesis-stimulating factor (ESF) called erythropoietin.

Deficient or reduced production of erythropoietin by the damaged or impaired kidney has been identified as the major cause of anemia [6, 7, 25, 27, 28, 34, 40, 43, 45, 50, 57, 70, 73, 76, 80, 100, 101]. Patients on maintenance hemodialysis are not able to produce a normal red cell mass; this failure is primarily the result of severe damage to the site of erythropoietin or REF production. Production of renal erythropoietin is suppressed either partially or completely, therefore stimulation of erythropoiesis will depend mainly upon erythropoietin provided by extrarenal sites [39, 73, 75, 78, 79] in order to maintain at least a subnormal level.

After bilateral nephrectomy, renal erythropoietin production is destroyed completely, while basic erythropoiesis maintains a hematocrit of about 10% [6, 25, 48]. This insufficient production of erythropoietin will explain the diminished erythropoiesis observed in dialysis patients by means of ferro-kinetic studies [30]. Erythropoietin inhibitors are discussed as responsible agents in erythropoietin deficiency; FISHER *et al.* [36] supposed them to block the effect of the hormone. In accordance with ESSERS *et al.* [35], we have found no erythropoietin inhibitors in the blood of patients with renal in-sufficiency. Clinical findings in bilaterally nephrectomized patients who are actually unable to produce renal inhibitors may help to explain the declining curves of hemoglobin and hematocrit as a result of primary erythropoietin deficiency.

It has been shown that kidney transplantation is followed by recovery of erythropoietin production and that, consequently, red cell production re-turns to its normal rate. DENNY *et al.* [18] and other authors [53, 74, 79] have shown in repeated tests that a transplanted kidney is capable of erythro-poietin production as early as 1 to 40 days after transplantation.

7.3. Treatment

The first and most urgent step in preventing anemia in patients on inter-mittent dialysis should be to reduce blood sampling to the inevitable minimum. Investigations of several authors [6, 26, 34] agree on estimates that some 1.4 to 3.1 l of blood are taken yearly from dialysis patients for the sole reason of diagnosis and research. This means a loss of blood easily comparable to the amount donated by regular blood donors. Such an artificial deprivation could be kept, however, at the inevitable minimum by taking samples only from the plasma with re-transfusion of cellular components.

Considering the hemolytic component of anemia in dialysis patients, splenec-tomy might appear as a potential remedy for anemia even without splenomegaly. But lowered immunologic activity after splenectomy would never justify such a drastic method simply to prolong the lifespan of red cells. Therefore, the decision in favour of surgery is called for by very few indications: spleno-megaly or splenic destruction of ^{51}Cr labeled red cells combined with an extremely short red cell life. The result of splenectomy is rarely spectacular or even satisfactory.

In the current management of anemia in patients on chronic intermittent dialysis, this procedure must always remain in the center of attention. A number of reports [6, 64, 65] have shown that an intensified regimen in dialysis may help to improve red cell production. Improvement of hematocrit appears as a result of increased erythropoiesis, and also of reduced hemolysis. This effect was demonstrated in ferrokinetic studies, but the mechanism of the improvement is not quite clear. In theory, the cause of improved marrow activity should be seen in the removal of uremic toxines. Toxines of medium molecular size seem to have an important influence on the pathogenesis of the uremic syndrome. This concept was subjected to clinical trials by BABB et al. [4], but the results failed to definitely localize anemia-specific toxines in this medium molecular range.

We shall have to await further observations regarding the use of highly permeable membranes to find out whether this therapeutic method will help dialysis patients to recover from anemia.

In this modified management of anemia, transfusion therapy is reduced as far as possible by providing an optimal environment for red cell production and by stimulating the bone marrow to a certain extra-activity. Moreover, chronic transfusion therapy of anemia in patients on permanent dialysis is associated with problems of hemosiderosis, depressed bone marrow activity, sensitization and immunologic response to isoantigens of blood cells and plasma proteins. It is essential that only washed and packed red blood cells are used. Frozen blood may permit a more liberal management of transfusion, but this is still not certain [83]. Most dialysis centers insist on reserving transfusion for cases with a very low hematocrit level, i.e. 10%, or when emergency signs of cardio-respiratory failure or cerebral hypoxia are present.

Until 1971, routine preparation of dialysis patients for transplantation would always include bilateral nephrectomy. But in view of the resulting

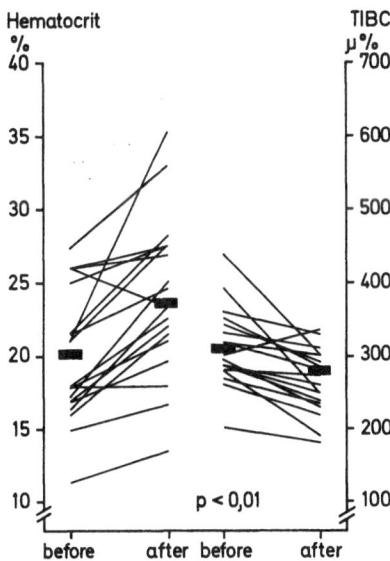

Fig. 12. Hematocrit and total iron binding capacity (TIBC) in 18 patients on permanent hemodialysis with iron deficiency, before and after administration of 1000 mg Fe-III i.v.

severe impairment of hematocrit it should be recommended that no other indication for nephrectomy be accepted than severe hypertension resisting any other treatment. Even malfunctioning kidneys are capable of producing a small amount of erythropoietin; therefore nephrectomy should be delayed until the moment of the actual transplantation.

As long as renal anemia had been treated with transfusion, iron substitution was unnecessary. But in the present dialysis system, loss of blood provokes a significant iron deficiency in almost every dialysed patient. Considering an average daily blood loss of 10 ml [6, 64], that would mean an extra loss of 2 mg iron which must be substituted. Since the normal iron loss is about 1–2 mg a day, the iron requirement is doubled and supplement iron is needed. Investigations of the dialysis patient's capacity to reabsorb iron have given different results, but most of them showed a decrease in iron absorption. The use of parenteral iron may be indicated to replenish depleted iron stores, or when patients claim oral iron intolerance. Administration of a total amount of 1 g iron resulted in a significant rise of hematocrit with simultaneous decrease of the total iron binding capacity in the serum (Fig. 12).

As a rule, supplementation of vitamin B_{12} is not required in dialysis patients because this vitamin is protein-bound and therefore not dialysable.

Folic acid is a dialysable co-enzyme needed for normal red cell production; its loss via dialysis fluid provoking severe folic acid deficiency has been described. A routine dietary supplement of 1 mg of folic acid seems to be useful.

Supplemental pyroxidine has not been recommended. But a supplement of histidine was recommended for patients on a strict low-protein diet [41]. There are, however, no convincing observations about the hematologic effects of these supplements. We want to emphasize that the restriction of protein intake should be relieved. The diet of dialysis patients should include high-quality proteins at the rate of 70 to 80 g a day.

In the specific erythropoiesis defect resulting from insufficient erythropoietin production, treatment is at present still unsatisfactory because purified human or animal erythropoietin is not available. On the other hand, it has been demonstrated that erythropoiesis is promoted by certain androgens capable of increasing renal and extrarenal erythropoietin production [38, 39, 73, 75, 76, 78]. The results of recent investigations have shown that androgens increase erythropoietin activity also in anephric patients [6, 93, 100]. Discussion continues about whether the stimulation might be caused by induction of stem cells.

A number of oral and parenteral androgen preparations are currently used in the treatment of anemia in dialysis patients, and impressive results have been reported from several renal centers [28, 37, 45, 50, 66, 88, 92, 93]. In anephric patients the effect is not as positive as in patients with kidney remnants. The use of androgens for treatment of aplastic anemia [91] is often associated with certain side effects, such as cholestasis, fluid retention, acne, hirsutism, and skin rash; but these symptoms fail to appear in patients with chronic renal disease. Nevertheless, in view of potential virilization in females [6], priapism in males [64, 65], hyperlipidemia [20, 69], and development of hepatocellular carcinoma [58], the therapeutic use of androgens should be strictly reserved to male patients with hematocrit below 15%, and to bilaterally nephrectomized patients.

Therapeutic replacement of exogenous erythropoietin seems to be the treatment of choice. Owing to the general shortage of erythropoietin, not more than a few clinical trials have been published until the present [21]. It was shown that 20–50 units of erythropoietin/kg per day will provoke reticulocyte production and a rise in hematocrit and red cell mass. Biochemical synthesis might offer a potential direct approach to mass production of erythropoietin [33]. We hope that the future will bring the development of natural or synthetic erythropoietin productions suited to human therapy.

7.4. Summary

Various factors are involved in the pathogenesis of anemia in dialysis patients. Reduced erythropoiesis is mainly attributed to erythropoietin deficiency. Stimulation of erythropoiesis may be promoted by androgens.

Parenteral substitution of iron is recommended in case of iron deficiency. As a rule, supplementation of vitamin B_{12} is not necessary, but administration of folic acid is recommended. Treatment of anemia in renal failure is rendered more effective by increased technical efficiency in hemodialysis permitting a relatively protein-rich diet. Blood transfusions are not necessary during routine treatment of dialysis anemia. Since bilateral nephrectomy will always provoke severe anemia, it should be reserved to special cases of severe hypertension.

Until now, no conservative therapy has been developed which would allow optimal treatment of anemia in dialysis patients. Successful renal transplantation still is, and will be, the best therapeutic intervention.

References

Sections 1–5

1. AHEARN, D. J., MAHER, J. F.: Heart failure as a complication of hemodialysis. Arteriovenous Fistula. Ann. Int. Med. **77**, 201–204 (1972)
2. ALFREY, A. C., LUEKER, R., GOSS, J. E., VOGEL, J. H. K., FARIS, T. D., HOLMES, J. H.: Control of arteriovenous shunt flow. J. Amer. Med. Ass. **214**, 884–888 (1970)
3. ASBURY, A. K., VICTOR, M., ADAMS, R. D.: Uremic polyneuropathy. Arch. Neurol. (Chicago) **8**, 413 (1963)
4. BAGDADE, J. D.: Disorders of carbohydrate and lipid metabolism in uremia. Nephron **14**, 153–162 (1975)
5. BAGDADE, J. D., PORTE, D., BIERMANN, E.: Hypertriglyceridemia. — A consequence of chronic renal failure. New Engl. J. Med. **279**, 181–185 (1968)
6. BAGDADE, J. D.: Uremic lipemia: Abnormal triglycerid transport in chronic renal failure. In: Uremia. Stuttgart: Georg Thieme, 1972
7. BAILEY, G. L., HAMPERS, C. L., MERRILL, J. R.: Reversible cardiomyopathy in uremia. Vol. XIII Trans. Amer. Soc. Artif. Int. Organs (1967)
8. BRASS, H., KRÜCKELS, E. D., MÜLLER, G., HEINTZ, R.: Pathomechanismen der Herzinsuffizienz bei Hämodialysepatienten. Dtsch. Med. Wschr. **96**, 1319–1324 (1971)
9. BUNDSCHU, H. G., LÜDERS, G., DÜRR, F.: Morphologische Veränderungen an Gonaden hämodialysierter chronisch nierenkranker Männer. Symp. Ges. Nephrol. Aachen: Heintz and Holzhüter, 1971, VIII
10. COHEN, A. D., GOWER, P. E., ROGERS, K. LL., PEGRUM, G. D., DE WARDENER, H. E.: Reproductive potential in males treated by chronic haemodialysis. Proceedings of the 10th Congress of the EDTA, Vol. **10** (1973)
11. COLEMAN, T. G., BOWER, J. D., LANGFORD, H. G., GUYTON, A. C.: Regulation of arterial pressure in the anephric state. Circulation, Vol. XLII, 509–514 (1970)
12. CRASWELL, P. W., HIRD, V. M., JUDD, P. A., BAILLOD, R. A., VARGHESE, Z., MOORHEAD, J. F.: Plasma renin activity and blood pressure in 89 patients receiving maintenance haemodialysis therapy. Brit. Med. J. **4**, 749–753 (1972)
13. CRASWELL, P. W., HIRD, V. M., BAILLOD, R. A., VARGHESE, Z., MOORHEAD, J. F.: Significance of high plasma renin activity in patients on maintenance haemodialysis therapy. Brit. Med. J. **2**, 741–743 (1973)
14. DOBBELSTEIN, H.: Die urämische Neuropathie in Abhängigkeit von Dialysedauer und -gerät. Klin. Wschr. **50**, 533–535 (1972)
15. FLOYD, M. D., AGYAR, D. R., HUDGSON, P., KERR, D. N. S.: Myopathy in chronic renal failure. Proc. Europ. Dial. Transpl. Ass. **6** (1969)
16. FRALEY, E. E., FELDMAN, B. H.: Renal hypertension. New Engl. J. Med. **287**, 550–552 (1972)
17. GURLAND, H. J., BRUNNER, F. P., v. DEHN, H., HÄRLEN, H., PARSONS, F. M., SCHÄRER, K.: Combined report on regular dialysis and transplantation in Europe, III, 1972. In: Proceedings of the European Dialysis and Transplant Association, **10**, London: Pitman Medical, 1973
18. HAMPERS, C. L., LOWRIE, E. G., SOELDNER, J. S., MERRILL, J. P.: Uremia and carbohydrate metabolism. In: Uremia. Stuttgart: Georg Thieme, 1972
19. HERON, J. R., KONOTEY-AHULU, F. I., SHALDON, S., THOMAS, P. K.: Nerve conduction in chronic renal failure treated by dialysis. Proc. Europ. Dial. Transpl. Ass. **2** (1965)
20. HÜBNER, W., DIEMER, A., FRIEBERG, J.: Das Verhalten der urämischen Hyperlipidämie und Glukosetoleranzstörung unter chronisch intermittierender Hämodialysebehandlung. Med. Welt **23**, 1415–1417 (1972)

21. JENNEKENS, F. G. I., VAN DER MOST, D., VAN SPIJK, E. J., Dorhout MESS: Nerve fiber degeneration in uremic polyneuropathy. Proc. Europ. Dial. Transpl. Ass. **6** (1969)

22. KENNEDY, A. C., LINTON, A. L., LUKE, R. G., RENFREW, S., DINWOODIE, A.: The pathogenesis and prevention of cerebral dysfunction during dialysis. Lancet **792** (1964)

23. KONOTHEY-AHULU, F. I. D., BAILLOD, R., COMTY, C. M., HERON, J. R., SHALDON, S., THOMAS, P. K.: Effects of periodic dialysis on the peripheral neuropathy of end-stage renal failure. Brit. Med. J. **2**, 1212 (1965)

24. KLÜTSCH, K., KULT, J., GROSSWENDT, J.: Die Hämodynamik regelmäßig hämodialysierter Patienten. Wissenschaftliche Information Fresenius, Aktuelle Nephrologie **1**, 47–63 (1972)

25. LINDNER, A., CHARRA, B., SHERRARD, D. J., SCHRIBNER, B. H.: Accelerated atherosclerosis in prolonged maintenance hemodialysis. New Engl. J. Med. **290**, 697–701 (1974)

26. LÜDERITZ, B., BOLTE, H. D.: Chronische Niereninsuffizienz und muskelzelluläre Erregbarkeit. In: Aktuelle Probleme der Dialyseverfahren und der Niereninsuffizienz. Friedberg: Bindernagel, 1971

27. PERKHOFF, G. T., THOMAS, C. L., NEWTON, J. C., SELLMANN, J. C., TYLER, F. H.: Mechanisms of impaired glucose tolerance in uremia and experimental hyperazotemia. Diabetes **7**, 375 (1958)

28. PIEHL, W., WILBRANDT, R., FREYLAND, M. D., FROTSCHER, U., MESSERSCHMIDT, W.: Herzbeuteltamponade bei terminaler Niereninsuffizienz. Dtsch. med. Wschr. **96**, 1249–1251 (1971)

29. PIPPIG, L.: Herz- und Kreislauffunktion bei Urämie. Arch. Klin. Med. **214**, 244–272 (1968)

30. SCHREINER, G. E., MAHLER, J. F.: Hemodialysis for chronic renal failure. Medical, moral and ethical, and socio-economic problems. Ann. Int. Med. **62**, 551 (1965)

31. SCHULZ, W., GESSLER, U.: Renale Hypertonie und bilaterale Nephrektomie. Nieren- und Hochdruckkrankheiten **6**, 258–261 (1973)

32. SIDDIQUI, J., KERR, D. N. S.: Complications of renal failure and their response to dialysis. Brit. Med. Bull. **27/2**, 153–159 (1971)

33. SILL, V., LANSER, K. G., BAUDITZ, W.: Einfluß der Anämie und der arteriovenösen Fistel auf die körperliche Leistungsfähigkeit der Dauerdialysepatienten. Z. Kardiologie **62**, 164–175 (1972)

34. SILL, V., TILSNER, V., BAUDITZ, W.: Beeinflussung der Hämodynamik durch arteriovenöse Fisteln bei Dialyse-Patienten. Dtsch. Med. Wschr. **94**, 1604–1607 (1969)

35. STERN, G., SMITH, H.: In: Research in muscular dystrophy. London: Ditman Medical, 1968

36. TENCKHOFF, H. A., BOEN, F. S. T., JEBSEN, R. H., SPIEGLER, J. H.: Polyneuropathy in chronic renal insufficiency. J. Amer. Med. Ass. **192**, 1121 (1965)

37. VERTES, V., CANGIANO, J. L., BERMAN, L. B., GOULD, A.: Hypertension in end-stage renal failure. New Engl. J. Med. **280**, 978 (1969)

38. WAGNER, H., BÖCKEL, K., HRUBESCH, M., SCHULZ, H., LOEW, H.: Hypogonadismus bei männlichen Dauerdialysepatienten. Aktuelle Probleme der Dialyseverfahren und der Niereninsuffizienz. In: Fifth Symposium, Innsbruck, Feb 1974. In press

39. WIEGAND, M. E., MEENTS, O., HEIDLAND, A.: Cochleovestibuläre Störungen bei Patienten mit terminaler Niereninsuffizienz. In: Aktuelle Probleme der Dialyseverfahren und Niereninsuffizienz. Friedberg: Bindernagel, 1971

40. ZUMKLEY, H., LOSSE, H., WESTERBOER, S.: Hypernatriämie als Ursache urämischer Encephalopathien. VI. Symposium Ges. Nephrologie, Wien, 1968

41. ZUMKLEY, H.: Differentialdiagnose renaler Encephalopathien. Med. Welt **23**, 555–559 (1972)

Section 6

1. ALBRIGHT, F., BURNETT, L. H., PARSON, W., REIFENSTEIN, E. C., ROOS, A.: Osteomalacia and late rickets. Various etiology met in the United States with emphasis on that resulting from specific form of renal acidosis, therapeutic indications for

each etiological subgroup, and relationship between osteomalacia and Milkman's syndrome. Medicine (Baltimore) **25**, 1946, 399–406

2. AVIOLI, L. V.: The therapeutic approach to hypoparathyroidism. Amer. J. Med. **57**, 1974, 34–42

3. AVIOLI, L. V., BIRGE, S. J., SLATOPOLSKY, E.: The Nature of Vitamin D Resistance of Patients with Chronic Renal Disease. Arch. Intern. Med. **124**, 1969, 451–454

4. AVIOLI, L. V., BIRGE, S. J., WON LEE, S., SLATOPOLSKY, E.: The metabolic fate of vitamin D_3–^{3}H in chronic renal failure. J. Clin. Invest. **47**, 1968, 2239–2252

5. AVIOLI, L. V., HADDAD, J. G.: Vitamin D: Current Concepts. Metabolism **22**, 1973, 507–531

6. AVIOLI, L. V., WON LEE, S., McDONALD, J. E., LUND, J., DeLUCA, H. F.: Metabolism of Vitamin D_3–^{3}H in Human Subjects: Distribution in Blood, Bile, Feces, and Urine. J. Clin. Invest. **46**, 1967, 983–992

7. BALL, J., GARNER, A.: Mineralisation of woven bone in osteomalacia. J. Path. Bact. **91**, 1966, 563–574

8. BELSEY, R. E., DeLUCA, H. F., POTTS, J. T.: A Rapid Assay for 25–OH–Vitamin D_3 Without Preparative Chromatography. J. Clin. Endocrin. Met. **38**, 1974, 1046–1061

9. BERLYNE, G. M.: Microcrystalline Conjunctival Calcification in Renal Failure. Lancet **I 1968**, 366–370

10. BERLYNE, G. M.: Red Eyes in Renal Failure. Lancet **I 1967**, 4–7

11. BERSON, S. A., YALOW, R. S.: Parathyroid hormone in plasma in adenomatous hyperparathyroidism, uremia and bronchogenic carcinoma. Sci. **154**, 1966, 90–7912

12. BINSWANGER, U., FISCHER, J., SCHENK, R., MERZ, W.: Osteopathie bei chronischer Niereninsuffizienz. Dtsch. med. Wschr. **96**, 1971, 1914–1919

13. BLUNT, J. W., DeLUCA, H. F., SCHNOES, H. K.: 25-Hydroxycholecalciferol. A Biologically Active Metabolite of Vitamin D_3. Biochemistry **7**, 1968, 3317–3322

14. BOYLE, I. T., GRAY, R. W., DeLUCA, H. F.: Regulation by Calcium of in vitro Synthesis of 1,25-Dihydroxycholecalciferol and 21,25-Dihydroxycholecalciferol. Proc. Nat. Acad. Sci. USA **68**, 1971, 2131–2134

15. BOYLE, I. T., GRAY, R. W., OMDAHL, J. L., DeLUCA, H. F.: The mechanism of adaption of intestinal calcium absorption to low dietary calcium. J. Lab. Clin. Med. **78**, 1971, 813

16. BRICKER, N. S., SLATOPOLSKY, E., REISS, E., AVIOLI, L. V.: Calcium, Phosphorus, and Bone in Renal Disease and Transplantation. Arch. Intern. Med. **123**, 1969, 543–553

17. CANER, J. E. Z., DECKER, J. L.: Recurrent Acute (? Gouty) Arthritis in Chronic Renal Failure Treated with Periodic Hemodialysis. Amer. J. Med. **36**, 1964, 571–582

18. CHASE, L. R., SLATOPOLSKY, E.: Secretion and Metabolic Efficacy of Parathyroid Hormone in Patients with Severe Hypomagnesemia. J. Cli. Endocr. Metab. **38**, 1974, 363–371

19. CLARKSON, E. M., LUCK, V. A., HYNSON, W. V., BAILEY, R. R., EASTWOOD, J. B., WOODHEAD, J. S., CLEMENTS, V. R., O'RIORDAN, J. L. H., DE WARDENER, H. E.: The effect of Aluminium Hydroxyde on Calcium, Phosphorus and Aluminium Balances, the Serum Parathyroid Hormone Concentration and the Aluminium Content of Bone in Patients with Chronic Renal Failure. Clin. Sci. **43**, 1972, 519–531

20. CLARKSON, E. M., McDONALD, S. J., DE WARDENER, H. E.: The Effect of a High Intake of Calcium Carbonate in Normal Subjects and Patients with Chronic Renal Failure. Clin. Sci. **30**, 1966, 425–438

21. COCHRAN, M., NORDIN, B. E. C.: Role of Acidosis in Renal Osteomalacia. Brit. Med. J. **2**, 1969, 276–279

22. CORRADINO, R. A., WASSERMAN, R. H.: Vitamin D_3: Induction of Calcium-Binding Protein in Embryonic Chick Intestine in vitro. Sci. **172**, 1971, 731–733

23. COUSINS, R. J., DeLUCA, H. F., GRAY, R. W.: Metabolism of 25-Hydroxycholecalciferol in Target and Nontarget Tissues. Bioch. **9**, 1970, 3649–3654

24. COUSINS, R. J.: DeLUCA, H. F., SUDA, T., CHEN, T., TANAKA, Y.: Metabolism and Subcellular Location of 25-Hydroxycholecalciferol in Intestinal Mucosa. Biochemistry **9**, 1079, 1453–1458

25. CRAWFORD, T., DENT, C. E., LUCAS, P., MARTIN, N. H.: Osteosclerosis Associated with Chronic Renal Failure. Lancet **II**, 1954, 981–989

26. Dambacher, M. A., Girad, J., Haas, H. G.: Die Vitamin D-Hormone. Neue Erkenntnisse über Stoffwechsel und Therapie. Der Internist **13**, 1972, 125–132

27. Delling, G.: Quantitative Auswertung von Skeletveränderungen bei chronischer Hämodialyse. Verh. Dtsch. Ges. f. Path. **56**. Tagung. 1972, 436–438

28. DeLuca, H. F.: The Role of Vitamin D and Its Relationship to Parathyroid Hormone and Calcitonin. Rec. Prog. Horm. Res. **27**, 1971, 479–516

29. DeLuca, H. F.: Parathyroid Hormone as a Trophic Hormone for 1,25-Dihydroxyvitamin D₃, the Metabolically Active Form of Vitamin D. New Engl. J. Med. **287**, 1972, 250–251

30. DeLuca, H. F.: 25-Hydroxycholecalciferol. The Probable Metabolically Active Form of Vitamin D₃: Its Identification and Subcellular Site of Action. Arch. Intern. Med. **124**, 1969, 442–450

31. DeLuca, H. F.: Neue Erkenntnisse über den Vitamin D-Stoffwechsel. Triangel **12**, 1974, 111–118

32. DeLuca, H. F., Avioli, L. V.: Treatment of Renal Osteodystrophy with 25-Hydroxycholecalciferol. Arch. Intern. Med. **126**, 1970, 896–899

33. Drescher, D., DeLuca, H. F.: Possible Precursor of Vitamin D Stimulated Calcium Binding Protein in Rats. Biochemistry **10**, 1971, 2308–2312

34. Drukker, W., Haagsma-Schouten, W. A. G., Alberts, G., Baarda, B.: Zit. nach: Ritz, E., Sieberth, H. G., und Krempien, B.: Ca-Stoffwechselstörungen bei chronischer Niereninsuffizienz. Klin. Wschr. **49**, 1971, 1305–1314

35. Duursma, S. A., Visser, W. J., Njio, L.: A quantitativ histological study of bone in 30 Patients with renal insufficiency. Calc. Tiss. Res. **9**, 1972, 216–221

36. Faser, D. R., Kodicek, E.: Unique Biosynthesis by Kidney of a Biologically Active Vitamin D Metabolite. Nature **228**, 1970, 764–766

37. Fournier, A. E., Arnaud, C. D., Johnson, W. J., Taylor, W. F., Goldsmith, R. S.: Etiology of Hyperparathyroidism and Bone Disease during Chronic Hemodialysis. II. Factors Affecting Serum Immunoreactive Parathyroid Hormone. J. Clin. Invest. **50**, 1971, 599–605

38. Friis, Th., Hahnemann, S., Weeke, E.: Serum Calcium and Serum Phosphorus in Uremia during Administration of Serum Phytate and Aluminium Hydroxide. Acta Med. Scand. **183**, 1968, 497–502

39. Friis, Th., Weeke, E.: Effect of Aluminium Hydroxyde upon Serum Calcium, Serum Phosphorus and Calcium Turnover in Uremic Patients. Acta Med. Scand. **187**, 1970, 41–46

40. Frolik, C. A., DeLuca, H. F.: 1,25-Dihydroxycholecalciferol: The Metabolite of Vitamin D Responsible for Increased Calcium Transport. Arch. Biochemistry and Bioph. **147**, 1971, 143–147

41. Frolik, C. A., DeLuca, H. F.: Metabolism of 26,27-³H-1,25-Dihydroxycholecalciferol. Fed. Proc. **31**, 1, 1972, 693

42. Garabedian, M., Holick, M. F., DeLuca, H. F., Boyle, I. T.: Control of 25-Hydroxycholecalciferol Metabolism by Parathyroid Glands. Proc. Nat. Acad. Sci. USA. **689**, 1972, 1673–1676

43. Garner, A., Ball, J.: Quantitative Observation on Mineralised and Unmineralised Bone in Chronic Renal Azotemie and Intestinal Malabsorption Syndrome. J. Path. Bact. **91**, 1966, 545–549

44. Gral, Th.: Medizinische Probleme der chronischen Hämodialyse. Med. Welt **10**, 1968, 637–642

45. Gray, R. W., Boyle, I., DeLuca, H. F.: Vitamin D Metabolism: The Role of Kidney Tissue. Sci. **172**, 1971, 1232–1234

46. Gray, R. W., Omdahl, J. L., Ghazarian, H. G., DeLuca, H. F.: 25(OH)-Vitamin D₃-Hydroxilation. Fed. Proc. **31**, 1972, 693

47. Hallick, R. B., DeLuca, H. F.: Metabolites of Dihydrotachysterol in Target Tissues. J. Biol. Chem. **247**, 1972, 91–97

48. Harrison, H. C., Harrison, H. E.: Comparison of Activity of 25-Hydroxycholecalciferol and Dihydrotachysterol in the Thyroparathyroidectomized Rat. Proc. Soc. Exper. Biol. Med. **136**, 1971, 411–414

49. Harrison, H. E., Harrison, H. C.: Dihydrotachysterol: a Calcium Active Steroid not Dependent upon Kidney Metabolism. J. Clin. Invest. **51**, 1972, 1919–1922

50. HARRISON, H. E., HARRISON, H. C.: Difference between Cholecalciferol and Dihydrotachysterol with Respect to Activation by Kidney. Fed. Proc. **31**, 1972, 226
51. HARTENBOWER, D. L., COBURN, J. W., REDDY, C. R., NORMAN, A. W.: Possible Role of Impaired Renal Production of 1,25-DiOH-Cholecalciferol in Causing Reduced Calcium Absorption in Chronic Uremia. Clin. Res. **20**, 1972, 595
52. HAUSSLER, M. R.: Studies on the Production of 25-Hydroxy-Vitamin D_3 and 1,25-Dihydroxy-Vitamin D_3 in vitro. Fed. Proc. **31**, 1972, 694
53. HAUSSLER, M. R., BOYCE, D. W., LITTLEDIKE, E. T., RASMUSSEN, H.: A Rapidly Acting Metabolite of Vitamin D_3. Proc. Nat. Acad. Sci. USA. **68**, 1971, 177–181
54. HEIDBREDER, E., HENNEMANN, H., HEIDLAND, A.: Renale Osteodystrophie. Med. Welt **25**, 1974, 736–744
55. HEINTZ, R., RENNER, D.: Über Hemmwirkungen des Serums von Kranken mit hepatorenalem Syndrom und mit chronischer Urämie auf Sauerstoffverbrauch und Kohlenhydratstoffwechsel von Nieren und Hirngewebe der Ratte. Klin. Wschr. **43**, 1965, 1167–1173
56. HENNING, H. V., QUELLHORST, E., SCHELER, F.: Myocardverkalkung als letale Komplikation bei chronischer Niereninsuffizienz. Med. Klin. **64**, 1969, 1591–1595
57. HERRATH, D. VON, KRAFT, D., GRIGOLEIT, H.-G., SCHAEFER, K.: Die Behandlung der urämischen Osteopathie. II. Die Wirkung von 5,6-trans-25-Hydroxycholecalciferol bei terminaler Niereninsuffizient. Dtsch. med. Wschr. **98**, 1973, 1379–1381
58. HERRATH, D. VON, SCHAEFER, K., KOCH, H. U., OPITZ, A., STRATZ, R.: Vitamin D-Stoffwechsel bei experimenteller Urämie. Zschr. ges. exp. Med. **155**, 1971, 315–324
59. HESCH, R.-D., GERLACH, W., HENNING, H. V., EMRICH, D., SCHELER, F., KATTERMANN, R.: Untersuchungen zur intestinalen ^{47}Ca-Absorption bei Gesunden und Patienten mit chronischer Niereninsuffizienz. Dtsch. med. Wschr. **97**, 1972, 1735–1742
60. HESCH, R.-D., HENNING, H. V., GERLACH, W., SCHELER, F.: Früherkennung von Störungen der intestinalen Ca-Absorption bei Niereninsuffizienz. Klin. Wschr. **49**, 1971, 115–118
61. HILL, L. F., VAN DEN BERG, C. J., MAWER, E. B.: Zit. nach HEIDBREDER, E., HENNEMANN, H., HEIDLAND, A.: Renale Osteodystrophie. Med. Welt **25**, 1974, 736–744
62. HITT, O., JAWORSKI, Z. F., SHIMIZU, A. G., FROST, H. M.: Tissue-level Bone Formation rates in Chronic Renal Failure, Measured by Means of Tetracycline Bone Labeling. Canad. J. Phys. Pharm. **48**, 1970, 824–828
63. HOLICK, M. F., DELUCA, H. F., AVIOLI, L. V.: Isolation and Identification of 25-Hydroxycholecalciferol From Human Plasma. Arch. Intern. Med. **129**, 1972, 56–61
64. HOLICK, M. F., GARABEDIAN, M., DELUCA, H. F.: 1,25-Dihydroxycholecalciferol: Metabolite of Vitamin D_3 Active on Bone in Anephric Rats. Sci. **176**, 1972, 1146–1147
65. HOLICK, M. F., SCHNOES, H. K., DELUCA, H. F.: Identification of 1,25-Dihydroxycholecalciferol, a Form of Vitamin D_3 Metabolically Active in the Intestine. Proc. Nat. Acad. Sci. USA **68**, 1971, 803–804
66. INGHAM, J. P., STEWART, J. H., POSEN, S.: Quantitative Skeletal Histology in Untreated End-stage Renal Failure. Brit. Med. J. **2**, 1973, 745–748
67. JOWSEY, J.: Die mikroradiographische Beurteilung der Knochenstruktur. Triangel **12**, 1974, 93–102
68. JOWSEY, J., MASSRY, S. G., COBURN, J. W., KLEEMAN, CH. R.: Microradiographic Studies of Bone in Renal Osteodystrophy. Arch. Intern. Med. **124**, 1969, 539–543
69. KAYE, M., CHATTERJEE, G., COHEN, G. F., SAGAR, S.: Arrest of Hyperparathyroid Bone Disease with Dihydrotachysterol in Patients Undergoing Chronic Hemodialysis. Ann. Intern. Med. **73**, 1970, 225–233
70. KAYE, M., SAGAR, S.: Effect of Dihydrotachysterol on Calcium Absorption in Uremia. Metabolism. **51**, 1972, 815–824
71. KAYE, M., SAGAR, S.: Dihydrotachysterol in Uremia. Clin. Res. **19**, 1971, 809
72. KIMBERG, V. D., BAERG, R. D., GERSHON, E.: The Nature of Vitamin D Resistance in Experimental Uremia. Arch. Intern. Med. **126**, 1970, 891–895
73. KODICEK, E., LAWSON, D. E. M., WILSON, P. W.: Biological Activity of a Polar Metabolite of Vitamin D_3. Nature **228**, 1970, 763–764
74. KORT, R.: Heparin-induzierte Mobilisation von Calcium und anorganischem Phosphat im Zusammenhang mit extraossären Verkalkungen bei chronischer Hämodialyse. Klin. Wschr. **49**, 1971, 684–692

75. Krawitt, E. L., Kunin, A. S.: Intestinal Calcium-Binding Protein and Rickets. Proc. Soc. Exp. Biol. Med. **136**, 1971, 530–533

76. Krempien, B., Ritz, E., Heuck, F.: Osteopathie bei Langzeithämodialyse. Histomorphometrische und microradiographische Untersuchungen. Verh. Dtsch. Ges. Path. 56. Tagung 1972, 439–442

77. Kuhlencordt, F., Bauditz, W., Lozano-Tonkin, C., Kruse, H.-P., Augustin, H. J., Rehpenning, W., Bartelheimer, H.: Osteopathien und Calcium-Phosphatstoffwechsel bei chronischer Hämodialyse. Klin. Wschr. **49**, 1971, 134–144

78. Kuhlencordt, F., Kruse, H.-P.: Was ist gesichert in der Therapie der Osteoporose und Osteomalacie? Internist **15**, 1974, 588–593

79. Lange, H., Gossmann, H. H.: Metastatische Verkalkungen während Peritonealdialyse im Terminalstadium einer chronischen Glomerulonephritis. Dtsch. med. Wschr. **92**, 1967, 296–300

80. Laubenthal, F., Reichenberger, M., Reinwein, D.: Vitamin-D-Intoxikation mit tödlichem Ausgang. Dtsch. med. Wschr. **100**, 1975, 412–415

81. Lawson, D. E. M., Faser, D. R., Kodicek, E., Morris, H. R., Williams, D. H.: Identification of 1,25-Dihydroxycholecalciferol, a New Kidney Hormone controlling Calcium Metabolism. Nature **230**, 1971, 228–230

82. Lefke, M., Sieberth, H. G., Firedmann, G.: Röntgenologische Veränderungen bei Calciumstoffwechselstörungen im Terminalstadium der Nierensinuffizienz. Dtsch. med. Wschr. **96**, 1971, 283–289

83. Litzow, J. R., Lemann, J., Jennon, E. J.: The Effect of Treatment of Acidosis on Calcium Balance in Patients with Chronic Azotemic Renal Disease. J. Clin. Invest. **46**, 1967, 280–286

84. Liu, S. H., Chu, H. I.: Studies of Calcium and Phosphorus Metabolism with Special Reference to Pathogenesis and Effects of Dihydrotachysterol. Medicine (Baltimore) **22**, 1943, 103–107

85. Lumb, G. A., Mawer, E. B., Stanbury, S. W.: The Apparent Vitamin D Resistance of Chronic Renal Failure. A Study of Physiology of Vitamin D in Man. Amer. J. Med. **50**, 1971, 421–441

86. Mallick, N. P., Berlyne, G. M.: Arterial Calcification after Vitamin-D Therapy in Hyperphosphataemic Renal Failure. Lancet **1968 II**, 1316–1320

87. Martin, D. L., Melancon, M. J., DeLuca, H. F.: Vitamin D Stimulated, Calcium-Depandent Adenosine Triphosphatase from Brush Borders of Rat Small Intestine. Bioch. Biophy. Res. Comm. **35**, 1969, 819–823

88. Mawer, E. B., Backhouse, J., Holman, C. A., Lumb, G. A., Stanbury, S. W.: The Distribution and Storage of Vitamin D and Its Metabolites in Human Tissues. Clin. Sci. **43**, 1972, 413–431

89. Mawer, E. B., Backhouse, J., Taylor, C. M., Lumb, G. A.: Failure of Formation of 1,25-Dihydroxycholecalciferol in Chronic Renal Insufficiency. Lancet **I 1973**, 626–631

90. Norman, A. W., Midgett, R. J., Myrtle, J. F., Nowicki, H. G.: Studies on Calciferol Metabolism. I. Production of Vitamin D Metabolit 4B from 25-OH-Cholecalciferol by Kidney Homogenates. Bioch. Biophy. Res. Comm. **42**, 1971, 1082–1087

91. Norman, A. W., Myrtle, J. F., Midgett, R. J., Nowicki, H. G.: 1,25-Dihydroxycholecalciferol: Identification of the Proposed Active Form of Vitamin D_3 in the Intestine. Sci. **173**, 1971, 51–54

92. Omdahl, J. L., Boyle, I. T., DeLuca, H. F.: Regulation of 25-Hydroxycholecalciferol Metabolism. Fed. Proc. **31**, 1972, 693–695

93. Omdahl, J. L., Holick, M., Suda, T., Tanaka, Y., DeLuca, H. F.: Biological Activity of 1,25-Dihydroxycholecalciferol. Biochemistry **10**, 1971, 2935–2940

94. Pak, Ch. Y. C., DeLuca, H. F., Chavez de Los Rios, J. M., Suda, T., Ruskin, B., Delea, C. S.: Treatment of Vitamin D-Resistant Hypoparathyroidism with 25-Hydroxycholecalciferol. Arch. Intern. Med. **126**, 1970, 239–247

95. Parfitt, A. M.: Soft-Tissue Calcification in Uremia. Arch. Intern. Med. **124**, 1969, 544–556

96. Parfitt, A. M.: Relation Between Parathyroid Cell Mass and Plasma Calcium Concentration in Normal and Uremic Subjects. Arch. Intern. Med. **124**, 1969, 269–273

97. Piazolo, P., Schleyer, M., Franz, H. E.: Das calciumbindende Protein in der menschlichen Darmschleimhaut bei Urämie. Klin. Wschr. **50**, 603–605 (1972)

98. PONCHON, G., DeLUCA, H. F.: The Role of the Liver in the Metabolism of Vitamin D. J. Clin. Invest. **48**, 1969, 1273–1279

99. PONCHON, G., KENNAN, A. L., DeLUCA, H. F.: Activation of Vitamin D by the Liver. J. Clin. Invest. **48**, 1969, 2032–2037

100. POTTS, J. T., REITZ, R. E., DEFTOS, L. J., KAYE, M., RICHARDSON, J. A., BUCKLE, R. M., AURBACH, G. D.: Secondary Hyperparathyroidism in Chronic Renal Disease. Arch. Intern. Med. **124**, 1969, 408–412

101. PUSCHETT, J. B., MORANZ, J., KURNICK, W. S.: Evidence for a Direct Action of Cholecalciferol and 25-Hydroxycholecalciferol on the Renal Transport of Phosphate, Sodium, and Calcium. J. Clin. Invest. **51**, 1972, 373–385

102. QUELLHORST, E., WILLMS, B., SCHELER, F.: Erfahrungen mit der intermittierenden Dialysebehandlung chronisch Nierenkranker. Verh. Dtsch. Ges. inn. Med. **72**, 1966, 407–411

103. RAISZ, L. G.: Physiologic and Pharmacologic Regulation of Bone Resorption. New Engl. J. Med. **282**, 1970, 909–913

104. RAISZ, L. G., TRUMMEL, C. L., HOLICK, M. F., DeLUCA, H. F.: 1,25-Dihydroxy-cholecalciferol. Sci. **175**, 1972, 768–769

105. RASMUSSEN, H., DeLUCA, H. F., ARNAUD, C., HAWKER, CH., von STEDINGH, M.: The Relationship Between Vitamin D and Parathyroid Hormone. J. Clin. Invest. **42**, 1963, 1940–1946

106. RASMUSSEN, H., WONG, M., BIKLE, D., GODDMAN, D. B. P.: Hormonal Control of the Renal Conversion of 25-Hydroxycholecalciferol to 1,25-Dihydroxycholecalciferol. J. Clin. Invest. **51**, 1972, 2502–2504

107. REISS, E., CANTERBURY, J. M., KANTER, A.: Circulating Parathyroid Hormone Concentration in Chronic Renal Insufficiency. Arch. Intern. Med. **124**, 1969, 417–422

108. RITZ, E.: Experimentelle Untersuchungen zum intestinalen Calciumtransport bei Urämie. Zschr. ges. exp. Med. **152**, 1970, 313–324

109. RITZ, E., ANDASSY, K., KREMPIEN, B.: Osteopathie bei Dauerdialyse. Med. Klin. **67**, 1972, 1132–1127

110. RITZ, E., KREMPIEN, B., ANDRASSY, K.: Niere und Knochensystem. Therapiewoche **28**, 1973, 2402–2403

111. RITZ, E., SIEBERTH, H. G., KREMPIEN, B.: Ca-Stoffwechselstörungen bei chronischer Niereninsuffizienz. Klin. Wschr. **49**, 1971, 1305–1314

112. ROTH, S. I., MARSHALL, R. B.: Pathology and Ultrastructure of the Human Parathyroid Glands in Chronic Renal Failure. Arch. Intern. Med. **124**, 1969, 397–407

113. RUSSEL, R. G. G. G., SMITH, R., WALTON, R. J., PRESTON, C., BASSON, R., HENDERSON, R. G., NORMAN, A. W.: 1,25-Dihydroxycholecalciferol and 1α'-Hydroxycholecalciferol in Hypoparathyroidism. Lancet II, 1974, 14–19

114. SCHAEFER, K., von HERRATH, D., KRAFT, D.: Vitamin D-Stoffwechsel und chronische Niereninsuffizienz. Dtsch. med. Wschr. **98**, 1973, 1338–1344

115. SCHAEFER, K., OPITZ, A.: Aktuelle Probleme azotämischer Knochenerkrankungen. Dtsch. med. Wschr. **95**, 1970, 84–88

116. SCHAEFER, K., OPITZ, A., STRATZ, R., KOCH, H.-U., von HERRATH, D.: Der Stoffwechsel von 25-hydroxycholecalciferol bei Gesunden und nephrektomierten Patienten. Dtsch. med. Wschr. **96**, 1971, 798–799

117. SCHAEFER, K., SCHAEFER, P., KOEPPE, P., OPITZ, A., HÖFFLER, D.: Untersuchungen zur Therapie der urämischen Osteopathie. Dtsch. med. Wschr. **94**, 1969, 70–72

118. SCHULZ, W., DELLING, G., SCHULZ, A., HEIDIER, R., GESSLER, U.: Vergleichende klinische und histomorphometrische Untersuchungen zum Ausmaß und zur Entwicklung der renalen Osteopathie. Nieren- und Hochdruckkrankheiten **1**, 1974, 169–174

119. SCHELLHORN, W.: „Kalkgicht" mit Nephrokalzinose, verursacht durch Langzeittherapie mit Dihydrotachysterin. Med. Klin. 1972, 1232–1237

120. SHERWOOD, L. M., HERRMANN, I., BASSET, C. A.: In Vitro Studies of Normal and Abnormal Parathyroid Tissue. Arch. Intern. Med. **124**, 1969, 426–430

121. SPANNAGEL, B., RITZ, E.: Intestinaler Ca-Transport bei experimenteller Urämie. Verh. Ges. Nephrologie 1970

122. STANBURY, S. W.: The Treatment of Renal Osteodystrophy. Ann. Intern. Med. **65**, 1966, 1133–1139

123. Stanbury, S. W.: Metabolic Studies of Renal Osteodystrophy. Medicine (Baltimore) 1962, **41**, 1–9

124. Stanbury, S. W., Lumb, G. A., Nicholson, W. F.: Elective subtotal parathyroidectomy for Renal Hyperparathyroidism. Lancet I, 1960, 793–798

125. Slatopolsky, E., Caglar, S., Pennell, J. P., Taggart, D. D., Canterbury, J. M., Reiss, E., Bricker, N. S.: On the Pathogenesis of Hyperparathyroidism in Chronic Experimental Renal Insufficiency in the Dog. J. Clin. Invest. **50**, 1971, 492–499

126. Suda, T., Hallick, R. B., DeLuca, H. F., Schnoes, H. K.: 25-Hydroxydihydro tachysterol. Synthesis and Biological Activity. Biochemistry **9**, 1970, 1651–1657

127. Tanaka, Y., Chen, T. C., DeLuca, H. F.: Dependence of 25-Hydroxycholecalciferol-Hydroxylase Regulation on RNA and Protein Synthesis. Arch. Biochem. Biophy. **152**, 1972, 291–298

128. Tanaka, Y., DeLuca, H. F.: Bone Mineral Mobilization Activity of 1,25-Dihydroxy-cholecalciferol, a Metabolite of Vitamin D. Arch. Biochem. Biophy. **146**, 1971, 574–578

129. Tanaka, Y., DeLuca, H. F., Omdahl, J., Holick, M. F.: Mechanism of Action of 1,25-Dihydroxycholecalciferol on Intestinal Calcium Transport. Proc. Nat. Acad. Sci. USA **68**, 1971, 1286–1288

130. Taylor, A. N., Wasserman, R. H.: Correlation between the Vitamin D-Induced Calcium Binding Protein and Intestinal Absorption of Calcium. Fed. Proc. **28**, 1969, 1834–1938

131. Terepka, A. R., Toribara, T. Y., Dewey, P. A.: The Ultrafiltrable Calcium of Human Serum. II. Variations in Disease States and under Experimental Conditions. J. Clin. Invest. **37**, 1958, 87–98

132. Trummel, C. L., Raisz, H. L., Blunt, J. W., DeLuca, H. F.: 25-Hydroxychole-calciferol: Stimulation of Bone Resorption in Tissue culture. Sci. **163**, 1969, 1450–1455

133. Tschöpe, W., Ritz, E., Bommer, J., Krempien, B., Andrassy, K., Mehls, O.: Wirbelkörperkollaps bei Dialyse-Osteopathie. Dtsch. med. Wschr. **98**, 1973 1471–1474

134. Wasserman, R. H., Taylor, A. N.: Die physiologische Bedeutung des Vitamin D-abhängigen calciumbindenden Proteins. Triangel **12**, 1974, 119–127

135. Wasserman, R. H., Taylor, A. N.: Evidence for a Vitamin D$_3$-Induced Calcium-Binding Protein in New World Primates. Proc. Soc. Exp. Biology Med. **136**, 1971, 25–28

136. Wong, R. G., Norman, A. W., Reddy, Ch. R., Coburn, J. W.: Biologic Effects of 1,25-Dihydroxycholecalciferol (a Highly Active Vitamin D Metabolite) in Actuely Uremic Rats. J. Clin. Invest. **51**, 1972, 1287–1291

137. Ziegler, R., Minne, H., Bellwinkel, S., Fröhlich, D.: Hypercalciämie-Syndrom und hypercalciämische Krise. Dtsch. med. Wschr. **98**, 1973, 276–283

138. Ziegler, R., Minne, H., Raue, F., Paar, G., Delling, G.: Beobachtungen zur Vitamin-D- und Dihydrotachysterin-Vergiftung. Dtsch. med. Wschr. **100**, 1975, 415–423

Section 7

1. Adamson, J. W., Eschbach, J., Finch, C. H.: The kidney and erythropoiesis. Am. J. Med. **44**, 725–733 (1968)

2. Alexanian, R.: Erythropoietin and erythropoiesis in anemic man following androgens. Blood **33**, 564–567 (1969)

3. Augustin, H. J., Kapoun, W., Kötter, C.: Der Einfluß von Testosteron auf die Anämie bei terminaler Niereninsuffizienz. Dtsch. med. Wschr. **98**, 2119–2122 (1973)

4. Babb, A. L., Popovich, R. P., Christopher, G. L., Scribner, B. H.: The genesis of the square-meter-hour hypothesis. Trans. Amer. Soc. Artif. Intern. Organs **17**, 81–89 (1971)

5. Becker, E.: Nierenkrankheiten. Bd. I. Jena: G. Fischer 1944

6. Blumberg, A.: Die renale Anämie. Bern-Stuttgart-Wien: Hans Huber 1972a

7. Blumberg, A.: Die Anämie bei chronischer Niereninsuffizienz. Schweiz. med. Wschr. **102**, 1044–1049 (1972b)

8. BLUMBERG, A., CHAPPIUS, L.: Die enterale Eisenresorption bei der chronischen Niereninsuffizienz unter Langzeit-Dialysebehandlung. Klin. Wschr. **49**, 41–46 (1971)
9. BOCK, H. E.: Die Blutarmut der Nierenkranken. Med. Welt **1**, 1–12 (1963)
10. BOCK, H. E., LÖHR, G. W., WALLER, H. D.: Beitrag zur Pathogenese der renalen Anämie. Schweiz. med. Wschr. **91**, 1213–1218 (1963)
11. BODDY, K., LAWSON, D. H., LINTON, A. L., WILL, G.: Iron metabolism in patients with chronic renal failure. Clin. Sci. **39**, 115–118 (1970)
12. BRIGHT, R.: Guy's Hospital Report **1**, 338 (1835)
13. BROWN, R.: Plasma erythropoietin in chronic uremia. Brit. Med. J. **2**, 1036–1039 (1965)
14. BÜCHNER, F.: Spezielle Pathologie Band II, p. 30. München: Urban & Schwarzenberg 1974
15. CARNOT, M. P., DEFLANDRE, C.: Sur l'activité hémopoiétique des différents organes au cours de la régénération du sang. C. R. Acad. Sci. Paris **143**, 432–435 (1906)
16. CONTRERA, J. F., GORDON, A. S.: The renal erythropoietic factor. Studies on its purification and properties. Ann. N.Y. Acad. Sci. **149**, 114–119 (1968)
17. CONTRERA, J. F., GORDON, A. S., WEINTRAUB, A. H.: Extraction of an erythropoietin producing factir from a particulate fraction of rat kidney. Blood **28**, 330–343 (1966)
18. DENNY, W. F., FLANIGAN, W. J., ZUKOWSKI, F.: Serial erythropoietin studies in patients undergoing renal homotransplantation. J. Lab. Clin. Med. **67**, 386–389 (1964)
19. DESFORGES, J. F., DAWSON, J. P.: The anemia of renal failure. Arch. Intern. Med. **101**, 326–332 (1958)
20. DOMBUK, D. H., LINDHOLM, D. D., UISHITA, J. A.: Lipid metabolism in uremia and the effects of dialysate glucose and oral androgen therapy. Trans. Amer. Soc. Artif. Intern. Organs **19**, 150–153 (1973)
21. VAN DYKE, D., POLLYCOVE, M., LAURENCE, J. H.: Erythropoietin therapy in the renoprival patient. In: Semi-annual report. Biology and Medicine, Donner Laboratory and Donner Pavilion, Lawrence Radiation Laboratory, p. 127. 1967
22. EDWARDS, M. S., PEGRUM, G. D., CURTIS, J. R.: Iron therapy in patients on maintenance hemodialysis. Lancet II, 1970, 491–493
23. ERSLEV, A. J.: Humoral regulation of red cell production. Blood **8**, 349–357 (1953)
24. ERSLEV, A. J.: Erythropoietic function in uremic rabbits. Arch. Intern. Med. **101**, 407–417 (1958)
25. ERSLEV, A. J.: Erythropoetic function of the kidney. In: Wessen, Physiology of the human kidney, pp 521–534 Grune & Stratton New York: 1969
26. ERSLEV, A. J.: Management of the anemia of chronic renal failure. Clin. Nephrology **2**, 174–178 (1974)
27. ERSLEV, A. J., KAZAL, L. A.: Renal erythropoietic factor. Lack of effect on hypertransfused mice. Blood **34**, 222–225 (1969)
28. ESCHBACH, J. W., ADAMSON, J..W.: Improvement in the anemia of chronic renal failure with fluoxymesterone. Arch. Intern. Med. **78**, 527–534 (1973)
29. ESCHBACH, J. W., COOK, J. D., FINCH, C. A.: Iron absorption in chronic renal disease. Clin. Sci. **38**, 191–196 (1970)
30. ESCHBACH, J. W., FINCH, C. H.: Anemia and hemodialysis. Proc. Fifth Internat. Congr. Nephrol. Stockholm, 1968, p. 165–175
31. ESCHBACH, J. W., FUNK, D., ADAMSON, J., KUHN, J., SCRIBNER, B. H., FINCH, C. A.: Erythropoiesis in patients with renal failure undergoing chronic dialysis. New Engl. J. Med. **276**, 653–658 (1967)
32. ESCHBACH, J. W., ADAMSON, J. W., COOK, J. D.: Disorders of red blood cell production in uremia. Arch. Intern. Med. **126**, 812–815 (1970)
33. ESPADA, J., LANGTON, A. A., DORADO, M.: Human erythropoietin. Studies on purity and partial characterization. Biochem. Biophys. Acta **285**, 427–433 (1972)
34. ESSERS, U.: Habilitationsschrift Aachen 1972
35. ESSERS, U., BRASS, A., SPICKER, K.: Die aplastische Anämie bei Niereninsuffizienz — eine inhibitorische Wirkung des Urämieserums auf Erythropoietin? Klin. Wschr. **48**, 92–95 (1970)
36. FISHER, J. W., HATCH, F. E., ROH, B. L., ALLESS, R. C., KELLEY, B. J.: Erythropoietin inhibitor in kidney extracts and plasma from anemic uremic human subjects. Blood **31**, 440–452 (1968)

37. Fried, W., Jonasson, O., Lang, C., Schwartz, F.: The hematologic effect of androgen in uremic patients. Ann. Intern. Med. **79**, 823–827 (1973)

38. Fried, W., Kilbridge, T.: Effect of testosterone and of cobalt on erythropoietin production by anephric rats. J. Lab. Clin. Med. **74**, 623–628 (1969)

39. Fried, W., Kilbridge, T., Krantz, S., McDonald, T. P., Lange, R. D.: Studies on extrarenal erythropoietin. J. Lab. Clin. Med. **73**, 244–248 (1969)

40. Gallagher, N. J., McCarthy, J. M., Lange, R. D.: Erythropoietin production in uremic rabbits. J. Lab. Clin. Med. **57**, 281–289 (1961)

41. Giordano, C., DeSanto, N. G., Rinaldi, S., Acove, D., Esposito, E., Gallo, B.: Histidine supplements in the treatment if uremic anemia. Proc. 10th Congr. Europ. Dialysis and Transplanation Assoc. Vienna, 1973, p. 160

42. Giovanetti, S., Giagnoni, P., Balestri, P. L., et al.: Red cell survival in chronic uremia: Its relationship with the spontaneous in vitro autohemolysis and with the degree of anemia. Experientia **27**, 739–741 (1966)

43. Gordon, A. S., Cooper, G. W., Zanjani, E. D.: The kidney and erythropoiesis. Sem. Haematol. **4**, 337–358 (1969)

44. Gordon, A. S., Zanjani, E. D.: Biogenesis of erythropoietin. Proc. Symposion Erythropoieticum, Prague, 1970

45. de Gowin, R. L., Lavender, A. R., Forland, M., Charleston, D., Gottschalk, A.: Erythropoiesis and erythropoietin in patients with chronic renal failure treated with hemodialysis and testosterone. Ann. Int. Med. **72**, 913–918 (1970)

46. Gray, S. J., Sterling, K.: The tagging of red cells and plasma proteins with radioactive chromium. J. Clin. Invest. **29**, 1604–1907 (1950)

47. Hampers, L., Streiff, R., Nathan, D. G., et al.: Megaloblastic hematopoiesis in uremia and in patients on longterm hemodialysis. New Engl. J. Med. **276**, 551–554 (1967)

48. Heilmann, E.: Das Verhalten des Erythropoietinspiegels im Serum bei verschiedenen Nierenerkrankungen. Verh. dtsch. Ges. inn. Med. **79**, 451–453 (1973)

49. Heilmann, E., Loew, H., Schullenbach, U.: Zur Frage der hämolytischen Komponente der Anämie bei Hämodialyse-Patienten. Kongreßbericht d. Ges. f. inn. Med., Hamburg, 1974a

50. Heilmann, E., Cicinnati, C., Müller, H.: Erythropoietin in polycythemic mice and dialysed patients treated with androgens. Kongreßber. Internat. Nephrologen-Kongreß, Vittel, 1974b

51. Heilmann, E.: Beziehungen zwischen Eisenbindungskapazität und den Eisenreserven im Knochenmark bei Dauerdialyse-Patienten. Ninth Symposion Ges. f. Nephrologie, Basel, 1973

52. Heilmann, E., Michael, C., Loew, H., Müller, H.: Untersuchungen zur Diagnose und Therapie des Eisenmangels bei Dauerdialyse-Patienten. Verh. dtsch. Ges. inn. Med. **80**, 679–681 1974c)

53. Hoffmann, G, G.: Human erythropoiesis following kidney transplantation. Ann. N.Y. Acad. Sci. **149**, 504–506 (1968)

54. Hughes-Jones, N. C., Mollison, P. C.: The interpretation of measurements with ^{51}Cr-labelled red cells. Clin. Sci. **15**, 207–212 (1956)

55. Hurst, G. A., Chanutin, A.: Organic phosphate compounds of erythrocytes from individuals with uremia. J. Lab. Clin. Med. **64**, 675–678 (1964)

56. Hyde, S. E., Sattler, J. H.: Red blood cell destruction in hemodialysis. Trans. Am. Soc. Artif. Int. Organs **15**, 50–52 (1969)

57. Jacobson, L. O., Goldwasser, E., Fried, W., Plzak, L. F.: Studies on erythropoiesis VII: The role of the kidney in the production of erythropoietin. Trans. A. Am. Physicians **70**, 633–634 (1957)

58. Johnson, F. L., Fengler, J. R., Lerner, K. G., Majerus, P. W., Siegel, M., Hartmann, J. R., Thomas, E. D.: Association of androgenic-anabolic steroid therapy with development of hepato-cellular carcinoma. Lancet **II**, 1273–1278 (1972)

59. Joist, J. H., Heller, A., Küttringhaus, U., et al.: Zur Frage der Entwicklung und Bedeutung eines Folsäuremangels bei fortgeschrittener chronischer Niereninsuffizienz. Klin. Wschr. **47**, 861–864 (1969)

60. Joske, R. A., McAlister, J. M., Polenkerd, T. A. J.: Isotope investigations of red cell production and destruction in chronic renal disease. Clin. Sci. **15**, 511–522 (1956)

61. Kasanen, A., Kallimaki, J. L.: Correlation of some kidney function tests with hemoglobin in chronic nephropathies. Acta med. Scand. **158**, 213–215 (1957)

62. Kaye, M.: The anemia assaciated with renal disease. J. Lab. Clin. Med. **52**, 83–100 (1958)

63. Keller, H. M.: Veränderungen der Erythrocyten und der roten Blutbildung bei Nierenkrankheiten. Handb. d. Inn. Medizin, 5. Aufl., Bd. VIII/2, p. 169 (1968)

64. Koch, K. M., Patyna, W. D., Shalden, S., Werner, E.: Anemia of the regular hemodialysis patient and its treatment. Nephron **12**, 405–419 (1974)

65. Koch, K. M., Werner, E., Patyna, W. D., Kaltwasser, P.: Die intestinale Eisen-adsorption bei fortgeschrittener Niereninsuffizienz. Der Einfluß der Hämodialyse-Behandlung. (In press)

66. Kraft, D., Freund, D., Karow, J.: Die Wirkung von Mesterolon auf die Erythro-poese chronisch hämodialysierter Patienten. Dtsch. med. Wschr. **99**, 1119–1125 (1974)

67. Kuroyanagi T.: Anemia associated with chronic renal failure with special reference to kinetics of erythron. Acta haematol. Jap. **24**, 48–67 (1961)

68. Lasker, N., Harvey, A., Baker, H.: Vitamin levels in hemodialysis and intermittent peritoneal dialysis. Trans. Amer. Soc. Artif. Intern. Organs **9**, 51–55 (1963)

69. Lindholm, D. D., Fisher, J. W., Vihira, J. A., Dombeck, D. H., Bonal, G., Lerthora, J.: Clinical effect of oral fluoxymesterone in patients with dialysis-controlled uremia. Trans. Amer. Soc. Artif. Intern. Organs **19**, 475–483 (1973)

70. Mackenzie, J. C., Ford, J. E., Waters, A. H., *et al.*: Erythropoiesis in patients undergoing regular dialysis treatment without transfusion. Proc. Europ. Dial. Transl. Ass. **5**, 172–175 (1968)

71. Maggiore, Q., Navalesi, R., Biagini, M., Balestri, P. L., Giagnoni, P.: Com-parative studies on uremic anemia in polycystic kidney disease and in other renal diseases. Proc. Europ. Dial. Transpl. Ass. **5**, 264–266 (1967)

72. Mertz, D. P., Koschnik, R.: Nephrogene Anämie und Nierenhämodynamik. Schweiz. med. Wschr. **95**, 83–88 (1965)

73. Mirand, E. A.: Extrarenal and renal control of erythropoietin production. Ann. N.Y. Acad. Sci. **149**, 94–96 (1968)

74. Mirand, A. E., Murphy, G. P., Steeves, R. A., *et al*: Erythropoietin activity in anephric, allotransplanted, unilaterally nephrectomiced, and intact man. J. Lab. Clin. Med. **73**, 121–128 (1969)

75. Mirand, E. A., Murphy, G. P., Steeves, R. A., Weber, H. W., Retief, F. P.: Extrarenal production of erythopoietin in man. Acta haemotol. **39**, 359–365 (1963)

76. Mirand, E. A., Prentice, T. C.: Presence of plasma erythropoietin in hypoxic rats with or without kidneys or spleen. Proc. Soc. Exper. Biol. Med. **96**, 49–51 (1957)

77. Morgan, J. M., Morgan, R. E.: Study of the effect of uremic metabolites on erythro-cyte glycolysis. Metabolism **13**, 629–632 (1964)

78. Murphy, G. P., Mirand, E. A., Kenny, G. M.: Renal and extrarenal erythropoietin in man. N.Y. State J. Med. **69**, 2007–2011 (1969)

79. Murphy, G. P., Mirand, E. A., Grace, J. T.: Erythropoietin activity in anephric ar renal allotransplanted man. Am. Surg. **170**, 581–583 (1969b)

80. Naets, J. P.: The role of the kidney in erythropoiesids. J. clin. Invest. **39**, 102–110 (1960)

81. Nathan, D. G., Beck, L. H., Hampers, C. G.: Erythrocyte production and meta-bolism in anephric and uremic man. Ann. N.Y. Acad. Sci. **149**, 539–543 (1968)

82. Neff, S. M., Kim, K. E., Persoff, M., Onesti, G., Swartz, C.: Hemodynamics of uremic anemia. Circulation **43**, 866–883 (1971)

83. Polesky, H. F., McCullough, J., Helgeson, M. A., Nelson, C.: Evaluation of methods for preparation of HLA-antigen poor blood. Transfusion **13**, 383–38 5(1973)

84. Prankerd, R. A. J.: The role of red cell enzymes in hemolysis. Brit. J. Haematol. **7**, 405–407 (1961)

85. Reissmann, C. R.: Studies on the mechanism of erythropoietic stimulation in para-biotic rats during hypoxia. Blood **5**, 372–380 (1950)

86. Reissmann, K. R., Nomura, T., Gunn, W. R., *et al.*: Erythropoietic response to anemia or erythropoietin injections in uremic rats. Blood **16**, 1411–1423 (1960)

87. Renner, H. D.: Zellstoffwechselstörungen bei Urämie. Habilitationsschrift, Aachen, 1968

88. RICHARDSON, J. R., jr., WEINSTEIN, M. B.: Erythropoietic response of dialysed patients to testosterone administration. Ann. Intern. Med. **73**, 403–407 (1970)

89. SASS, M. D., VORSANGER, E., SPEAR, P. W.: Enzyme activity as an indicator of red cell age. Clin. Chim. Acta (Amsterd.) **10**, 21–23 (1964)

90. SCRIBNER, B. H., BURRI, R., CONES, J.E. Z., *et al.*: The treatment of chronic uremia by means of intermittent hemodialysis: a preliminary report. Trans. Amer. Soc. Artif. Intern. Organs **6**, 114–119 (1960)

91. SHAHIDI, N. T.: Androgens and erythropoiesis. New Engl. J. Med. **289**, 72–80 (1973)

92. SHALDON, S., KOCH, K. M., OPPERMANN, F., PATYNA, W. D., SCHOEPPE, W.: Testosterone therapy for anemia: 25 patients in maintenance dialysis. Brit. Med. J. **3**, 212–215 (1971a)

93. SHALDON, S., PATYNA, W. D., KALTWASSER, P., WERNER, E., KOCH, K. M., SCHOEPPE, W. E.: The use of testosterone in bilateral nephrectomized dialysis patients. Trans. Amer. Soc. Artif. Intern. Organs **17**, 104–107 (1971b)

94. SHAW, A. B.: Hemolysis in chronic renal failure. Brit. Med. J. **II**, 213–216 (1967)

95. SILL, V., LANSER, K. G., BAUDITZ, W.: Einfluß der Anämie auf die körperliche Leistungsfähigkeit von Dauerdialyse-Patienten. Z. Kardiol. **62**, 164–175 (1973)

96. STEWART, J. H.: Hemolytic anemia in acute and chronic renal failure. Quart. J. Med. **36**, 85–105 (1967)

97. VOLHARD, F.: Die doppelseitigen hämatogenen Nierenerkrankungen. In: Handbuch d. Inn. Medizin, 2. Aufl. Berlin: Springer 1931

98. WERNER, E., FINK-ROSSKAMP, P., OPPERMANN, F., PATYNA, W. D., KOCH, K. M., SCHOEPPE, W.: Die Bestimmung des individuellen Gesamtblutverlustes bei der chronischen Hämodialyse als Grundlage für die optimale Eisensubstitution. Tenth Intern. Jahrestagg d. Ges. Nuklearmedizin, Freiburg, 1972

99. WHITEHEAD, V. M., COMPTY, C. H., POSER, G. A., *et al.*: Homeostasis of folic acid in patients undergoing maintenance hemodialysis. New Engl. J. Med. **279**, 970–974 (1968)

100. YPERSELE DE STRITOU, C. van, VANDENBROUCKE, J. N., STRAGIER, A.: Anemia in maintenance hemodialysis. Klin. Nephrologie **1**, 2/I, p. 26–33 (1972)

101. ZANJANI, E. D., CONTRERA, J. F., GORDON, A. S., COOPER, G. W., WONG, K. K., KATZ, R.: The renal erythropoietic factor (REF) III. Enzymatic role in erythropoietin production. Proc. Soc. Exper. Biol. New York **125**, 505–508 (1967)

Subject Index

The numbers set in *italics* refer to those pages on which the respective catch-word is discussed in detail

accelerated serum sickness 14
acidosis, renal 247, 253
acroosteolysis 253
active serum sickness *14*, 18
acute exsudative proliferative glomerulo-
    nephritis 73
— glomerulonephritis *46*, 48, 50, *52*, 53,
    54, 58, *69*, 96, 164
— —, diffuse 48, 52
— —, "elapsed" 52
— lipid nephrosis *49*
— poststreptococcal nephritis 70, 71, 72
— proliferative glomerulonephritis *118*,
    121, 131
— renal failure 162, 164, 165, 170, 176,
    177, 178, 182, 183, 184, 188, 190, 192,
    193, 196, 197
— serum sickness 2, 3, 26
— — — nephritis 3, 4, *14*, 30, 174
aldosterone effect, renal 230
— secretion 216, 228, 230
Aleutian disease virus 21
— mink disease 21, 28, 138
alkaline phosphatase level 254
allergic vasculitis 183
Alport's syndrome 98, *131*
aluminium hydroxide 252, 253, 254
amines, vasoactive 26
aminonucleoside nephrosis in rats 110
amyloidosis 53, *91*, 94
anaphylactoid purpura *91*, 130
androgens 264
anemia 240, 241, *256*
—, renal, treatment *262*
angiitis, necrotizing 14
—, systemic 21
angiotensin I 216, 221
angiotensin II 204, 206, 207, 208, 209,
    214, 216, 218, 220, 221, 222, 223, 224,
    225, 226, 227, 230
— analogues 218, 225, 226, 229
— antagonists 204, 209, 218, 219, 225,
    226, 228, 229, 230
— antibodies 204, 226
— inhibitors 207, 211, 218, 226

angiotensinogen 216
antibodies, autologous 7, 12
—, nephrotoxic 61
anticoagulant treatment 12, 25
anti-GBM antibodies 3
antigen-antibody complexes 2, 3, 4, 14,
    17, 22, 23, 26, 27, 28, 29, 30, 34
— — interaction 2, 3, 25, 31, 34
— — reaction 187
antikidney sera 2
antisera, fluorochrome-labeled *63*
antitissue sera, heterologous 3
arteriosclerotic induration 45
arthritis, uremic 253
Arthus type inflammation 29
atherosclerosis 240, 243
ATP'ase, calcium dependent 250
atrophic glomerulonephritis, chronic 54
autologous antibodies 7, 12
— anti-GBM antibodies 12
— (second) phase of Masugi nephritis
    2, 3, *7*, 11, 25, 32, 33
axon degeneration 245
azathioprine 157, 162, 170, 173, 175, 176,
    178, 179, 184, 186, 190, 191, 195
azoospermia in chronic uremia 246
azotemia 248, 256, 257
azotemic hyperparathyroidism 246
— osteomalacia 246

benign recurrent hematusia 130
Berger's disease 129
bilirubin, indirect 257
blood coagulability, pathologic 240
bone disease, renal, clinical syndrome
    253
— —, —, roentgenological appearance
    253
— —, —, therapy *254*
— — in chronic uremia *246*
— — under chronic hemodialysis
    treatment *252*
— mineralization, disturbed 246, 248
— resorption 247
bovine serum albumin (BSA) 3, 15, 16, 18

"Bright's disease" 45
BSA = bovine serum albumin 3, 15, 16, 18

calcifications, metastatic 253
calcium absorption 248
— —, intestinal 248, 249, 250, 251, 254, 255
— gluconate 255
— metabolism 252
— mobilization from the bone 248, 251, 252
capillary thrombosis 129
capsulitis, proliferative 48
carbohydrate intolerance in chronic uremia 243
carbon tetrachloride 143
cardiac hypertrophy 203
cardiomyopathy 241, 243
cardiovascular alterations in chronic uremia 240
catecholamines 221
catecholamine secretion 216
cholesterol 243, 244
chorionic gonadotropin 246
chronic atrophic glomerulonephritis 54
— glomerulonephritis 46, 47, 50, 52, 53, 54, 58, 115, 131
— — diffuse 48, 52
— —, "smooth type" 47, 50
— — with granulation 47, 50
— — without granulation 47, 50
— hog cholera 23
— indurative nephritis 45
— lobular glomerulonephritis 54
— mixed glomerulonephritis 54
— nephritis without induration 45
— parenchymatous nephritis 45
— sclerosing glomerulonephritis 52, 54, 57
— serum sickness 2, 21, 27
— — — nephritis 18, 20, 28
— uremia and anemia 256
— — and bone disease 246
— — and carbohydrate metabolism 243
— — and cardiovascular system 240
— — and fat metabolism 243
— — and gonadal dysfunction 246
— — and polyneuropathy 245
complement 3, 5, 7, 14, 21, 24, 25, 26, 29, 70, 83, 89, 91, 117, 171
— activation 75
— deficient animals 10
— fixation 7, 25
— sequence 75
congenital syphilis 48, 117
Coxsackie virus B 95
crescent formation 12, 17, 22, 23, 31, 32, 33, 46, 48, 49, 52, 54, 55, 57, 58, 66, 93, 111, 115, 118, 123, 124, 130, 181, 193

crescentic glomerulonephritis 66
crescents, diffuse 158, 182, 188
—, focal 158, 181, 183, 188, 193
cross-reacting antibodies 3
cryoglobulins 95
cyclophosphamide therapy 176
cytotoxic effect 95
— therapy 157, 159, 160, 164, 168, 169, 171, 172, 176, 178, 179, 182, 187, 190, 191, 197

degenerative glomerulonephritis 18
demyelinisation, segmental 245
dense-deposit disease 78, 126
diabetes mellitus 53, 117, 243
diabetic glomerulosclerosis 69, 98
diacetylbenzidine 111
diffuse endocapillary glomerulonephritis 56, 58
— glomerulonephritis, acute 48, 52
— —, chronic 48, 52
dihydrotachysterol 255, 256
dihydroxycholecalciferol 248, 249, 250, 251, 255
direct immunofluorescence 64
disseminated intravascular coagulation 140
duck NTAbs 8, 9, 10, 11, 25

"elapsed" acute glomerulonephritis 52
Ellis' types of glomerulonephritis 49
embolic glomerulonephritis, focal 130
embolism type of glomerulonephritis 48
endocapillary glomerulonephritis 56, 58, 158, 172, 178, 188, 190, 191, 193, 195, 196
— proliferative glomerulitis 51
— — glomerulonephritis 69
endocarditis 48, 130, 131, 164
end-stage glomerulonephritis 54
epithelioid cells 7, 9, 30
erythrocytic enzymes 257, 258
erythropoiesis 256, 257
— defect 264
erythropoietin 257, 261, 264
— activity 264
— inhibitors 261
— production 264
ethionine 143
experimental radiation nephritis 111
extracapillary glomerulonephritis 47, 50, 51, 54, 56, 57, 66, 121
— proliferative glomerulitis 51
extracellular volume 208, 211, 222
extramembranous glomerulonephritis 82, 166
— —, chronic 70
exudative glomerulonephritis 48, 54, 56, 57, 59, 73

family nephropathies 53
fat metabolism in chronic uremia 243
fibrinolytic activity 31
fibrosis, focal 86
—, global 86
first phase of Masugi nephritis 2, 3, 4,
  5, 8, 12, 24, 29, 31
fluorescein isothiocyanate 63
fluorescence microscopy 8, 18, 22, 24, 65
fluorescent antibody method 3
fluorine 255
— intoxication 252
fluorochrome-labeled antisera 63
focal fibrosis 86
— glomerular sclerosis 110, 111, 115,
  122, 123
— embolic glomerulonephritis 130
— glomerulitis 53
— glomerulonephritis 50, 53, 55, 56, 57,
  126
— —, types (Churg) 54
— glomerulosclerosis 55, 56
— hyalinosis 56, 86
— necrotizing glomerulonephritis 129
— nephritis 47, 51, 53, 58, 59
— —, glomerular 53
— proliferative glomerulonephritis 127
— — — with IgA 75
— sclerosing glomerulonephritis 131,
  158, 162, 188, 189, 191, 192, 195, 196,
  197
— sclerosis 48, 58, 86
— segmental sclerosing glomerulonephritis
  57, 86
— — sclerosis 86
— suppurative glomerulonephritis 127
folic acid 256, 260, 263, 264
foreign serum 2
— — antigen 2
Freund's adjuvant 3, 12, 13, 20
furosemide (Lasix) 204, 205, 211, 212,
  213, 215, 219, 229
— diuresis 206, 211, 215, 220, 223,
  227, 230

giant cells 9, 30
global fibrosis 86
glomerular basement membrane antigens
  12
— — —, glycoprotein antigen 14
— — —, rupture 9, 12, 33
— focal nephritis 53
— sclerosis, focal 110, 111, 115, 122,
  123
glomerulitis, endocapillary proliferative
  51
—, extracapillary proliferative 51
—, focal 53
—, lobular 51
—, membranoproliferative 54

glomerulonephritis, acute 46, 48, 50,
  52, 53, 54, 58, 69, 96, 164
—, — diffuse 48, 52
—, —, "elapsed" 52
—, — exsudative proliferative 73
—, — membranous 160
—, — proliferative 118, 121, 131
—, chronic 18, 46, 47, 50, 52, 53, 54,
  58, 115, 131
—, — atrophic 54
—, — diffuse 48, 52
—, —, extramembranous 70
—, — lobular 54
—, — mixed 54
—, — sclerosing 52, 54, 57
—, —, "smooth type" 47, 50
—, —, with granulation 47, 50
—, —, without granulation 47, 50
—, crescentic 66
—, classification of Bohle 51, 57
—, — of Cameron 55
—, — of Earle 53
—, — of Fahr 49
—, — of Glyda 54
—, — of Habib 50, 53
—, — of Heptinstall 53
—, — of Kincaid-Smith 55
—, — of Kinoshita 52
—, — of Thoenes 56
—, — of Zollinger 52, 57, 58
—, degenerative 18
—, diffuse endocapillary 56, 58
—, — mesangiocapillary 56
—, — proliferative 131
—, Ellis' types 49
—, embolism type 48
—, endocapillary 158, 172, 178, 188,
  189, 190, 193, 195, 196
—, — proliferative 69
—, extracapillary type 47, 50, 51, 54,
  56, 57, 66, 121
—, extramembranous 82, 166
—, exudative type 48, 54, 56, 57, 59, 73
—, focal 50, 53, 55, 56, 57, 126
—, — embolic 130
—, — necrotizing 129
—, — proliferative 75, 127
—, — sclerosing 131, 158, 162, 188,
  189, 191, 192, 195, 196, 197
—, — segmental sclerosing 57, 86
—, — suppurative 127
—, —, types (Churg) 54
—, hemorrhagic type 48
—, hypocomplementemic 124
—, — persistent 78
—, IgA mesangioproliferative 75
—, immunologically induced 5
—, intracapillary type 47, 50, 56, 57, 66
—, —, minimal proliferative 160
—, lobular 54, 59, 78, 124

glomerulonephritis, membranoproliferative
  56, 57, 58, 73, *78*, 91, *124*, 158, *170*,
  188, 189, 192, 193, 195, 196, 197
—, membranous   19, 20, 27, 51, 53, 55,
  56, 57, *82*, *113*, 166
—, mesangial   121
—, mesangiocapillary   *78*, 124, 131, 136,
  138
—, mesangioproliferative   54, 57, 58, *69*,
  75, 158, 159, *176*, 188, 189, 190, 192,
  193, 195, 196
—, —, with diffuse crescents   158, 192,
  195, 196
—, —, with focal crescents   158, *181*,
  192, 193, 195, 196, 197
—, minimal proliferative intercapillary
  160
—, mixed membranous   *78*
—, necrotizing   56, 57, 58, *66*, 131, 158,
  182, *186*, 188, 189, 190, 192, 194
—, peracute   50, 51, *182*
—, perimembranous   158, *166*, 171, 188,
  189, 192, 195, 196, 197
—, postacute   50, 51
—, postinfectious   *69*, 80
—, poststreptococcal   16, 34, 53, 57, 58,
  69, 75, 80, 96, 120, 121, 122, 123, 158,
  159, 177, 178, 179, 181, 185, 189, 190
—, progressive   *30*
—, proliferative   2, 14, 17, 18, 23, 27, 28,
  48, 51, 53, 54, 55, 56, 70, 73, 131
—, —, acute   54
—, —, chronic   54
—, —, sclerosing   56
—. rapidly progressive   53, 54, 56, *66*, 70,
  121, *181*, *182*, 190, 193, 195, 196, 197
—, recurrent   95
—, "resolving"   *69*, 75
—, sclerosing   52, 54, 57
—, subacute   *46*, *49*, 50, 52, 54, *66*, *182*
—, — diffuse   52, 58
—, subchronic   *47*, 50, 52, *176*
— associated with infection   *21*
— and viral infections   *23*
— in Aleutian disease of mink   21
— in mice   *22*
— in plasmodium infection   23
— of mixed membranous-proliferative
  type   53
— of several days duration   46
— — — weeks' or months duration   46
— of systemic diseases   *133*
glomerulonephropathy, idiopathic membranous   *82*
glomerulopathy, focal segmental sclerosing
  86
glomerulosclerosis, diabetic   69, 98
—, focal   55, 56
—, hepatic   126
glucose assimilation   243

glycine   110
Goldblatt hypertension   203, 208, 209,
  210, 211, 222
gonadal dysfunction in chronic uremia
  246
gonadotropin, chorionic   246
Goodpasture's syndrome   56, 66, 67, 68,
  69, 70, 95, 122, 123, 131, 183, 184, 186
guanidine   257, 258

Habu snake poisoning   31, 32
hematocrit   206, 208, 211, 212, 220, 241,
  242, 256, 261, 262, 263, 264
hematopoietin   261
hematuria, benign recurrent   130
—, recurrent   *75*
hemodialysis treatment, intermittent
  239
hemolysis   256, 257, 262
hemolytic uremic syndrome   126, *138*
hemorrhagic type of glomerulonephritis
  48
hemosiderosis   263
heparin   240, 252
— therapy   184, 185, 187, 190, 191, 195
hepatic glomerulosclerosis   126, *142*
hepatitis, acute viral   142
— antigen   64, 95
hepatocellular carcinoma   264
"hereditary nephritis"   98, *131*
herpes virus   146
heterologous (first) phase of Masugi
— utilization, pathologic   240
  nephritis   2, 3, 4, *5*, 8, 12, 24, 29, 31
Heymann nephritis   *20*, 28, 83, 118
histidine   263
hog cholera, chronic   23
homologous antibodies   25
host antibody   7, 14
hyalinosis, focal   54, 56, *86*
—, segmental   55, 56
hydroxylysine   110
hydroxyproline   110
hypercalcemia   252, 256
— syndrome   255
hyperlipemia   240, *243*, 264
hyperparathyroidism   246, 254
—, azotemic   246
—, hypocalcemic   251
—, primary   250
—, secondary   240, 256
hyperphosphatemia   *247*, 251, 256
hyperphosphatemia   *247*, 251, 256
hyperplasia of the parathyroid gland
  251
hypertension   48, 49, 52, 118, 124, 140,
  157, 159, 162, 164, 169, 170, 172, 177,
  180, 188, 190, 192, *193*, 194, 195, 196,
  197, *203*, *240*, 264
—, malignant   140, 179, 241

hypertriglyceridemia 243, 244, 245
hypertrophy, cardiac 203
hyperuricemia 243
hypocalcemia 247
hypocalcemic hyperparathyroidism 251
hypocomplementemia 171
hypocomplementemic glomerulonephritis
  124
— persistent glomerulonephritis *78*
hypogonadism in chronic uremia *246*
hypophosphatemia 249, 255

idiopathic membranous glomerulonephropathy *82*
IgA-IgG mesangial nephropathy *75*
IgA mesangioproliferative glomerulonephritis *75*
— nephropathy *128*, 130
immunofluorescence 3, 14, 18, 21, 62, 63,
  64
— microscopy 120
—, technique *63*, 186
immunsuppressive therapy *157*, 159,
  160, 164, 168, 171, 172, 176, 178, 179,
  182, 187, 197
indirect bilirubin 257
indomethacin therapy 157, 158, 160,
  161, 164, 165, 168, 171, 172, 178, 179,
  187, 190, 191, 197
induration, arteriosclerotic 45
initial phase of Masugi nephritis 2, 3, 4,
  5, 8, 12, 24, 29, 31
insulin level 243
— resistance in uremia 243
interstitial nephritis 46
— —, acute 58
— —, chronic 58
intestinal calcium absorption 248, 249,
  250, 251, 254, 255
intracapillary type of glomerulonephritis
  47, 50, 56, 57
intravascular coagulation 25, 26, 31
— thrombosis 130, 139
iron binding capacity, total 263
— deficiency 258, 259, 260, 263
— substitution 263
ischemic nephritis 48

juxtaglomerular apparatus 214, 215,
  224, 230
— index 214, 221

kidney antigens 2
— —, heterologous 2
— —, homologous 2

lactate-dehydrogenase 257
LE cell phenomenon 21, 22
lipoid nephrosis *49*, 86, *108*, *160*, 162
liver cirrhosis 142

— damage, toxic 142
lobular glomerulitis 51
— glomerulonephritis 54, 59, *78*, *124*
— —, chronic 54
Looser's zones 253
loss of hearing in chronic uremia 245
lupus erythematosus 21, 22, 53, 56, 82,
  90, 93, 95, 115, 117, 118, 122, 126, 131,
  133, 171, 181
lupus-like nephritis 2, 21
luteotropic hormones 246
lymphocytic choriomeningitis virus 23

macroglobulinemia Waldenström 82
macula densa 123
magnesium 252
— concentration in the serum 251
malaria 95
malarial antigen 24
malignant hypertension 140, 179
— nephrosclerosis 68, 98
Masugi nephritis 2, 3, 4, *5*, 17, 24, 29,
  31, 33, 124
— —, first phase (initial phase) 2, 3, 4,
  5, 8, 12, 24, 29, 31
—, heterologous (initial) phase 2, 3, 4,
  5, 8, 12, 24, 29, 31
— —, phases *2*
— —, second (autologous) phase 2, 3, *7*,
  11, 25, 32, 33
— — in rabbits *8*, 17, 32
measles antigen 95
membranoproliferative glomerulitis 54
— glomerulonephritis 56, 57, 58, 73,
  78, 91, 158, *170*, 188, 189, 191, 192,
  193, 195, 196, 197
membranous glomerulonephritis 19, 20,
  27, 51, 53, 55, 56, 57, *82*, *113*, *166*
— —, acute 160
— glomerulonephropathy, idiopathic
  82
— nephropathy 19, 20, 27, 28, 55, 110,
  113, 121, 131, 135
mesangial glomerulonephritis 121
— nephropathy, IgA-IgG *75*
mesangiocapillary glomerulonephritis *78*,
  124, 131, 136, 138
— —, diffuse 56
mesangioproliferative glomerulonephritis
  54, 57, 58, *69*, *75*, 158, 159, *176*, 188,
  189, 190, 192, 193, 195, 196
— — with diffuse crescents 158. *182*,
  188, 189, 192, 195, 196
— — with focal crescents 158, 178, *181*,
  183, 188, 189, 192, 193, 195, 196, 197
mesangiolysis 9, 31, 32
mesangium-centrilobular location 80, 81
— circumferencial areas 80
metastatic calcifications 253
mineralization of the osteoid 248

minimal change disease *108*
mixed glomerulonephritis, chronic 54
— membranous glomerulonephritis 78
monocytic accumulation 7, 8, 9, 11, 14,
    18, 29, 30
motor nerve conduction 245
misaic theory 203
muscle wasting in chronic uremia 245
myopathy, uremic 245

nail patella syndrome 132, 133
necrotizing angiitis 14
— glomerulonephritis 56, 57, 58, *66*,
    131, 158, 182, *186*, 188, 189, 192, 195,
— —, focal 129
"nephritic syndrome" 118, 121
nephritis, acute poststreptococcal 70, 71,
    72, 158, 159
—, chronic indurative 45
—, — perenchymatous 45
—, —, without induration 45
—, diffuse 45
—, focal 47, 51, 53, 58, 59
—, "hereditary" 98, *131*
—, interstitial 46
—, ischemic 48
—, lupus-like 2, 21
—, nephrotoxic (Masugi) 2, 3, 4, *5*, 17,
    24, 29, 31, 33
—, parenchymatous 45, 47, 48
—, primary indurative 45
—, secondary indurative 45
—, toxic 48, 50
—, classification of Löhlein *46*
—, classification of Senator *45*
—, classification of Volhard *47*
nephrocirrhosis 45
nephropathy, membranous 19, 20, 27,
    28, 55, 110, *113*, 121, 131, 135
—, preeclamptic *143*
nephrosclerosis, malignant 68, 98
nephrosis 46, 47, 49, 53, 56
nephrotic syndrome 20, 28, 50, 53, 58,
    89, 95, 98, 108, 110, 111, 113, 115,
    116, 117, 124, 125, 135, 157, 158, *160*,
    162, 163, 164, 165, 166, 167, 170, 171,
    172, 177, 179, 187, 188, 190, 191, 192,
    193, 194, 196
nephrotoxic antibodies (NTAbs) 2, 3, 5,
    7, 8, 25, 31, 61
— effect 66, 89
— guinea pig IgG₁ 7
— nephritis (Masugi nephritis) 2, 3, 4,
    5, 17, 24, 29, 31, 33
— rabbit IgG 4, 8
— sera 2
NIL-disease 100
nitrogen-mustard therapy 187
NTAbs = nephrotoxic antibodies 2, 3,
    5, 7, 8, 25, 31

oligospermia in chronic uremia 246
"one-shot" serum sickness 2, 14, 15, 26
osteoblastic activity 254
osteoclasia 254, 256
osteodystrophy, renal 246, 255
osteoid, mineralization 248
osteomalacia 253, 255
—, azotemic 246
—, renal 248
osteoporosis 247
osteosclerosis 247, 253

paralysis in chronic uremia 245
parathyroid gland, hyperplasia 251
— hormone 246, 247, 248, 249, *250*,
    252, 253, 254, 255
— — activity 247
— — synthesis 251, 252
parathyroidectomy 249, 250, 256
parenchymatous nephritis 45, 47, 48
passive serum sickness 14, *17*, 27, 29
penicillamine 117
penicillin treatment 176
peracute glomerulonephritis 50, 51, *182*
periarteriitis nodosa 53, 98, 122
pericardial effusion 243
pericarditis 241, 243
periglomerulitis 186
perimembranous glomerulonephritis 158,
    166, 171, 188, 189, 191, 192, 195, 196,
    197
peritonitis 48
phases of Masugi nephritis *2*
phosphatase level, alkaline 254
phosphate mobilization 252
— resorption 247, 252
— retention 247
plasma renin 241
— — activity 203, 204, 206, 208, 211,
    212, 214, 216, 218, 220, *221*, 241
— — —, normal 203, 204
— — level 213, 214
— sodium concentration 208, 211, 222,
    241
— testosterone 246
— triglycerides 244, 245
plasmodium 95
— infections 23
pneumococcal infections 49
pneumonia 48
polyarteritis 130
polyneuropathy in chronic uremia 240,
    241, *245*
post-heparin lipolytic activity 245
postinfectious glomerulonephritis *69*, 80
poststreptococcal glomerulonephritis
    69, 75, 80, 96, 120, 121, 122, 123, 177,
    178, 179, 181, 185, 189, 190
— nephritis, acute 70, 71, 72, 158, 159
pre-eclamptic nephropathy *143*

primary hyperparathyroidism 250
progressive glomerulonephritis *30*
proliferative capsulitis 48
— glomerulitis, endocapillary 51
— extracapillary glomerulitis 51
— glomerulonephritis 2, 14, 17, 18, 23,
   27, 28, 48, 51, 53, 54, 55, 56, 70, 73, *75*,
   131
— —, acute 54, *118*, 121
— —, — exudative 73
— —, chronic 54
— —, diffuse 131
— —, focal *127*
— sclerosing glomerulonephritis 56
properdin 64
— depression 82
— system 75
protein-diet 263, 264
postacute glomerulonephritis 50, 51
puromycin 110
purpura, anaphylactoid *91*
pyelonephritis 58
pyridoxine 256, 260, 263

rabbit Masugi nephritis *8*, 17, 32
— NTAbs 5, 12, 24, 25
radiation nephritis *140*
— —, experimental 111
rapidly progressive glomerulonephritis
   53, 54, 56, *66*, 70, 121, *181*, *182*, 190,
   193, 195, 196, 197
recurrent glomerulonephritis 95
— hematuria *75*
"red eye syndrome" 253
renal acidosis 247, 253
— aldosterone effect 230
— anemia, treatment *262*
— bone disease, classification 246
— — —, clinical syndrome *253*
— — —, roentgenological appearance
   253
— — —, therapy *254*
— erythropoietic factor 261
— failure, acute 162, 164, 165, 170, 176'
   177, 178, 182, 183, 184, 188, 190, 192,
   193, 196, 197
— osteodystrophy 246
— transplantation 240, 265
— vein thrombosis 117
renin 203, *215*, 225
— activity 216, 222, 224, 241
— —, normal 203, 204
— release 204, 220, 221, 223
— —, renal 216, 221, 222, 224
— preinhibitor 225
— secretion 226
— angiotensin effects 229
— — system 203, 229, 241
"resolving" glomerulonephritis *69*, 75
"restles leg syndrome" 245

reticulocytosis 257
rheumatic fever 127
"rugger jersey" spine 253

sarcoidosis 57
scarlet fever nephritis 46
schistosoma infections 23
Schönlein-Henoch's purpura 56, *91*, 94,
   131, 181
sclerosing glomerulonephritis, chronic
   52, 54, 57
sclerosis, focal 48, 58, *86*
—, segmental 56
second phase of Masugi nephritis 2, 3,
   7, 11, 25, 32, 33
secondary hyperparathyroidism 240, 256
secretion of sexual hormone 240
segmental hyalinosis 55, 56
— sclerosis 56
sepsis 48
septicemia 127
serum calcium concentration 248, 249,
   251, 254
— complement level 70
— insulin 243, 245
— phosphate level 247, 249, 251, 252,
   254
— sickness 34
— —, acute 2, 3, 26
— —, chronic 2, 21, 27
— — inflammations 2
— — nephritis 32, 33, 120, 121, 174
— triglycerides 244, 245
sexual hormone, secretion 240
sheep nephritis 3
— NTAbs 11, 12
Shwartzman phenomenon 140
skin, changes in chronic uremia 240
smooth type of chronic glomerulonephritis 47, 50
sodium concentration in plasma 208,
   211, 222, 241
specific host antibodies 2, 3
splenectomy 262
staphylococcal infections 48, 118
Staphylococcus aureus 127
Steblay nephritis *12*
steroid therapy 157, 160, 162, 164, 168,
   169, 170, 171, 172, 178, 179, 182, 184,
   186, 187, 190, 191, 195, 197
streptococcal infections 46, 49, 69, 73,
   118, 172, 179
streptococci antigens 64
subacute bacterial endocarditis 130
— diffuse glomerulonephritis 52, 58
— glomerulonephritis 46, *49*, 50, 52, 54,
   66, *182*
subchronic glomerulonephritis *47*, 50,
   52, *176*
syphilis, congenital 48, 117

systemic angiitis 21
— diseases *133*

testicular insufficiency 246
testosterone in plasma 246, 267
thrombocapillaritis (Löhlein) 53, 57, 130
thrombosis of afferent arterioles 48
— of glomerular capillaries 48
thrombotic microangiopathy 53
— thrombocytopenic purpura 138
thyroglobulin 95
tissue calcification 252, 253
tonsillitis 46, 171, 175, 183, 184
total iron binding capacity 263
toxic liver damage 142
— nephritis 48, 50
toxines, uremic 257
transfusion therapy 262, 263, 264
transplantation *145*
transplant-glomerulopathy 95, *145*
— rejection 95
treponemal antigens 95
tubulus antigens 64
tumor antigens 95

uremia, chronic, and anemia *256*
—, —, and bone disease *246*
—, —, and carbohydrate metabolism *243*
—, —, and cardiovascular system *240*

—, —, and fat metabolism *243*
—, —, and gonadal dysfunction *246*
—, —, and polyneuropathy *245*
uremic arthritis 253
— myopathy, specific 245
— toxines 257

vasculitis 22
—, allergic 183
vasoactive amines 26
vertigo in chronic uremia 245
vibratory sensitivity 245
viral hepatitis, acute 142
vitamin D 246, 255
— — metabolism 246
— D_3 metabolism *248*
— — metabolites 251, 255
— D resistence 254
— B_{12} 256, 260, 263, 264
volume, extracellular 208, 211, 222

Waldenström's macroglobulinemia 82
warfarin 12
Wegener's granulomatosis 53, 56, 122, 130, 186
wire-loop glomerular lesions 21, 22, 134, 135, 137

yeast 128

Index to Volumes 51—60

Current Topics in Pathology

Volume 51

K. BENIRSCHKE, Spontaneous Chimerism in Mammals: A Critical Review 1
P. J. FITZGERALD, B. CAROL, Quantitative Autoradiography: Statistical Study of
the Variance, Error and Sensitivity of the Labeling Index (Thymidine-H³ and
DNA Synthesis) 62
W. REMMELE, A. HINRICHS, Renal Siderosis. Morphology, Etiology, Pathogenesis
and Differential Diagnosis. With Special Reference to Traumatic Hemolytic-
Anemia 97
M. MARIN-PADILLA, Morphogenesis of Anencephaly and Related Malformations . . 145
G. A. PADGETT, J. M. HOLLAND, W. C. DAVIS, J. B. HENSON, The Chediak-Higashi
Syndrome: A Comparative Review 175

Volume 52

Z. LOJDA, P. FRIČ, J. JODL, V. CHMELÍK, Cytochemistry of the Human Jejunal
Mucosa in the Norm and in Malabsorption Syndrome 1
M. WANKE, Experimental Acute Pancreatitis 64
J. WIENER, Ultrastructural Aspects of Delayed Hypersensitivity 143

Volume 53

R. BÄSSLER, The Morphology of Hormone Induced Structural Changes in the Female
Breast 1
K. JELLINGER, F. SEITELBERGER, Spongy Degeneration of the Central Nervous
System in Infancy 90
H. HAMPERL, The Myothelia (Myoepithelial Cells). Normal State; Regressive
Changes; Hyperplasia; Tumors 161

Volume 54

A. TAKEUCHI, Penetration of the Intestinal Epithelium by Various Microorganisms 1
J. K. FRENKEL, Toxoplasmosis. Mechanisms of Infection, Laboratory Diagnosis
and Management 28
A. VOLKMAN, A Current Perspective of Monocytopoiesis 76
D. E. SCARBOROUGH, The Pathogenesis of Thrombosis in Artificial Organs and
Vessels 95
P. PFITZER, Nuclear DNA Content of Human Myocardial Cells 125

Volume 55

D. H. BOWDEN, The Alveolar Macrophage 1
R. L. NAEYE, The Anthracotic Pneumoconioses 37
J. HURLIMANN, Immunoglobulin Synthesis and Transport by Human Salivary
Glands. (Immunological Mechanisms of the Mucous Membranes.) 69
H. LIETZ, C-Cells: Source of Calcitonin. A Morphological Review 109
R. A. GOYER, Lead and the Kidney 147

Volume 56

E. ALTENÄHR, Ultrastructural Pathology of Parathyroid Glands   1
F. HUTH, A. SOREN, W. KLEIN, Structure of Synovial Membrane in Rheumatoid
   Arthritis   55
K. CHRISTOV, R. RAICHEV, Experimental Thyroid Carcinogenesis 79
D. G. SHEAHAN, Current Aspects of Bacterial Enterotoxins   115

Volume 57

H. U. ZOLLINGER, J. MOPPERT, G. THIEL, H.-P. ROHR, Morphology and Pathogenesis
   of Glomerulopathy in Cadaver Kidney Allografts Treated with Antilymphocyte
   Globulin   1
H. A. AZAR, E. A. MOSCOVIC, S. G. ABUNASSAR, J. S. McDOUGAL, Some Aspects of
   Sarcoidosis   49
H. F. OTTO, The Interepithelial Lymphocytes of the Intestinum. Morphological
   Observations and Immunological Aspects of Intestinal Enteropathy. 81
K. SALFELDER, M. MENDELOVICI, J. SCHWARZ, Multiple Deep Fungus Infections:
   Personal Observations and a Critical Review of the World Literature 123

Volume 58

H. P. ROHR, U. N. RIEDE, Experimental Metabolic Disorders and the Subcellular
   Reaction Pattern (Morphometric of Hepatocyte Mitochondria)   1
G. FREYTAG, G. KLÖPPEL, Insulitis — A Morphological Review 49
O. KLINGE, Cytologic and Histologic Aspects of Toxically Induced Liver 91
G. DELLING, Age-Related Bone Changes (Histomorphometric Investigation of the
   Structure of Human Cancellous Bone 117
G. MOLZ, Perinatal and Newborn Deaths (Necropsy Findings in 970 Term, Preterm
   and Small-for-Date Births)   149

Volume 59

J. TORHORST, Studies on the Pathogenesis and Morphogenesis of Glomerulonephrosis   1
I. DAMJANOV, D. SOLTER, Experimental Teratoma 69
W. MEIER-RUGE, Hirschsprung's Disease: Its Aetiology, Pathogenesis and Differ-
   ential Diagnosis   131
U. N. RIEDE, Experimental Aspects of Growth Plate Disorders   181

Volume 60

F. HUTH, M. KOJIMAHARA, T. FRANKEN, P. RHEDIN, K. A. ROSENBAUER, Aortic
   Alterations in Rabbits Following Sheathing with Silastic and Polyethylene Tubes   1
K. BÜRKI, J. C. SCHAER, P. GRÉTILLAT, R. SCHINDLER, Radioactively Labeled
   Iododeoxyuridine in the Study of Experimental Liver Regeneration 33
G. ALTSHULER, P. RUSSELL, The Human Placental Villitides. A Review of Chronic
   Intrauterine Infection   63
H. MITSCHKE, W. SAEGER, Ultrastructural Pathology of the Adrenal Glands in
   Cushing's Syndrome   113
N. BÖHM, W. SANDRITTER, DNA in Human Tumors: A Cytophotometric Study . . 151